FOREBRAIN AREAS INVOLVED IN PAIN PROCESSING

British Library Cataloguing in Publication Data
A catalogue record for this book is available from the British Library.
ISBN 2-7420-0093-3

Éditions John Libbey Eurotext
127, avenue de la République, 92120 Montrouge, France.
Tél : (1) 46.73.06.60

John Libbey and Company Ltd
13, Smiths Yard, Summerley Street, London SW18 4HR, England.
Tel : (1) 947.27.77

John Libbey CIC
Via L. Spallanzani, 11, 00161 Rome, Italy.
Tel : (06) 862.289

© John Libbey Eurotext, 1995, Paris.

Il est interdit de reproduire intégralement ou partiellement le présent ouvrage — loi du 11 mars 1957 — sans aurtorisation de l'éditeur ou du Centre français du Copyright, 6 *bis*, rue Gabriel-Laumain, 75010 Paris.

FOREBRAIN AREAS INVOLVED IN PAIN PROCESSING

J.M. BESSON
G. GUILBAUD
H. OLLAT

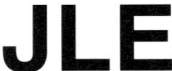

ACKNOWLEDGEMENTS

This book contains the presentations made at the Symposium on "Forebrain areas involved in pain processing" held in Dinard, France, 29-31 May 1995.

This Symposium was organized with the cooperation of the "Association pour la Neuro-Pharmacologie" and in collaboration with l' "Institut de Recherche International Servier".

Illustration de couverture :
Edvard Munch, le cri, 1893 ;
Photo Bridgeman-Giraudon,
Munch-Museum / Munch Ellingsen Group - ADAGP, Paris, 1995

Contents

List of contributors VII
Preface IX

1. The organization of spinothalamic tract circuitry in the macaque and the role of GABA information processing
   H.J. Ralston III, P.T. Ohara, X.W. Meng, D.D. Ralston 1

2. Supraspinal projections of lamina I neurons
   A.D. Craig 13

3. The spino-parabrachio -amygdaloid and -hypothalamic nociceptive pathways
   J.F. Bernard, H. Bester, J.M. Besson 27

4. The spino-hypothalamic tract
   G.J. Giesler Jr 49

5. Thalamic processing of sensory-discriminative and affective-motivational dimensions of pain
   M.C. Bushnell 63

6. Thalamic and cortical processing in rat models of clinical pain
   G. Guilbaud, J.M. Benoist 79

7. Thalamic anatomy and physiology of pain perception: connectivity, somato-visceral convergence and spatio-temporal dynamics of nociceptive information coding
   A.V. Apkarian 93

8. The region postero-inferior to the human thalamic principal sensory nucleus (Vc) may contribute to the affective dimension of pain through thalamo-corticolimbic connections
   F.A. Lenz 119

9. The role of excitatory amino acid receptors in thalamic nociception
   S.A. Eaton, T.E. Salt 131

10. Brain neural images of persistent pain states in rats using 2-DG autoradiography
    D.D. Price, J. Mao, D.J. Mayer 143

11. Hindbrain structures involved in pain processing as revealed by the evoked expression of immediate early genes in freely behaving animals
    D. Menétrey 155

12. Potential role of orbital and cingulate cortices in nociception
    J.O. Dostrovsky, W.D. Hutchison, K.D. Davis, A. Lozano 171

13. Cortical nociceptive mechanisms. A review of neurophysiological and behavioral evidence in the primate
    W.K. Dong, E.H. Chudler 183

14. The role of pain in cingulate cortical and limbic thalamic mediation of avoidance learning
    M. Gabriel, A. Poremba 197

15. The forebrain network for pain: an emerging image
    K.L. Casey, S. Minoshima 213

16. Cortical and thalamic imaging in normal volunteers and patients with chronic pain
    A.K.P. Jones, S.W.G. Derbyshire 229

17. Central pain syndromes
    J. Boivie, A. Österberg 239

18. Are there still indications for destructive neurosurgery at supraspinal levels for the relief of painful syndromes ?
    J. Gybels, B. Nuttin 253

19. Motor cortex stimulation for deafferentation pain relief in various clinical syndromes and its possible mechanism
    T. Tsubokawa 261

List of contributors

Apkarian A.V., Department of Neurosurgery, Computational Neuroscience Program at SUNY Health Science Center, Syracuse, NY 13210, USA.
Benoist J.M., Unité 161 INSERM, 2, rue d'Alésia, 75014 Paris, France.
Bernard J.F., Unité de Recherches de Physiopharmacologie du Système Nerveux, INSERM U 161 and EPHE, 2, rue d'Alésia, 75014 Paris, France.
Besson J.M., Unité de Recherches de Physiopharmacologie du Système Nerveux, INSERM U 161 and EPHE, 2, rue d'Alésia, 75014 Paris, France.
Bester H., Unité de Recherches de Physiopharmacologie du Système Nerveux, INSERM U 161 and EPHE, 2, rue d'Alésia, 75014 Paris, France.
Boivie J., Department of Neurology, University Hospital, S-581 85 Linköping, Sweden.
Bushnell M.C., Département de Stomatologie and Centre de Recherche en Sciences Neurologiques, Université de Montréal, Montréal PQ H3C 3J7, Canada.
Casey K.L., (1) Departments of Neurology and Physiology, University of Michigan, (2) Neurology Research Laboratories, Veteran's Affairs Medical Center, Ann Arbor, Michigan 48105, USA.
Chudler E.H., Departments of Anesthesiology and Psychology and Multidisciplinary Pain Center, University of Washington School of Medicine, Seattle, WA 98195, USA.
Craig A.D., Division of Neurobiology, Barrow Neurological Institute, 350 West Thomas Road, Phoenix AZ 85013, USA.
Davis K.D., Department of Physiology and Division of Neurosurgery, University of Toronto, Toronto ON M5S 1A8, Canada.
Derbyshire S.W.G., MRC Cyclotron Unit, Hammersmith Hospital, Ducane Road, London W12 OHS, UK.
Dong W.K., Departments of Anesthesiology and Psychology and Multidisciplinary Pain Center, University of Washington School of Medicine, Seattle, WA 98195, USA.
Dostrovsky J.O., Department of Physiology and Division of Neurosurgery, University of Toronto, Toronto ON M5S 1A8, Canada.
Eaton S.A., Department of Visual Science, Institute of Ophtalmology, 11-43 Bath Street, London EC1V 9EL, UK.
Gabriel M., Beckman Institute for Advanced Science and Technology, University of Illinois, Urbana, IL 61801, USA.
Giesler J.G. Jr, Department of Cell Biology and Neuroanatomy, University of Minnesota, 4-135 Jackson Hall, Minneapolis MN 55455, USA.
Guilbaud G., Unité 161 INSERM, 2, rue d'Alésia, 75014 Paris, France.
Gybels J., Laboratory of Experimental Neurosurgery and Neuroanatomy, KUL University of Leuven, Provisorium I, Minderbroedersstraat 17, B-3000, Leuven, Belgium.

Hutchinson W.D., Department of Physiology and Division of Neurosurgery, University of Toronto, Toronto ON M5S 1A8, Canada.
Jones A.K.P., (1) University of Manchester Rheumatic Diseases Centre, Clinical Sciences Building, Hope Hospital, Eccles Old Road, Salford, M6 8HD, UK.
Lenz F.A., Department of Neurosurgery, Johns Hopkins Hospital, Baltimore, MD 31287-7713, USA.
Lozano A., Department of Physiology and Division of Neurosurgery, University of Toronto, Toronto ON M5S 1A8, Canada.
Mao J., Department of Anesthesiology, Medical College of Virginia, Richmond VA 23298, USA.
Mayer D.J., Department of Anesthesiology, Medical College of Virginia, Richmond VA 23298, USA.
Menétrey D., INSERM U 161, 2, rue d'Alésia, 75014 Paris, France.
Meng X.W., W.M. Keck Foundation Center for Integrative Neuroscience, University of California, San Francisco CA 9414, USA.
Minoshima S., Department of Internal Medicine, Division of Nuclear Medicine, University of Michigan, Ann Arbor, Michigan 48105, USA.
Nuttin B., Laboratory of Experimental Neurosurgery and Neuroanatomy, and Department of Neurosurgery, KUL University of Leuven, Provisorium I, Minderbroedersstraat 17, B-3000, Leuven, Belgium.
Ohara P.T., W.M. Keck Foundation Center for Integrative Neuroscience, University of California, San Francisco CA 9414, USA.
Österbreg A., (1) Department of Neurology, University Hospital, S-581 85 Linköping, (2) Department of Geriatrics and Rehabilitation, Motala Hospital, S-591 85 Motala, Sweden.
Poremba A., Beckman Institute for Advanced Science and Technology, University of Illinois, Urbana, IL 61801, USA.
Price D.D., Department of Anesthesiology, Medical College of Virginia, Richmond VA 23298, USA.
Ralston D.D., W.M. Keck Foundation Center for Integrative Neuroscience, University of California, San Francisco CA 9414, USA.
Ralston H.J. III, W.M. Keck Foundation Center for Integrative Neuroscience, University of California, San Francisco CA 9414, USA.
Salt T.E., Department of Visual Science, Institute of Ophtalmology, 11 - 43 Bath Street, London EC1V 9EL, UK.
Tsubokawa T., University Reasearch Center, Department of Neurological Surgery, Nihon University School of Medicine, 30-1, Oyaguchi Kami-machi, Itabashi-ku, Tokyo 173, Japan.

Preface

Although the informations on spinal dorsal horn mechanisms in pain processing are still much more documented than those concerning the "brain" level, evidence on the involvement of "brain structures", thalamus, hypothalamus, amygdala, cortex, has been accumulated over the last 15 years. As in other domains, this progress is due to a large amount of studies based on multidisciplinary approaches associating classical and modern methods of investigations for anatomical, physiological, pharmacological, behavioural, radiological aspects. In fact, most data compiled in this book have been obtained with combined technics, and thus, have more functional significance. For instance, nociceptive behaviours have been correlated with electrophysiology, or immunocytochemical labelling of nuclear proteins expressed in the central nervous system and coded by immediate early genes (*c-fos, c-jun, krox*). The use of animal models of clinical pain, the clinical observations performed by clinicians of various specialities, (neurologists, neurosurgeons, etc.) associated with the new technics of the radiological imagery have improved the validity of several basic data. These new data have enlighted the role of several structures such as thalamic nuclei, and several cortical areas, not only in the sensory discriminative but also in the emotional, cognitive… components of pain. Indeed, beside the classical pain pathways, others newly described, such as the spino-ponto-amygdalian, or the spino-hypothalamic pathways, have been extensively considered, and the putative role of insular and cingular cortex have been emphasized. Data on the intimate role of neuromediators and neuromodulators at the brain level are still scarce, behavioural studies are limited and should be extended. Obviously, all the reported studies do not work out all the problems arisen by pain and its treatment. However, they do provide new insight and new perspectives to explore pain processing at the brain level in animals and in humans.

J.M. Besson, G. Guilbaud, H. Ollat

The organization of spinothalamic tract circuitry in the macaque and the role of GABA information processing

H.J. RALSTON III, P.T. OHARA, X.W. MENG, D.D. RALSTON

*Department of Anatomy, W.M. Keck Foundation Center for Integrative Neuroscience,
University of California, San Francisco, California, USA.*

The spinothalamic tract (STT) of the primate carries information arising from peripheral noxious stimuli, and conveys the stimuli to various regions of the somatosensory thalamus, where the STT afferents activate thalamic neurons that then transmit this information to the cerebral cortex. In this present paper, we will review our knowledge about the thalamic circuitry involved in the processing of noxious information and will suggest some mechanisms by which altered thalamic circuitry may be involved in pain syndromes that often follow injury to the central nervous system.

STT projections from spinal cord neurons carry noxious information, as well as those evoked by non-noxious stimuli, from cutaneous and deep structures and terminate in several regions of the somatosensory thalamus [1]: the ventroposterolateral nucleus (VPLc), the posterior group (PO/SG) and, in the intralaminar nuclei, chiefly the centrolateral nucleus (Cl). There is now evidence [2, 3] that the «nociceptive specific» STT neurons of lamina I of the dorsal horn send their axons in the most lateral regions of the STT and have a predominant termination in PO/SG, which has recently been postulated as a major thalamic center for the processing of noxious stimuli in humans [2, 4]. The axons of «wide-dynamic range» (WDR) STT cells of lamina V travel in the ventrolateral aspect of the STT and have a predominant termination in VPLc [2]. The STT afferents to VPLc form "parcellated bursts" [5] and occupy a subcomponent of VPLc where they are overlapped by the more abundant lemniscal afferents. Thus, it is anticipated that some of the neurons of VPLc would exhibit exclusively non-noxious response properties, in that they would be driven only by ML afferents that project to the entire extent of the nucleus. Other VPLc neurons would be expected to exhibit convergent properties, being activated by both ML and STT afferents, or by the numerous dorsal horn STT neurons that receive convergent input from both noxious and non-noxious primary afferents (WDR). Physiological studies of macaque thalamic neurons [6] found that more than half of the VPLc neurons responded exclusively or preferentially to noxious mechanical stimuli, the remainder responding in varying degrees to non-noxious or to noxious stimuli.

Several studies [7] of the neuronal and synaptic organization of the thalamus of monkey and of cat have revealed a complex circuitry for processing afferent information. Thalamic nuclei contain two neuronal cell types:
- the thalamocortical relay cell, usually about 20 µm to 40 µm in cell body diameter, which projects to functionally related regions of the cerebral cortex and which constitutes approximately 75-90% of the total complement of neurons,
- the interneuron (local circuit neuron) which represents approximately 10-25% of the total neuronal population and which exhibits γ-aminobutyric acid immunoreactivity (GABA-ir).

When stained by the Golgi method or labeled by the intracellular iontophoresis of horseradish peroxidase (HRP), the interneurons have been shown to be morphologically distinct from relay cells, being approximately 10-15 µm in cell body diameter, and to possess complex dendritic appendages. The thalamocortical relay cells lack these dendritic appendages.

When examined by electron microscopy, medial lemniscal (ML) and spinothalamic tract (STT) terminals exhibit a similarly morphology, in that they contain rounded synaptic vesicles and are relatively large, resulting in their designation as RL-type synaptic terminals. The RL-type medial lemniscal terminals contact the dendrites of relay cells, as well as being presynaptic to vesicle-containing profiles that, in turn, contact the relay cell dendrites to form a triadic synaptic relationship. These postsynaptic vesicle-containing profiles have been shown to be the dendritic appendages of interneurons, to be GABA-ir and to be presynaptic, and have thus been called presynaptic dendrites [8]. These relationships between ML afferent, relay cell and GABA-ir appendages presumably serve a fundamental aspect of information transfer in the thalamus, in which the afferent axon transmits an excitatory message to the relay cell and to the GABAergic appendages, resulting in feed-forward GABAergic inhibition of the relay cell by the interneuronal dendritic appendages.

The most thorough study of the functional properties of the GABAergic presynaptic dendritic appendages of interneurons in processing afferent information in the thalamus is that of Paré *et al.* [9]. These authors examined the interactions of mammillary body afferent axons with relay cells and presynaptic dendrites in the cat anterior nuclear complex. They described a triphasic series of inhibitory postsynaptic potentials (IPSPs) in relay cells following stimulation of mammillothalamic afferents: a short latency, brief duration IPSP (designated a) that they concluded was due to feed-forward inhibition mediated by the triadic synaptic relationships between mammillary afferents, interneuronal presynaptic dendrites and relay cells; and two longer latency, more prolonged IPSPs (designated A and B) that they assumed were evoked by the axons of interneurons. They showed that a and A were mediated by $GABA_A$ receptors, and that the B IPSP was due to activation of $GABA_B$ receptors. Given the small size of the interneuron and its dendritic appendages and the consequent high input resistance, they concluded that afferent stimulation was probably very effective in evoking release of GABA from the presynaptic dendrites. They suggested that the short duration IPSPs in relay cells resulting from afferent activation of presynaptic dendrites would promote effective information transfer by the relay cells by reducing postsynaptic summation, leading to the rapid return of the relay cell to its resting potential to permit higher frequency of information transfer. Assuming that the findings of Paré et al. are applicable to the primate somatosensory thalamus, it is likely that the information transfer between STT afferents and relay cells, relatively unmodulated by GABAergic presynaptic dendrites (see below), is substantially different than that evoked by stimulation of the ML.

Lemniscal and spinal projections to the thalamus are modulated in the dorsal horn and dorsal column nuclei, respectively, and then are subject to modulation in the thalamus. We have recently demonstrated [10] that the thalamic circuitry serving the pathways carrying non-noxious and noxious information, respectively, is fundamentally different, and we suggest some functional consequences that may result from these differences in circuitry. The substantial majority of lemniscal terminals form synaptic contacts with GABA-ir presynaptic dendrites (Figure 1) and the dendritic shafts of thalamocortical relay neurons. In contrast, most STT terminals (about 85%) form simple axodendritic synapses with relay cell dendrites (Figure 2), but have few synaptic relationships with GABA-ir presynaptic dendrites. Thus, there is little potential for immediate disynaptic GABAergic modulation of the STT activation of relay cells. Most STT axons convey information arising from noxious stimuli, and we suggest that it is this population of STT afferents that do not have their excitatory inputs modulated by GABA-containing interneurons.

Individual dendritic segments of thalamocortical relay neurons receive projections from either medial lemniscal (ML) or spinothalamic tract (STT) afferent axons. Approximately 84% of ML projections mediating non-noxious information to VPLc of the thalamus are involved in complex circuitry with GABA-ir interneurons, presumably modulating the effects of the ML input upon relay neurons, resulting in a rapid return of the relay cell to its resting membrane potential to permit high frequency following of the afferent input. In contrast, 85% of spinal projections to VPLc, primarily transmitting information perceived by the cortex as noxious, lack interactions with GABA-ir interneurons and form simple axodendritic synapses upon thalamocortical relay cells. The relative lack of GABAergic modulation of the STT information would presumably result in the transmission of a different type of thalamocortical signal by neurons

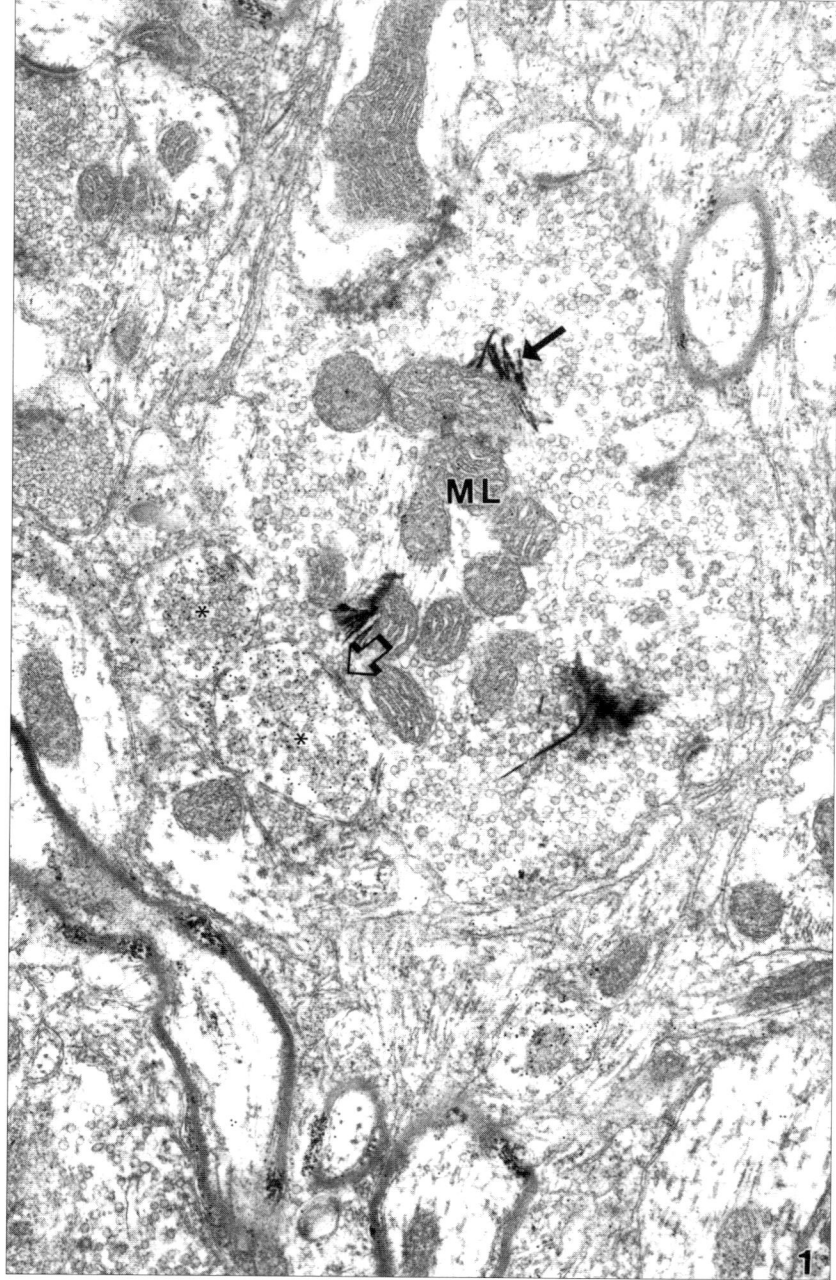

Figure 1. Medial lemniscal terminal (ML), containing HRP reaction product (dark arrow) transported from the contralateral dorsal column nuclei, contacts (open arrow) a GABA immunoreactive presynaptic dendrite (*) that contains 10 nm gold particles that are conjugated to the GABA antibody.

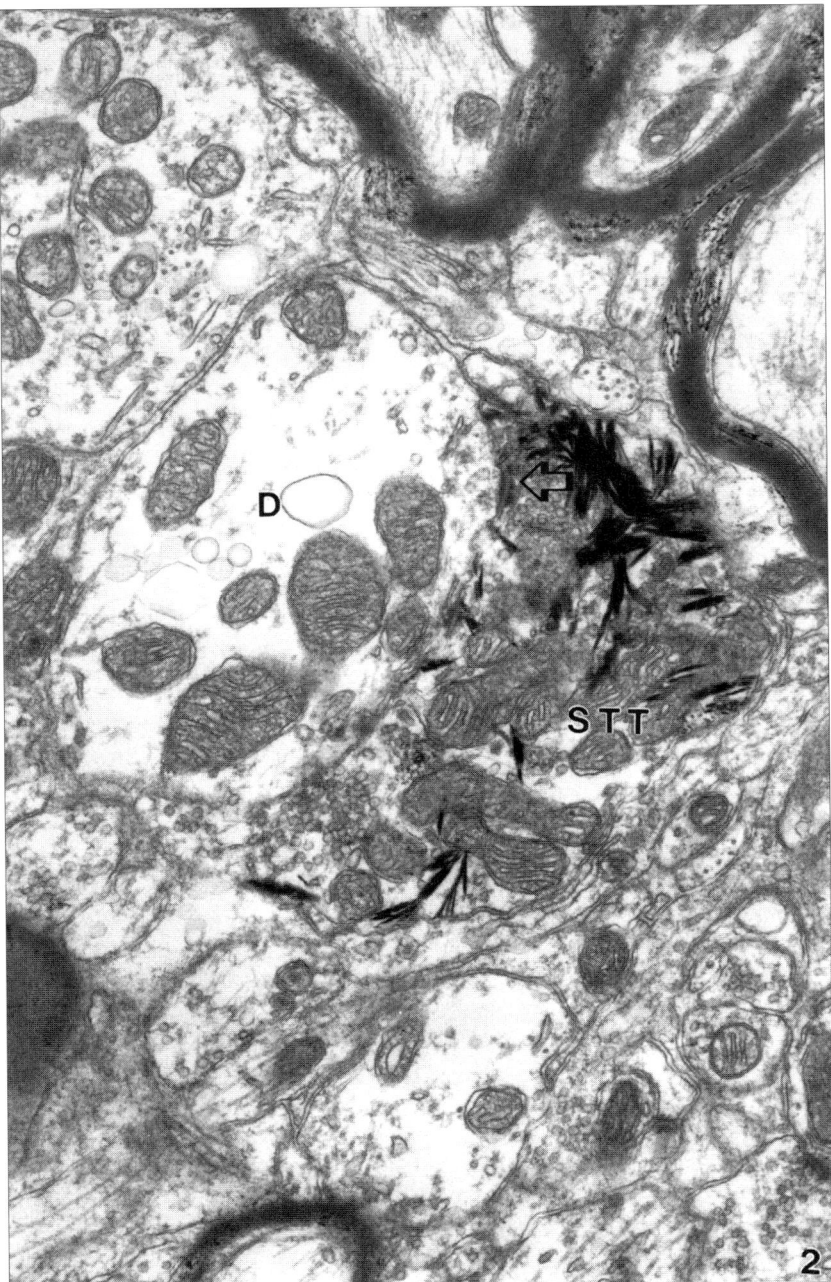

Figure 2. STT terminal, containing HRP reaction product transported from the spinal cord, contacts (open arrow) a dendrite (D) of a thalamocortical projection neuron. Note that the projection neuron contains no GABA immunoreactivity.

activated by STT, compared to ML, afferents. Because the majority of spinal afferents carry noxious messages, we propose that it is this information that lacks thalamic GABAergic modulation before being transmitted to the cortex.

Our findings raise an hypothesis concerning the genesis of the thalamic pain syndrome [11], also known as central post-stroke pain, which is characterized by severe pain and abnormalities in somatic sensibility. The central nervous system lesion, usually vascular in origin, is not necessarily located in the thalamus, but may involve diverse regions of the diencephalon, brainstem or spinal cord, and appears to be associated with central somatosensory deafferentation, particularly of the spino-thalamo-cortical pathways [12]. One possible explanation for these painful syndromes following central lesions may be the reorganization of thalamic circuitry in response to afferent injury. It has been observed that, after lesions of lemniscal afferents to the thalamus, there is a reduction of GABA-ir presynaptic dendrites within VPLc (personal communication, J. Wells), without apparent changes in the numbers of the interneurons themselves. In another study, chronic deafferentation of the cord following extensive dorsal rhizotomy has been shown to result in transneuronal degeneration of the dorsal column nuclei, leading to decreases in $GABA_A$ receptors in VPLc [13] without a reduction of GABA-ir interneurons. These examples indicate that central nervous system degeneration can lead to changes in thalamic GABAergic presynaptic dendritic appendages and postsynaptic $GABA_A$ receptors. Paré et al. [9] have shown that the presynaptic dendritic appendages, acting via postsynaptic $GABA_A$ receptors, play a major role in setting the firing properties of thalamic neurons. In addition, Roberts et al. [14] have demonstrated that alterations in inhibitory interactions mediated by $GABA_A$ receptors may participate in pathological pain states, following central nervous system injury. In our study we have shown that ML inputs conveying non-noxious information have substantial interactions with GABA-ir interneurons; STT afferents, most of which carry noxious information, have significantly less interactions with GABA-ir interneurons. The nature of the signals from relay neurons to cortex would be different, depending upon whether the input was GABA modulated or not. Our findings suggest that, in the primate thalamic transmission system, changes in the normal GABAergic circuitry following injury may cause the cortex to misinterpret non-noxious signals which are normally GABA modified in the thalamus to arise from non-modified noxious stimuli, potentially resulting in central pain states.

Given the overlap of the terminal arbors of ML and STT axons in VPLc, it is possible that some VPLc relay neurons receive convergent input from these two afferent systems, conveying fundamentally different sensory modalities. This creates a potential problem for the cerebral cortical neurons that are the recipients of information from such thalamocortical relay cells. However, the differences between the two afferent systems in synaptic interactions with GABAergic interneurons may result in distinct firing properties of relay neurons receiving ML and STT input, depending upon the degree of GABA modulation of the afferent signal, so that the cortex could distinguish between non-noxious and noxious information carried by convergent afferents upon thalamocortical cells. On the other hand, Rausell et al. [15] have suggested that macaque VPL neurons receiving either ML or STT input are spatially separated and characterized by the presence of different calcium-binding proteins (parvalbumin or calbindin D28k, respectively). Their conclusions suggest that there is little or no convergent input of the ML and STT afferents onto single VPLc cells, and therefore, the information relayed to the cortex is transmitted by separate populations of thalamocortical neurons.

3-D reconstructions of ML or STT afferents reveal that a given segment of the relay cell dendritic arbor receives labeled terminals from one or the other source [10]; for instance, RL profiles contacting a particular dendritic segment are labeled after dorsal column nuclei injection or after spinal cord injection (Figure 3), respectively. This is in contrast to thalamic convergence studies in the rat, in which degenerating lemniscal and HRP-labeled spinal terminals are found to be adjacent to one another, synapsing upon the same segment of dendrite in VPL [16]. The rat VPL is fundamentally different than that of the monkey in another respect, in that GABA-ir interneurons are essentially absent in this nucleus in the rat.

Peripheral or central somatosensory deafferentation in adult animals has been shown to cause substantial reorganization in the somatosensory thalamus. In an examination of macaques surviving more than 12 years after peripheral deafferentation of the upper extremity, there is a profound transneuronal degeneration of the ipsilateral dorsal column nuclei, and a loss of axons and neurons staining for the calcium-binding protein, parvalbumin, but not of calbindin 28-kDa, and a marked decrease of $GABA_A$ receptors in the contralateral thalamus [13]. There is a particular interest in the consequences of injury to the spinothalamic tract (Figure 4), as lesions of this pathway are believed to play a seminal role in the genesis of central post-stroke pain in humans [12]. Patients exhibiting this pain syndrome have been found to have abnormal bursting responses of thalamic neurons [17], which mirror neuronal hyperactivity demonstrated in the cat with STT lesions [18], in which cells have been shown to exhibit hyperactive responses to both innocuous and noxious peripheral stimulation. These responses can be blocked by MK-801, an antagonist of the NMDA receptor, leading to the suggestion that the recruitment of NMDA receptors plays a role in deafferentation pain. The changes in response characteristics of thalamic neurons following partial interruption of afferent input can occur acutely, as well as in chronic situations. Anesthetic block of afferent information from mystacial vibrissae can substantially alter the receptive fields and response properties of thalamic neurons [19]. Taken together, all this evidence indicates that the somatosensory afferent pathways, in particular the somatosensory thalamus, are capable of substantial plastic changes, and some of these changes may be maladaptive in that they lead to central pain syndromes.

We are now analyzing the GABAergic circuitry of the macaque thalamus with confocal scanning microscopy, because this technique permits us to examine the entire extent of thalamic neurons and their dendritic arbors and the distribution of GABA-containing profiles of presynaptic dendrites and axon terminals that are in apposition to them. Following extracellular microinjections [20] of a tracer such as biotinylated

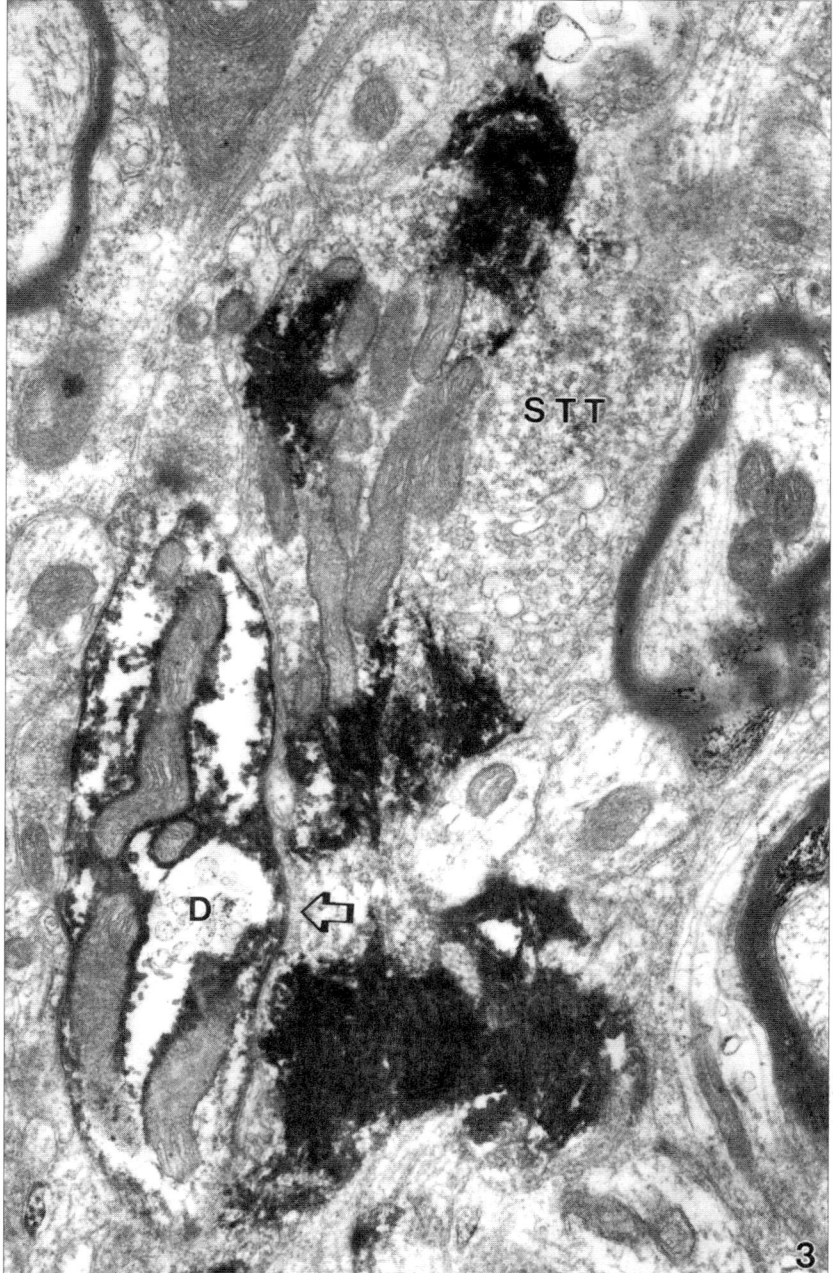

Figure 3. STT terminal, containing HRP reaction product transported from the spinal cord, synapses (open arrow) upon a dendrite (D) of a thalamocortical projection neuron that has been labeled with an intracellular injection of HRP. An analysis of such labeled neurons permits a description of the synaptic relationships of individual thalamic arbors.

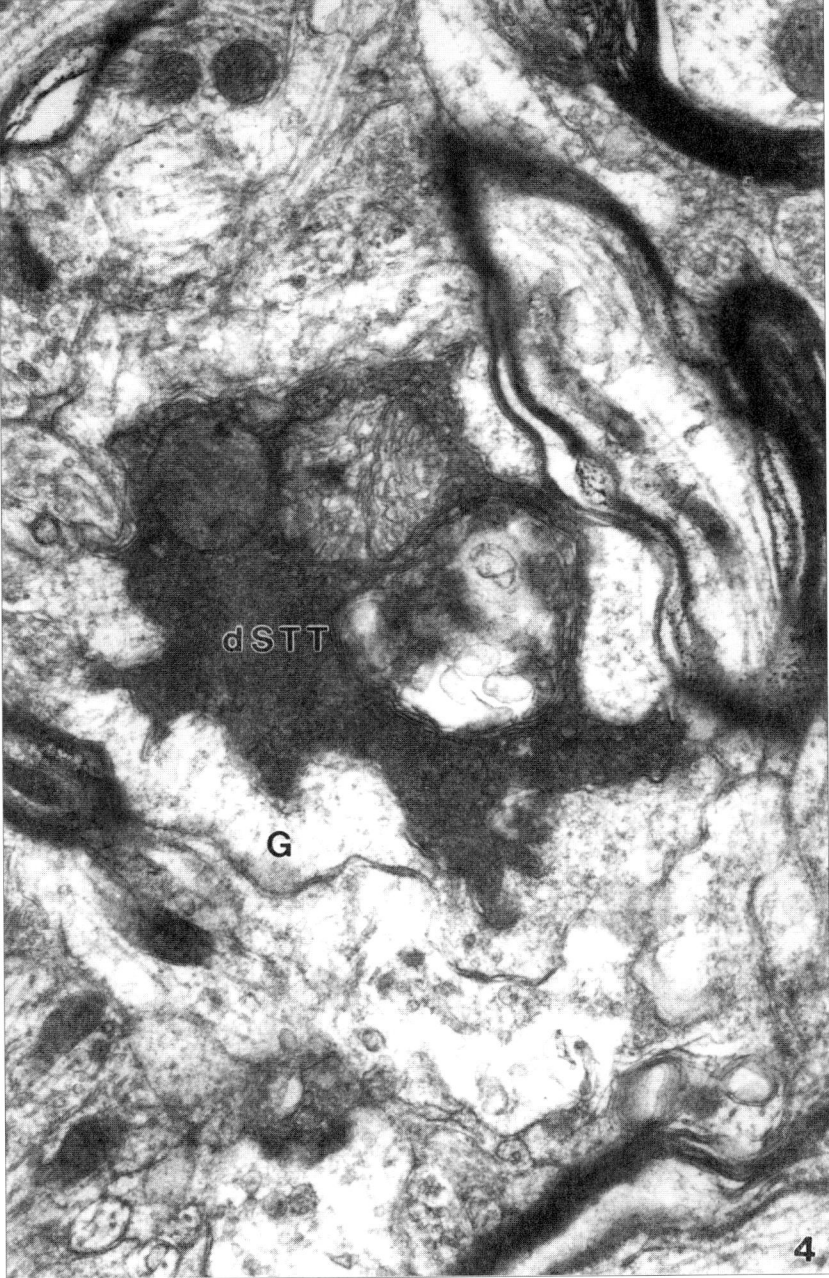

Figure 4. A degenerating STT (dSTT) terminal 3 days following an ipsilateral high cervical anterolateral cordotomy. The degenerating structure is being phagocytosed by a glial cell process (G).

dextran amine (BDA) into physiologically defined areas of the macaque somatosensory thalamus, serial sections are reacted with fluorescently-labeled compounds to demonstrate individual neurons and the GABA-immunoreactive terminals that are in apposition to them (Figure 5). These relationships between GABAergic synapses and thalamic neurons can be quantified, and we are using this method to determine whether changes in the GABA circuitry of the thalamus may underlie alterations in thalamic information processing that may be related to central deafferentation pain syndromes in humans.

In summary, we have shown that non-noxious information carried by the medial lemniscus is subject to substantial GABA modulation in the somatosensory thalamus, and that noxious information conveyed by the spinothalamic tract has relatively little

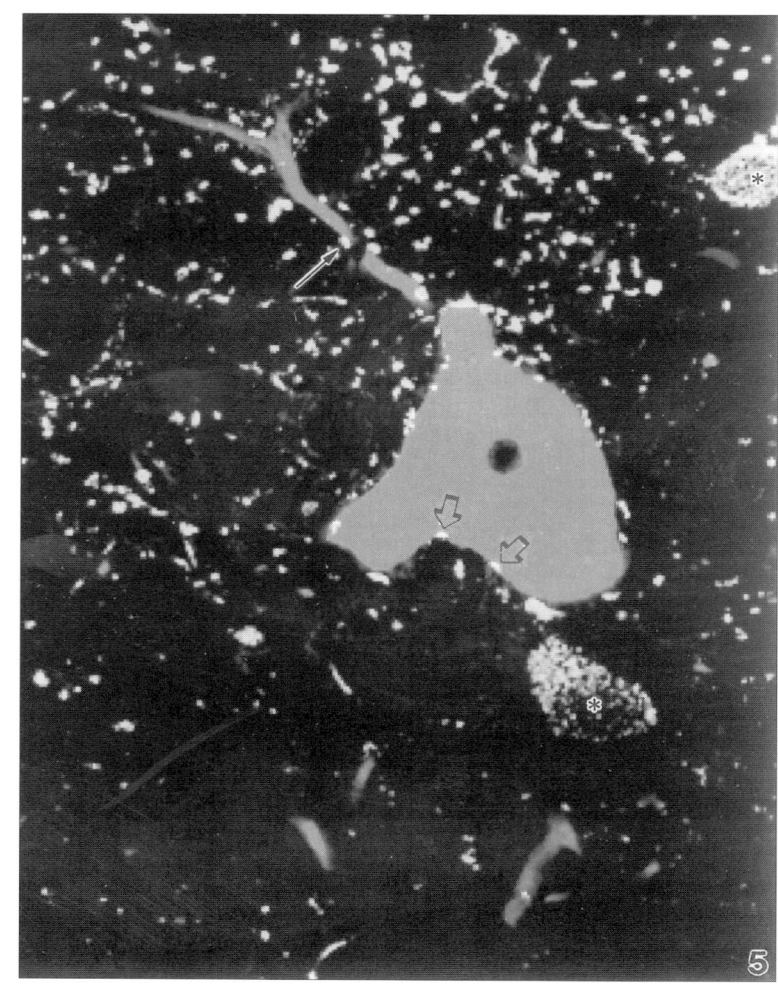

Figure 5. Confocal scanning micrograph. A thalamocortical projection neuron in VPL has been labeled with Texas red (red pseudo color), and GABA anti-body conjugated to fluorescene (green pseudo color). GABA immunoreactive structures can been seen to be in close apposition to the neuron, and are presumed axosomatic and axodendritic synapses (arrows). The confocal method permits a quantitative analysis in changes in synaptic populations following deafferentation. Optical image thickness: 1.5 μm. (See appendix for colour figures.)

thalamic GABA modulation. We suggest that deafferentation lesions of the STT may result in thalamic sprouting of the ML to occupy the deafferented sites on thalamic neurons, thus forming synaptic contacts that are not GABA modulated. This results in a misinterpretation by the brain that an innocuous, normally GABA-modified, stimulus has arisen from a noxious injury, leading to the perception of pain following a non-painful input. Studies of plastic changes in the primate thalamus following STT deafferentation should determine whether this hypothesis is correct, and may lead to more effective therapies for central pain states in humans.

Acknowledgements

We thank Antonia Milroy for her electron microscopic and immunocytochemical preparations, and Sandra Canchola for her histological and photographic materials. Supported by grants NS 23347 and NS 21445 from the National Institutes of Health.

References

1. Boivie J. An anatomical reinvestigation of the termination of the spinothalamic tract in the monkey. *J Comp Neurol* 1979 ; 186 : 343-70.
2. Ralston HJ III, Ralston DD. The primate dorsal spinothalamic tract: evidence for a specific termination in the posterior nuclei (Po/SG) of the thalamus. *Pain* 1992 ; 48 : 107-18.
3. Craig AD. Spinal distribution of ascending lamina I axons anterogradely labeled with *Phaseolus vulgaris* leucoagglutinin (PHA-L) in the cat. *J Comp Neurol* 1991 ; 313 : 377-93.
4. Craig AD, Bushnell MC, Zhang ET, Blomqvist A. A thalamic nucleus specific for pain and temperature sensation. *Nature* 1994 ; 372 : 770-3.
5. Mehler WR. The anatomy of the so-called "pain tract" in man: an analysis of the course and distribution of the ascending fibers of the fasciculus anterolateralis. In : French JD, Porter RW, eds. *Basic research in paraplegia*. Springfield, Illinois : Charles C. Thomas, 1962 : 26-55.
6. Chung JM, Lee KH, Surmeier DJ, Sorkin LS, Kim J, Willis WD. Response characteristics of neurons in the ventral posterior lateral nucleus of the monkey thalamus. *J Neurophysiol* 1986 ; 56 : 370-90.
7. Ralston HJ III. Local circuitry of the somatosensory thalamus in the processing of sensory information. *Prog Brain Res* 1991 ; 87 : 13-28.
8. Ralston HJ III. Evidence for presynaptic dendrites and a proposal for their mechanism of action. *Nature* 1971 ; 230 : 585-7.
9. Paré D, Dossi RC, Steriade M. Three types of inhibitory postsynaptic potentials generated by interneurons in the anterior thalamic complex of cat. *J Neurophysiol* 1991 ; 66 : 1190-204.
10. Ralston HJ III, Ralston DD. Medial lemniscal and spinal projections to the Macaque thalamus: an electron microscopic study of differing GABAergic circuitry serving thalamic somatosensory mechanisms. *J Neurosci* 1994 ; 14 : 2485-502.
11. Dejerine J, Roussy G. La syndrome thalamique. *Rev Neurol* 1906 ; 14 : 521-32.
12. Boivie J, Leijon G, Johansson I. Central post-stroke pain; a study of the mechanisms through analyses of the sensory abnormalities. *Pain* 1989 ; 37 : 173-85.

13. Rausell E, Cusick CG, Taub E, Jones EG. Chronic deafferentation in monkeys differentially affects nociceptive and nonnociceptive pathways distinguished by specific calcium-binding proteins and down-regulates gamma-aminobutyric acid type A receptors at thalamic levels. *Proc Natl Acad Sci USA* 1992 ; 89 : 2571-5.
14. Roberts WA, Eaton SA, Salt TE. Widely distributed GABA-mediated afferent inhibition processes within the ventrobasal thalamus of rat and their possible relevance to pathological pain states and somatotopic plasticity. *Exp Brain Res* 1992 ; 89 : 363-72.
15. Rausell E, Bae CS, Viñuela A, Huntley GW, Jones EG. Calbindin and parvalbumin cells in monkey VPL thalamic nucleus: distribution, laminar cortical projections, and relations to spinothalamic terminations. *J Neurosci* 1992 ; 12 : 4088-111.
16. Ma W, Peschanski M, Ralston HJ III. The differential synaptic organization of the spinal and lemniscal projections to the ventrobasal complex of the rat thalamus. Evidence for convergence of the two systems upon single thalamic neurons. *Neurosci* 1987 ; 22 : 925-34.
17. Lenz FA, Kwan HC, Dostrovsky JO, Tasker RR. Characteristics of the bursting pattern of action potentials that occurs in the thalamus of patients with central pain. *Brain Res* 1989 ; 496 : 357-60.
18. Koyama S, Katayama Y, Maejima S, Hirayama T, Fujii M, Tsubokawa T. Thalamic neuronal hyperactivity following transection of the spinothalamic tract in the cat: involvement of N-methyl-D-aspartate receptor. *Brain Res* 1993 ; 612 : 345-50.
19. Nicolelis MAL, Lin RCS, Woodward DJ, Chapin JK. Induction of immediate spatiotemporal changes in thalamic networks by peripheral block of ascending cutaneous information. *Nature* 1993 ; 361 : 533-6.
20. Pinault D. Golgi-like labeling of a single neuron recorded extracellularly. *Neurosci Lett* 1994 ; 170 : 255-60.

2

Supraspinal projections of lamina I neurons

A.D. CRAIG

Division of Neurobiology, Barrow Neurological Institute, Phoenix, USA.

The sensations of pain and temperature are associated with the ascending projections of the spinothalamic tract (STT) on the basis of lesions in humans [1-5], and experimental studies in animals have verified that many STT cells have nociceptive and thermoreceptive response properties [2, 6]. With the goal of providing insight into the central neural mechanisms for pain and temperature sensation, this laboratory has pursued the anatomical identification of the thalamic terminations of the nociceptive and thermoreceptive components of the STT. Previous studies of STT terminations based on the use of silver degeneration or transport of radioactive amino acids or HRP have provided evidence of the overall distribution of STT axons [7-13] (*see* chapter by HJ Ralston, this volume). The use of modern anterograde tracers such as PHA-L and labeled dextrans provides the ability to identify the projections of individual components of the STT. By combining the results of these hodological studies with physiological, cytoarchitectonic, and immunohistochemical evidence, it has been possible to identify an ascending spino-thalamo-cortical pathway for pain and temperature sensibility in monkeys. As recently reported in *Nature* [14], comparative functional anatomical evidence indicates that a homologous pathway is present in humans.

A focus on the lamina I STT projection

The STT originates in three main groups of cells found contralaterally in lamina I, lamina V, and lamina VII. Almost one half of the STT in monkey and cat originates in lamina I of the dorsal horn [15-17]. This component of the STT is of particular interest for pain and temperature sensation for several reasons.

First, lamina I receives small-diameter Aδ and C fiber primary afferent input from essentially all tissues of the body, skin, muscle, joint, teeth, cornea, and viscera (*see* [18, 19]). Such fibers are activated by changes in the physiological status of the tissues and organs of the body, such as (noxious) mechanical or thermal stress or damage, changes in temperature, muscle exercise, chemical or metabolic stimuli such as pH, pCO_2, glucose concentration, hypoxia, osmolarity, or interstitial inflammatory agents [1, 20-24]. The projections of lamina I neurons distribute such afferent activity in a modality selective manner to spinal and brainstem sites involved in homeostasis and autonomic control [25], as well as to the thalamus.

Second, lamina I contains a unique concentration of nociceptive and thermoreceptive STT neurons that includes at least three classes of cells with distinct physiological characteristics [26-33]: **NS**, or nociceptive-specific cells, that respond only to pinch and/or noxious heat; **COLD**, or thermoreceptive-(cooling)-specific cells, that respond monotonically to innocuous cooling from about normal skin temperature (34 °C) down to about noxious cold (15 °C); and **HPC**, or multimodal nociceptive cells, that respond to noxious heat, pinch, and noxious cold (from about normal room temperature (23 °C) down to at least 0° C). These three classes of lamina I STT cells have also been differentiated in the cat on the basis of their distinct conduction velocities [26, 33], their axonal distributions in the thalamus [34], and the shapes of their somata [35]: NS cells are fusiform, COLD cells are pyramidal, and HPC cells are multipolar. In the monkey, the same three classes of cells are present (JO Dostrovsky, AD Craig, unpublished observations), but some nociceptive lamina I STT cells have WDR response properties (sensitive to both low- and high-threshold stimuli) [28, 30, 36].

Third, the spinal course of the ascending axons of lamina I STT cells has been demonstrated in the middle of the contralateral lateral funiculus in cat and monkey [37, 38]. This is the critical location for temperature sensibility in cats [39] and for pain and temperature sensibility in humans [4, 5, 40]. Recent observation of a distinct bundle of calbindin-positive fibers in this same location in humans has provided further support of this correlation (A Blomqvist, AD Craig, unpublished observations), because this immunohistochemical marker labels both lamina I cells and lamina I spinothalamic terminations (*see* below).

Identification of a specific lamina I STT termination site in monkey

Lamina I STT terminations have been identified in the thalamus of macaque monkeys in which restricted injections of the anterograde tracers PHA-L or labeled dextrans were made into lamina I in the cervical or the lumbosacral enlargement [37,41]. In such cases, terminations occur in a variety of thalamic nuclei; the distribution of terminal labeling seen in one case with a PHA-L injection in lamina I at the C7 segment is shown in Figure 1. The three main termination sites are: the ventral caudal part of the medial dorsal nucleus (MDvc), the ventral posterior inferior n. (VPI), and a portion of the region usually described as the suprageniculate / posterior complex (SG/PO; *see* chapter by HJ Ralston, this volume). Of these, the lamina I STT terminations in the latter site are the most dense and extensive. They comprise compact clusters of profuse terminal arbors with large bouton complexes. Based on the pattern of lamina I terminal labeling, it has been possible to distinguish this site cytoarchitectonically as a distinct nucleus within the SG/PO region that has clusters or lobules of medium-sized ovoid and polygonal cells which stain moderately darkly with a Nissl stain. It extends rostrally from the level of the magnocellular portion of the medial geniculate, and it adjoins anteriorly the basal part of the ventral medial nucleus (VMb). For this structural reason, it has been termed the posterior part of the ventral medial nucleus, or VMpo; furthermore, this designation is consonant with its cortical projection to insular cortex, in parallel with that of VMb [42, 43] (*see* below), rather than to the somatosensory cortices to which the main somatosensory VP nuclei project.

The cytoarchitectonic delineation of VMpo is definitively supported by an immunohistochemical marker. Many lamina I somata are calbindin-immunoreactive [44], and it was found that an antibody against 28kD calbindin produces labeling of a dense, compact terminal fiber plexus in the macaque. In double-labeled material, anterogradely PHA-L-labeled lamina I STT terminations were found to be coextensive with the calbindin-positive fiber zone in the same or adjacent sections, and double-labeled lamina I terminals immunoreactive for calbindin were seen. The extent of the calbindin-positive fiber plexus coincides with the cytoarchitectonic borders of VMpo. Other calbindin-positive regions were observed in the thalamus, but these can be differentiated from VMpo by intervening unlabeled zones, weaker staining with a different appearance, or the presence of many calbindin-positive cells.

By making simultaneous injections into lamina I of different fluorescent dextrans at different levels of the cord, it was found that the lamina I terminations in VMpo are topographically organized, with trigeminal input most anteriorly and lumbosacral input most posteriorly. Preliminary retrograde labeling evidence obtained with iontophoretic injections of CTb (cholera toxin subunit B), which is not confounded by fiber of passage uptake [45], indicates that nearly all STT cells that project to VMpo are located in lamina I (E-T Zhang, AD Craig, unpublished observations).

The physiological characteristics of VMpo are consistent with the properties of its lamina I STT input. Recordings made with tungsten microelectrodes in barbiturate-anesthetized monkeys have revealed that VMpo contains clusters of nociceptive- or thermoreceptive-specific neurons [46]. Nearly all (91%) of 87 characterized neurons in VMpo were specifically sensitive to noxious or thermal (cold) stimuli. That is, VMpo neurons generally have properties like NS and COLD lamina I STT cells. The VMpo cells have small receptive fields that are topographically organized antero-posteriorly, similar to the anatomical findings, and their discharge rates grade with stimulus intensity above threshold.

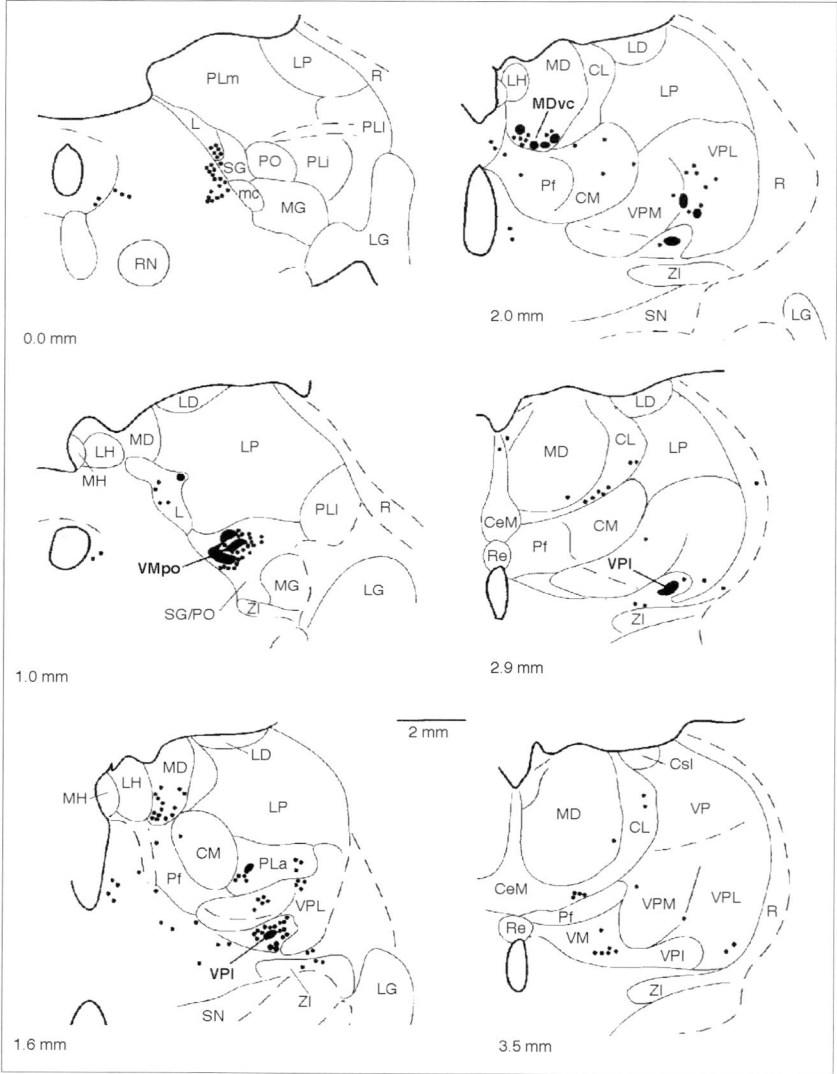

Figure 1. The distribution in frontal sections of PHA-L-labeled cervical lamina I terminations in the thalamus of a cynomolgus macaque monkey. The three main termination sites, VMpo, MDvc, and VPI, are highlighted. Numbers indicate distance anterior from the most posterior section in mm. Abbreviations: CeM = central medial n., CL = central lateral n., CM = centre median, Csl = central superior lateral n., H = habenula, L = n. limitans, LD = lateral dorsal n., LG = lateral geniculate n., LH = lateral habenula n., LP = lateral posterior n., MD = medial dorsal n., MDvc = ventral caudal part of the medial dorsal n., MG = medial geniculate n., MH = medial habenula n., Pc = paracentral n., Pf = parafascicular n., Pla = anterior pulvinar n., Plm = medial pulvinar n., PV = paraventricular (thalamic) n., R = reticular n., Re = reuniens n., RN = red n., SG/PO = suprageniculate / posterior complex, Sth = subthalamic n., VA = ventral anterior n., VLa = anterior part of the ventral lateral n., VLp = posterior part of the ventral lateral n., VM = ventral medial n., VMb = basal part of the ventral medial n., VMpo = posterior part of the ventral medial n., VPI = ventral postrior inferior n., VPLp = posterior part of the ventral posterior lateral n., VPM = ventral posterior medial n.

Thus, these findings in the macaque monkey indicate that VMpo is a specific, topographic lamina I STT projection target that could serve as a thalamic relay nucleus for nociception and thermoreception. It should be emphasized that the available evidence indicates that lamina I STT projections in the cat and rat are organized differently [47, 48]. Lamina I input to the ventral aspect of VMb in the cat may be analogous, but there is not a distinct, topographic nucleus present.

The cortical projection of VMpo

New studies in this laboratory have identified the cortical projection of VMpo. Large, pressure injections and small, iontophoretic injections of PHA-L, or red (TRITC) or green (FITC) fluorescent 10,000MW dextran have been made into VMpo under physiological guidance, and anterogradely labeled terminations have been observed in the ipsilateral cortex. In the particular case shown in Figure 2, an injection of red dextran was made into the portion of VMpo in which nociceptive-specific neurons with receptive fields on the hand were recorded (Figure 2, lower left). An injection of green dextran was made into the most rostral portion of VMpo in which nociceptive and thermoreceptive neurons with receptive fields on the face were recorded (Figure 2, upper left). This rostral injection overlapped into VMb, the gustatory relay nucleus. Dense terminal labeling was found in the middle layers (layers 3/4) of the anterodorsal insula and the fundus of the superior limiting sulcus from both injections. The results in this and similar cases demonstrate that VMpo projects in a topographic fashion to the agranular insula posterior to the gustatory cortex. There is an additional projection to the middle of the posterior insula. There is also weak input to the lateral precentral cortex, and discrete patches of labeling occur in the topographically appropriate parts (trigeminal and cervical, in this case) parts of the SI cortex at the area 3a/3b border, within the fundus of the central sulcus.

Correlative anatomical findings in the human brain

The location of VMpo in monkeys is consistent with descriptions of the general region in the human thalamus in which infarcts can produce analgesia and thermanesthesia [49-51], in which stimulation has evoked painful or thermal sensations [52, 53], and in which a few nociceptive neurons have recently been recorded [54]. This region of the human thalamus has been denoted as VCpc (parvicellular part of the ventral caudal nucleus) or as VC portae by Hassler [55, 56], but a distinct nucleus that could be compared with VMpo in the macaque has not been identified. With the use of the immunohistochemical marker calbindin and cytoarchitecture, it was possible to identify a nucleus homologous to VMpo in the human. A dense calbindin-positive fiber plexus was found in the human posterior thalamus that unmistakably resembles that observed in VMpo in the macaque monkey. Calbindin-positive fibers were observed entering this plexus from the spinal lemniscus, and a distinct bundle of calbindin-

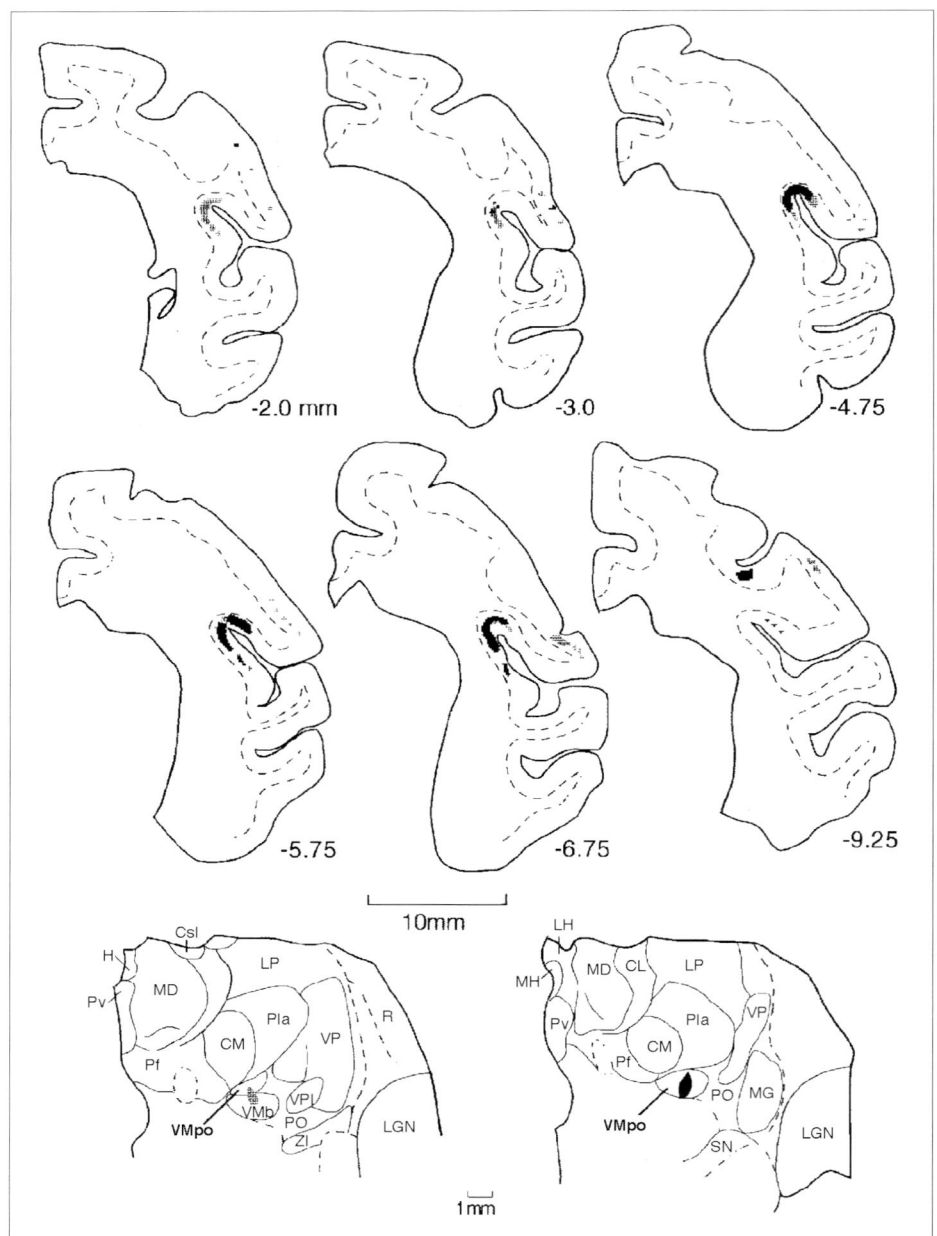

Figure 2. The distribution in frontal sections of cortical terminations from two different injections of labeled 10,000MW dextran. An injection of TRITC-labeled dextran (marked with black) was made in the center (cervical) part of VMpo, and an injection of FITC-labeled dextran (marked with light gray) was made in the rostral (trigeminal) part of VMpo, which overlapped into VMb. The main cortical projection of VMpo is to the antero-dorsal insula. Numbers indicate distance posterior from the anterior limit of the insula in mm. Abbreviations as in Figure 1.

positive fibers was observed in the middle of the lateral funiculus in upper spinal segments (A Blomqvist, AD Craig, unpublished observations). This calbindin fiber plexus is localized in a cytoarchitectonically distinct nucleus whose location is homologous to VMpo in the macaque monkey. The location of VMpo in the human thalamus is shown in Figure 3.

Correlative physiological findings in the human brain

The location of VMpo posterior to the main somatosensory representation of the face in VC (or VP) in the human thalamus fits well with the physiological data available in humans. Reports from two groups have demonstrated that threshold electrical stimulation can produce a localized sensation of pain or of cold in awake motor-disorder

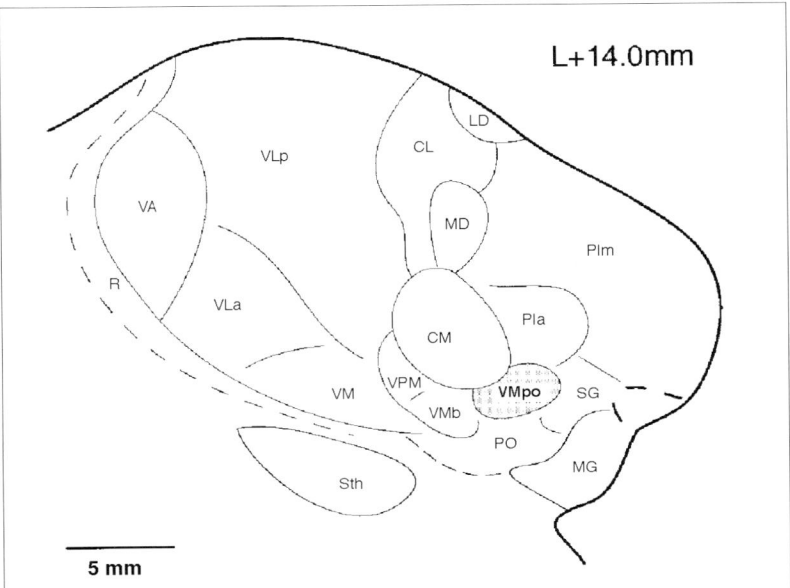

Figure 3. A cytoarchitectonic drawing of a sagittal section of a human thalamus at approximately lateral 14.0 mm, showing the location of VMpo.
Abbreviations: CeM = central medial n., CL = central lateral n., CM = centre median, CsI = central superior lateral n., H = habenula, L = n. limitans, LD = lateral dorsal n., LG = lateral geniculate n., LH = lateral habenula n., LP = lateral posterior n., MD = medial dorsal n., MDvc = ventral caudal part of the medial dorsal n., MG = medial geniculate n., MH = medial habenula n., Pc = paracentral n., Pf = parafascicular n., Pla = anterior pulvinar n., Plm = medial pulvinar n., PV = paraventricular (thalamic) n., R = reticular n., Re = reuniens n., RN = red n., SG/PO = suprageniculate / posterior complex, Sth = subthalamic n., VA = ventral anterior n., VLa = anterior part of the ventral lateral n., VLp = posterior part of the ventral lateral n., VM = ventral medial n., VMb = basal part of the ventral medial n., VMpo = posterior part of the ventral medial n., VPI = ventral postrior inferior n., VPLp = posterior part of the ventral posterior lateral n., VPM = ventral posterior medial n.

patients from a region just posterior and inferior to the main face and hand representation of somatosensory thalamus [52, 53]. Lenz and his colleagues [54] have recently described recordings from nociceptive neurons in this region of the human thalamus. These findings refine the earlier reports by Hassler and Riechert [55] and Halliday and Logue [57]. The location of VMpo just posterior to CM in the human thalamus is also consistent with the possibility that lesions of this region made years ago may have produced pain relief in part by involvement of this nucleus [58-60].

Recent studies of pain-evoked activity (local cerebral blood flow) in the human brain by several groups with the technique of positron emission tomographic imaging (PET) have illuminated several sites [61-64]. These include the posterior thalamus, the anterior insula, the SI and SII cortices, and the anterior cingulate cortex. Among these, the most significant increase in activity over that evoked by non-noxious mechanical stimulation was located in the anterior insula by one recent study [64]. The projection of VMpo to the anterior insula provides a sound anatomical substrate to explain this PET activity in the human brain. The corollary lamina I STT projections to MDvc, which projects to the anterior cingulate, and to VPI, which projects to SII, could explain the PET activity observed in these regions.

Conclusions

These observations identify VMpo as an homologous thalamic nucleus in humans and macaque monkeys. It is a lamina I STT thalamic nucleus that relays specific pain and temperature activity. The existence of this nucleus provides direct evidence supporting the specific nature of human pain and temperature sensibilities, and its cortical projection to the insula supports the functional association of pain and temperature with the limbic system.

The existence of a posterolateral thalamic relay nucleus for pain and temperature sensation was first postulated by Head and Holmes in 1911 [49]. They examined patients with the Dejerine-Roussy thalamic pain syndrome, associated with infarcts in the posterolateral thalamus, and found that the ongoing, burning dyesthetic pain was referred paradoxically to a peripheral zone of analgesia and thermanesthesia. They inferred that this indicated the existence of a specific sensory relay in this region of thalamus for pain and temperature. The identification of VMpo explains the analgesia and thermanesthesia observed in such thalamic pain syndrome patients in which lesions in this region of thalamus occurred due to infarcts of the thalamo-geniculate artery. In such patients, the peripheral zone of thermanesthesia and analgesia can, on the basis of the presently described observations, be ascribed to the loss of the specific pain and temperature representation in VMpo and the insula. This is consistent also with the observations of Biemond [65] on patients with parieto-insular lesions, and also with an anterior insula lesion case discussed by Berthier et al. [66]. However, such patients experience a burning dyesthetic pain that is referred to the peripheral zone of thermanesthesia and analgesia. Thus, activity in another region of the brain must account for such experiences. Accordingly, it has been proposed that the loss of the specific thermal representation in VMpo and the insula results in the disinhibition of the lamina I pathway *via* MDvc to the anterior cingulate [47, 67]. The observations described in this article are consistent with this proposal (as discussed in greater detail elsewhere).

Acute pain is not a simple sensation, because it also generates a strong effect that signals an emergency condition in which the integrity of the body is threatened and the survival of the individual animal may be at stake. It demands attention, it motivates action, and it heightens awareness and memory. It activates sympathetic and neuroendocrine reflex mechanisms. It engages specific responses at all levels of the neuraxis that promote the maintenance of the organism. Similarly, thermoreceptive, visceroreceptive, and putative metaboreceptive afferent activity carried by ascending lamina I axons also evoke strong, characteristic emotions of pleasantness or unpleasantness that reflect the status of the body, that is, of the need for homeostatic or behavioral adjustment to ensure the integrity and well-being of the animal. Like pain, these modalities can also demand attention and color memories, and they can activate autonomic, limbic and sensori-motor systems. In addition, pain, temperature, metabolic, vasomotor, tickle, itch, genital, and other enteroceptive sensations (or "feelings" from the body itself) typically are relatively poorly localizable, and display spatial summation, radiation, and temporal persistence. These are, in fact, the characteristics of the "common sensation" ("Gemeingefühl") discussed by Sherrington [68] as the sense of the physical body, or the "material me".

The projections of lamina I demonstrated in cat and monkey provide a substrate to support these characteristics. Propriospinal lamina I projections to the thoracolumbar sympathetic nuclei provide a substrate for spinal sympathetic reflexes [25]. Lamina I projections to the brainstem terminate in pre-autonomic regions that generate generalized homeostatic responses, in general visceral integrative sites that can activate ascending pathways to the hypothalamus and the amygdala, and in the periaqueductal gray, which can affect homeostasis, motivational state, and behavioral responses [19]. Finally, as described in this article, lamina I spino-thalamo-cortical projections reach the limbic system at the insular and anterior cingulate cortices, in addition to providing input to the somatosensory system. These components of the limbic system are classically associated with motivation, affect, and emotion. Thus, primary afferent input relevant to the integrity and "well-being" of the physical body itself reaches, *via* lamina I, all levels associated with the reactions evoked by changes in the status of the body. The lamina I projection system can therefore be viewed as a general homeostatic afferent system. From this perspective, the specific, topographic lamina I projection to the insular cortex *via* VMpo can be the basis for a cortical sensory map of the physical status of the body. The VMpo projection field lies adjacent to the VMb projection field, which is the cortical representation of gustation and other visceral activity relayed by the solitarius/parabrachial pathway [69]. Together, the VMpo and VMb cortical fields thus contain sensory representations of the body that parallel, respectively, the organization of the efferent sympathetic and parasympathetic systems.

Finally, the insula is also the main route by which every somatosensory information reaches the limbic system [70], and it is intimately involved in the processing of emotion [66, 71, 72]. In his recent book "Descartes' Error", the neurologist Antonio Damasio [72] has postulated that the insula and the adjacent somatosensory cortical fields are integral for the mental generation of the image of the self that underlies the basic emotional states, and that this is required for the motivation to make rational decisions affecting survival and quality of life. This argument suggests the notion that the specific and topographic lamina I pathway *via* VMpo to the anterodorsal insula could, by providing the afferent sensory representation of the status of the physical body, be an integral component of the generation of emotion.

Acknowledgements

Warm gratitude is expressed to the collaborators, colleagues, and friends who have contributed to these data and ideas: A. Blomqvist, M.C. Bushnell, J.O. Dostrovsky, Z.-S. Han, and E.-T. Zhang. Thanks are expressed to T. Fleming, K. Krout, E. O'Campo Perez, and A. Sinnott for technical support. This laboratory is supported by NIH grant NS25616 and by the James R. Atkinson Memorial Pain Research Fund administered by the Barrow Neurological Foundation.

References

1. Perl ER. Pain and nociception. In : Darian-Smith I, ed. *Handbook of physiology*, Section 1, *The nervous system, Volume III, Sensory processes*. Bethesda : American Physiological Society, 1984 : 915-75.
2. Willis WD. *The pain system*. Basel : Karger, 1985.
3. Noordenbos W, Wall PD. Diverse sensory functions with an almost totally divided spinal cord. A case of spinal cord transection with preservation of part of one anterolateral quadrant. *Pain* 1976 ; 2 : 185-95.
4. Foerster O. *Die Leitungsbahnen des Schmerzgefuhls und die chirurgische Behandlung der Schmerzzustande*. Berlin : Urban und Schwarzenberg, 1927.
5. Kuru M. *The sensory paths in the spinal cord and brain stem of man*. Tokyo : Sogensya, 1949.
6. Besson JM, Chaouch A. Peripheral and spinal mechanisms of nociception. *Physiol Rev* 1987 ; 67 : 67-186.
7. Mehler WR. Some neurological species differences - *a posteriori*. *Ann N Y Acad Sci* 1969 ; 167 : 424-68.
8. Berkley KJ. Spatial relationships between the terminations of somatic sensory and motor pathways in the rostral brainstem of cats and monkeys. I. Ascending somatic sensory inputs to lateral diencephalon. *J Comp Neurol* 1980 ; 193 : 283-317.
9. Boivie J. An anatomical reinvestigation of the termination of the spinothalamic tract in the monkey. *J Comp Neurol* 1979 ; 186 : 343-70.
10. Jones EG, Burton H. Cytoarchitecture and somatic sensory connectivity of thalamic nuclei other than the ventrobasal complex in the cat. *J Comp Neurol* 1974 ; 154 : 395-432.

11. Ganchrow D. Intratrigeminal and thalamic projections of nucleus caudalis in the squirrel monkey (*Saimiri sciureus*): a degeneration and autoradiographic study. *J Comp Neurol* 1978 ; 178 : 281-312.
12. Apkarian AV, Hodge CJ. Primate spinothalamic pathways: III. Thalamic terminations of the dorsolateral and ventral spinothalamic pathways. *J Comp Neurol* 1989 ; 288 : 493-511.
13. Burton H, Craig AD Jr. Spinothalamic projections in cat, raccoon and monkey: a study based on anterograde transport of horseradish peroxidase. In : Macchi G, Rustioni A, Spreafico R, eds. *Somatosenory integration in the thalamus*. New York : Elsevier, 1983 : 17-41.
14. Craig AD, Bushnell MC, Zhang ET, Blomqvist A. A thalamic nucleus specific for pain and temperature sensation. *Nature* 1994 ; 372 : 770-3.
15. Willis WD, Kenshalo DR Jr, Leonard RB. The cells of origin of the primate spinothalamic tract. *J Comp Neurol* 1979 ; 188 : 543-74.
16. Craig AD Jr, Linington AJ, Kniffki KD. Cells of origin of spinothalamic tract projections to the medial and lateral thalamus in the cat. *J Comp Neurol* 1989 ; 289 : 568-85.
17. Apkarian AV, Hodge CJ. Primate spinothalamic pathways: I. A quantitative study of the cells of origin of the spinothalamic pathway. *J Comp Neurol* 1989 ; 288 : 447-73.
18. Panneton WM. Primary afferent projections from the upper respiratory tract in the muskrat. *J Comp Neurol* 1991 ; 308 : 51-65.
19. Craig AD. Distribution of brainstem projections from spinal lamina I neurons in the cat and the monkey. *J Comp Neurol* 1995 ; (in press)
20. Vallet PG, Baertschi AJ. Spinal afferents for peripheral osmoreceptors in the rat. *Brain Res* 1982 ; 239 : 271-74.
21. Pickar JG, Hill JM, Kaufman MP. Dynamic exercise stimulates group III muscle afferents. *J Neurophysiol* 1994 ; 71 : 753-60.
22. Kress M, Koltzenburg M, Reeh PW, Handwerker HO. Responsiveness and functional attributes of electrically localized terminals of cutaneous C-fibers *in vivo* and *in vitro*. *J Neurophysiol* 1992 ; 68 : 581-95.
23. Steen KH, Reeh PW, Anton F, Handwerker HO. Protons selectively induce lasting excitation and sensitization to mechanical stimulation of nociceptors in rat skin, *in vitro*. *J Neurosci* 1992 ; 12 : 86-95.
24. MacIver MB, Tanelian DL. Activation of C fibers by metabolic perturbations associated with tourniquet ischemia. *Anesthesiology* 1992 ; 76 : 617-23.
25. Craig AD. Propriospinal input to thoracolumbar sympathetic nuclei from cervical and lumbar lamina I neurons in the cat and the monkey. *J Comp Neurol* 1993 ; 331: 517-30.
26. Craig AD Jr, Kniffki KD. Spinothalamic lumbosacral lamina I cells responsive to skin and muscle stimulation in the cat. *J Physiol (Lond)* 1985 ; 365 : 197-221.
27. Cervero F, Tattersall JEH. Somatic and visceral inputs to the thoracic spinal cord of the cat: marginal zone (lamina I) of the dorsal horn. *J Physiol (Lond)* 1987 ; 383 : 383-95.
28. Price DD, Dubner R, Hu JW. Trigeminothalamic neurons in nucleus caudalis responsive to tactile, thermal, and nociceptive stimulation of monkey's face. *J Neurophysiol* 1976 ; 39 : 936-53.
29. Dostrovsky JO, Hellon RF. The representation of facial temperature in the caudal trigeminal nucleus of the cat. *J Physiol (Lond)* 1978 ; 277 : 29-47.
30. Ferrington DG, Sorkin LS, Willis WD. Responses of spinothalamic tract cells in the superficial dorsal horn of the primate lumbar spinal cord. *J Physiol (Lond)* 1987 ; 388 : 681-703.
31. Christensen BN, Perl ER. Spinal neurons specifically excited by noxious or thermal stimuli: marginal zone of the dorsal horn. *J Neurophysiol* 1970 ; 33 : 293-307.
32. Craig AD, Hunsley SJ. Morphine enhances the activity of thermoreceptive cold-specific lamina I spinothalamic neurons in the cat. *Brain Res* 1991 ; 558 : 93-7.

33. Craig AD, Serrano LP. Effects of systemic morphine on lamina I spinothalamic tract neurons in the cat. *Brain Res* 1994 ; 636 : 233-44.
34. Dostrovsky JO, Craig AD. Antidromic identification of nociceptive lamina I cell terminations in the cat thalamus. *Soc Neurosci Abstr* 1993 ; 19 : 1572.
35. Han ZS, Craig AD. Morphological characteristics of physiologically identified lamina I cells in cats. *Soc Neurosci Abstr* 1994 ; 20 : 547.
36. Price DD, Hayes RL, Ruda M, Dubner R. Spatial and temporal transformations of input to spinothalamic tract neurons and their relation to somatic sensations. *J Neurophysiol* 1978 ; 41 : 933-47.
37. Craig AD. Spinal distribution of ascending lamina I axons anterogradely labeled with *Phaseolus vulgaris* leucoagglutinin (PHA-L) in the cat. *J Comp Neurol* 1991 ; 313 : 377-93.
38. Ralston HJ III, Ralston DD. The primate dorsal spinothalamic tract: evidence for a specific termination in the posterior nuclei (Po/SG) of the thalamus. *Pain* 1992 ; 48 : 107-18.
39. Norrsell U. Unilateral behavioural thermosensitivity after transection of one lateral funiculus in the cervical spinal cord of the cat. *Exp Brain Res* 1983 ; 53 : 71-80.
40. Nathan PW, Smith MC. Clinico-anatomical correlation in anterolateral cordotomy. In : Bonica JJ, ed. *Advances in pain research and therapy*, vol. 3. New York : Raven Press, 1979 : 921-6.
41. Craig AD. Organization of lamina I terminations in the posterior thalamus of the cynomolgus monkey. *Soc Neurosci Abstr* 1992 ; 18 : 385.
42. Friedman DP, Murray EA. Thalamic connectivity of the second somatosensory area and neighboring somatosensory fields of the lateral sulcus of the macaque. *J Comp Neurol* 1986 ; 252 : 348-73.
43. Pritchard TC, Hamilton RB, Morse JR, Norgren R. Projections of thalamic gustatory and lingual areas in the monkey, *Macaca fascicularis. J Comp Neurol* 1986 ; 244 : 213-28.
44. Antal M, Freund TF, Polgár E. Calcium-binding proteins, parvalbumin- and calbindin-D 28k-immunoreactive neurons in the rat spinal cord and dorsal root ganglia: a light and electron microscopic study. *J Comp Neurol* 1990 ; 295 : 467-84.
45. Luppi PH, Fort P, Jouvet M. Iontophoretic application of unconjugated cholera toxin B subunit (CTb) combined with immunohistochemistry of neurochemical substances: a method for transmitter identification of retrogradely labeled neurons. *Brain Res* 1990 ; 534 : 209-24.
46. Bushnell MC, Craig AD. Nociceptive- and thermoreceptive-specific neurons in a discrete region of the monkey lateral thalamus. *Soc Neurosci Abstr* 1993 ; 19 : 1073.
47. Craig AD. Supraspinal pathways and mechanisms relevant to central pain. In: Casey KL, ed. *Pain and central nervous system disease: the central pain syndromes*. New York : Raven Press, 1991 : 157-70.
48. Iwata K, Kenshalo DR Jr., Dubner R, Nahin RL. Diencephalic projections from the superficial and deep laminae of the medullary dorsal horn in the rat. *J Comp Neurol* 1992 ; 321 : 404-20.
49. Head H, Holmes G. Sensory disturbances from cerebral lesions. *Brain* 1911 ; 34 : 102-254.
50. Leijon G, Boivie J, Johansson I. Central post-stroke pain-neurological symptoms and pain characteristics. *Pain* 1989 ; 36 : 13-25.
51. Bogousslavsky J, Regli F, Uske A. Thalamic infarcts: clinical syndromes, etiology, and prognosis. *Neurology* 1988 ; 38 : 837-48.
52. Lenz FA, Seike M, Richardson RT, Lin YC, Baker FH, Khoja I, Jaeger CJ, Gracely RH. Thermal and pain sensations evoked by microstimulation in the area of human ventrocaudal nucleus. *J Neurophysiol* 1993 ; 70 : 200-12.
53. Dostrovsky JO, Wells FEB, Tasker RR. Pain sensations evoked by stimulation in human thalamus. In : Inoka R, Shigenaga Y, Tohyama M, eds. *Processing and inhibition of nociceptive information*, International Congress Series 989. Amsterdam : Excerpta Medica, 1992 : 115-20.

54. Lenz FA, Seike M, Lin YC, Baker FH, Rowland LH, Gracely RH, Richardson RT. Neurons in the area of human thalamic nucleus ventralis caudalis respond to painful heat stimuli. *Brain Res* 1993 ; 623 : 235-40.
55. Hassler R, Riechert T. Klinische und anatomische Befunde bei stereotaktischen Schmerzoperationen im Thalamus. *Arch Psychiatry* 1959 ; 200 : 93-122.
56. Hassler R. Dichotomy of facial pain conduction in the diencephalon. In : Hassler R, Walker AE, eds. T*rigeminal neuralgia*. Philadelphia : Sanders, 1970 : 123-38.
57. Halliday AM, Logue V. Painful sensations evoked by electrical stimulation in the thalamus. In : Somjen GG, ed. *Neurophysiology studied in man*. Amsterdam : Excerpta Medica, 1972 : 221-30.
58. White JC, Sweet WH. *Pain and the neurosurgeon: a forty-year experience*. Springfield : Thomas, 1969.
59. Richardson DE. Thalamotomy for intractable pain. *Confinia Neurol* 1967 ; 29 : 139-45.
60. Craig AD. Supraspinal pathways and integration of pain and temperature. In : Boivie J, Hansson P, Lindblom U, eds. *Touch, temperature, and pain in health and disease. Progress in pain research and management*, Vol.3. Seattle : IASP Press 1994 ; (in press).
61. Talbot JD, Marrett S, Evans AC, Meyer E, Bushnell MC, Duncan GH. Multiple representations of pain in human cerebral cortex. *Science* 1991 ; 251 : 1355-8.
62. Jones AKP, Brown WD, Friston KJ, Qi LY, Frackowiak RSJ. Cortical and subcortical localization of response to pain in man using positron emission tomography. *Proc R Soc Lond (Biol)* 1991 ; 244 : 39-44.
63. Casey KL, Minoshima S, Berger KL, Koeppe RA, Morrow TJ, Frey KA. Positron emission tomographic analysis of cerebral structures activated specifically by repetitive noxious heat stimuli. *J Neurophysiol* 1994 ; 71 : 802-7.
64. Coghill RC, Talbot JD, Evans AC, Meyer E, Gjedde A, Bushnell MC, Duncan GH. Distributed processing of pain and vibration by the human brain. *J Neurosci* 1994 ; 14 : 4095-108.
65. Biemond A. The conduction of pain above the level of the thalamus opticus. *Arch Neurol Psychiatry* 1956 ; 75 : 231-44.
66. Berthier ML, Starkstein SE, Leiguarda RC. A symbolia for pain: a sensory-limbic disconnection syndrome. *Ann Neurol* 1988 ; 24 : 41-9.
67. Craig AD, Bushnell MC. The thermal grill illusion: unmasking the burn of cold pain. *Science* 1994 ; 265 : 252-5.
68. Sherrington CS. Cutaneous sensations. In : Schäfer EA, ed. *Text-book of physiology*. Edinburgh : Pentland, 1900 : 920-1001.
69. Yasui Y, Breder CD, Saper CB, Cechetto DF. Autonomic responses and efferent pathways from the insular cortex in the rat. *J Comp Neurol* 1991 ; 303 : 355-74.
70. Schneider RJ, Friedman DP, Mishkin M. A modality-specific somatosensory area within the insula of the rhesus monkey. *Brain Res* 1993 ; 621 : 116-20.
71. Lane R, Reimann EM, Ahern GL, Schwartz GE, Davidson RJ, Axelrod B, Yun LS. Neuroanatomical correlates of happiness, sadness, and disgust. *Human Brain Mapping Supple* 1995 ; 1: 212 (abstract).
72. Damasio AR. *Descartes' error*. New York : Putnam, 1993.

3

The spino-parabrachio -amygdaloid and -hypothalamic nociceptive pathways

J.F. BERNARD, H. BESTER, J.M. BESSON

Unité de Recherches de Physiopharmacologie du Système Nerveux, INSERM U 161 and EPHE, Paris, France.

The powerful new anatomical tracing techniques have not only allowed a better visualization of the "classical" ascending pain pathways (origins and terminals), but also revealed numerous "novel" ascending tracts which participate in pain integration. Thus, there is increasing evidence that nociception is not related to a unique system of pathways or relay nuclei.

Among the so called "pain pathways", the spinothalamic tract seems to be highly implicated in sensory-discriminative aspects of pain. The functional roles of other ascending pathways such as the spino-cervico-thalamic tract, the postsynaptic dorsal column fibers and the various components of the spinoreticular and spino-reticulo-thalamic tracts are poorly understood. Recent studies provided evidence of new pain pathways such as the spino-hypothalamic tract (*see* Burstein, this volume) and the spino-parabrachio -amygdaloid and -hypothalamic pathways, the latter two being the subject of this report. Both electrophysiological and anatomical characteristics of these two pathways lead us to suggest they are strongly implicated in the affective-emotional and autonomic aspects of pain.

The parabrachial (PB) area is a group of cells surrounding the brachium conjunctivum in the dorsolateral pons (pontine PB (pPB) division) up to the mesencephalon where it continues into the mesencephalic PB (mPB) division. The coronal plane, where the inferior colliculus merges with the pons, used as the reference plane (Pr), permits the clear identification of the pPB division (caudal to the Pr), and the mPB division (rostral to the Pr). Initial observations [1, 2] have shown that the lateral PB area receives projections from neurons located in the superficial lamina I of the dorsal horn of the spinal cord, which contains a high proportion of neurons receiving noxious inputs (see ref in [3]). In addition, lamina I neurons projecting to the PB area have been shown to be specifically driven by noxious stimuli [4-6]. However, despite these latter studies, the importance and the location of terminal fibres in the PB area originating from the spinal laminae were not completely known. These observations very recently led us to perform an extensive and detailed anatomical investigation of the spino-parabrachial projections [7] that is reported in the the first section of this chapter.

Since PB neurons project to various brainstem and forebrain structures, with the central nucleus of the amygdala being a major target of neurons located in the PB area receiving spinal projections, we postulated the existence of a new pain pathway, the spino-parabrachio-amygdaloid tract. In fact we have shown that WGA-HRP injected in the PB area simultaneously labeled neurons in the superficial dorsal horn and terminals in the central nucleus of the amygdala [8]. A parallel study performed in our laboratory [9] observed synaptic contacts between spinal afferents and PB neurons retrogradely labeled from the amygdala. These observations led us to perform an extensive electrophysiological investigation (several hundred neurons) to determine the response to noxious events of the PB neurons projecting to the amygdala. Since the hypothalamus is the major target of a second PB region that also receives spinal projection, we postulated the existence of a second new pain pathway, the spino-parabrachio-hypothalamic tract. Similar electrophysiological investigation was performed on PB neurons antidromically driven from the hypothalamus. The second and third section of this report refer to specific electrophysiological investigations of these pain pathways, with parallel anatomical investigations of the projections of the PB-amygdaloid and PB-hypothalamic efferents which corroborate the former physiological findings.

The spino-parabrachial pathway

The high density of the projection, originating from the superficial dorsal horn to the PB was already suggested by several anatomical studies using retrograde tracer [1, 8, 10-12]. Our recent investigation using restricted injection of *Phasoleus vulgaris* leucoagglutinin (PHA-L), an anterograde and very sensitive tracer, in different laminae of the spinal cord [7] demonstrated that two areas of the cervical enlargement project to the PB area in different ways, namely:

- the superficial laminae (I, II, see example of injection in Figure 1), which showed a very dense projection with a clear contralateral predominance at the coronal level where the inferior colliculus merges with the pons, to a restricted "superficial" portion of the PB area, namely the lateral crescent area, the dorsal lateral, the superior lateral (PBsl) and the outer portion of the external lateral PB subnuclei (Figure 2). Less dense

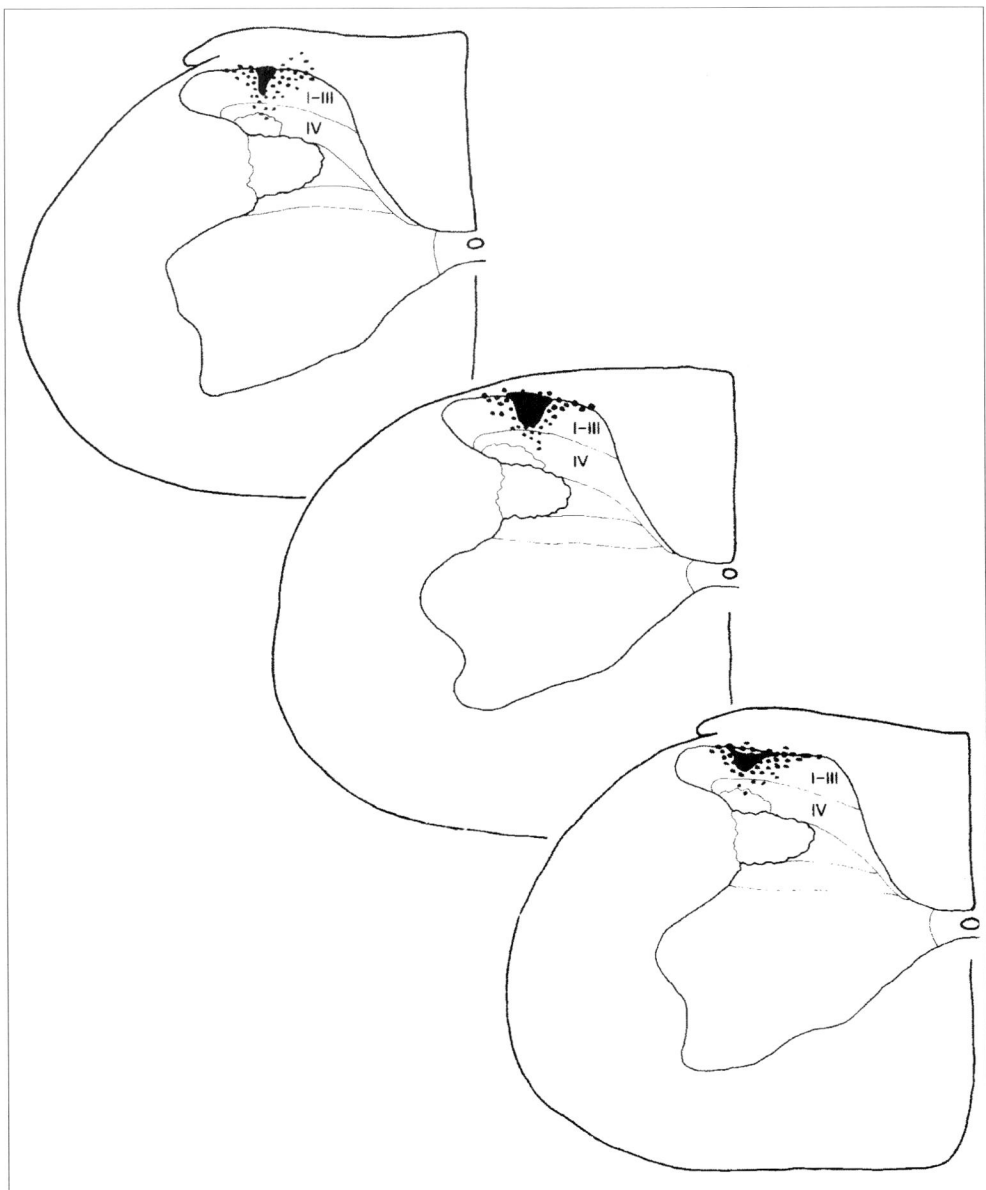

Figure 1. Series of camera lucida drawings of coronal sections of the cervical enlargement, illustrating the extent of the PHA-L injection sites in superficial laminae. Note the dense core of the injection site centred in laminae I and II and the numerous labelled cells in these laminae. Scale bar = 1 mm. From [7].

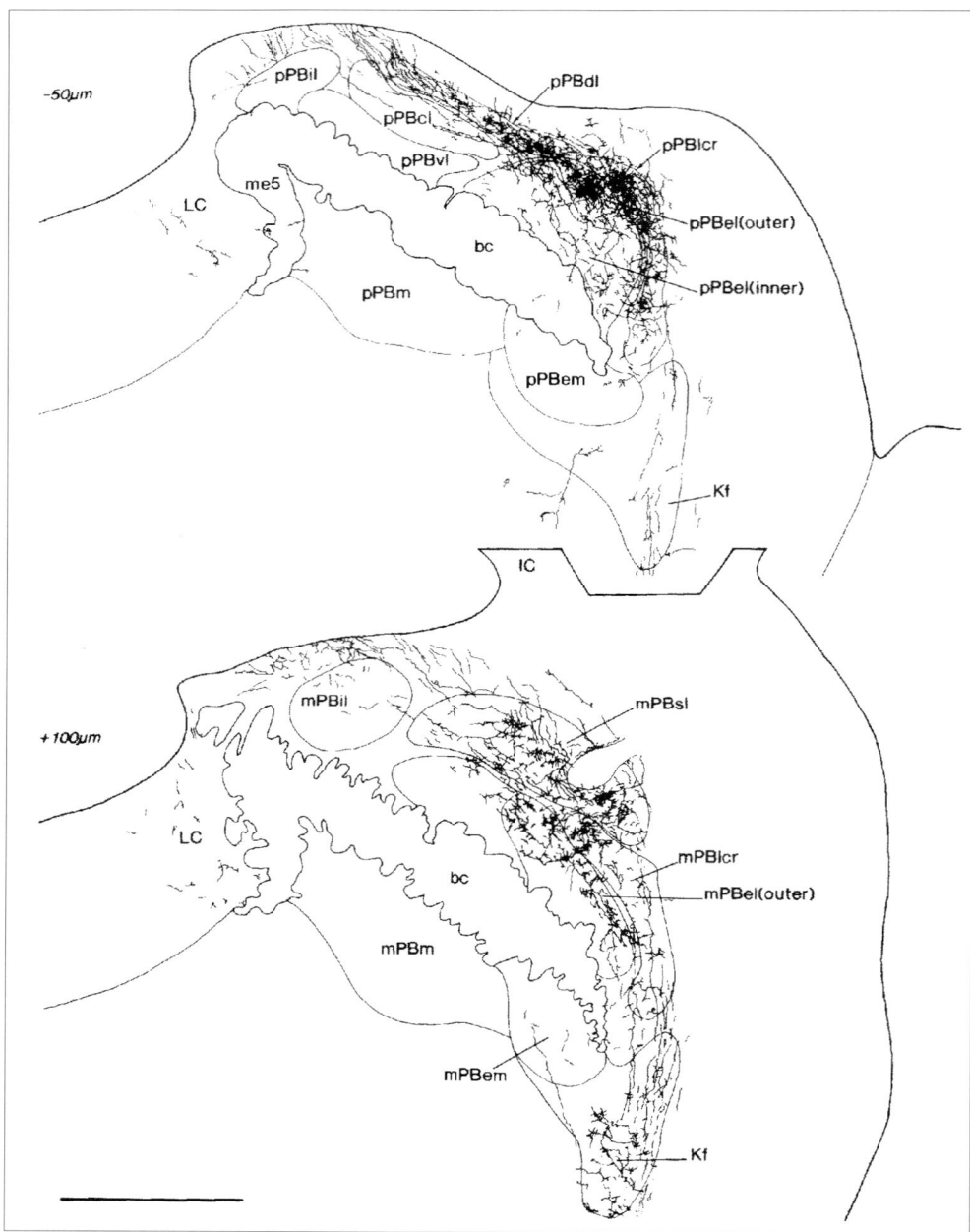

Figure 2. Camera lucida drawings of coronal sections, illustrating (from caudal to rostral) the spread of labelled terminals in the contralateral pPB area following an injection in the superficial laminae of the cervical enlargement (*see* Figure 1). The gap between coronal sections is 150 μm. Distance of each PB section caudal (-) or rostral (+) to the Pr is indicated in μm. Scale bar = 500 μm. For abbreviations, *see* separate list. Modified from [7].

projections were observed in the Kölliker-Fuse nucleus (KF) and in the ventrolateral/lateral quadrant of the caudal and mid PAG. By contrast, the labelling was weak or absent in the other PB subnuclei and the outer adjacent regions; in particular, no or very little labelling was found in the cuneiform nucleus. The PB area appeared to be the supraspinal target which received the densest projection from laminae I and II of the dorsal horn. Projections were less dense in the PAG and the thalamus, and markedly less dense in other sites such as the ventrolateral medulla, the subnucleus reticularis dorsalis, the nucleus of the solitary tract and the hypothalamus ;
- the reticular portion of lamina V, the medial portion of laminae IV - VI up to X and lamina VIII, showed bilateral projections with a medium to high density onto a very restricted portion of the PB area, namely the internal lateral PB subnucleus. A lesser projection was also observed in the adjacent portion of the PBsl, the KF and the lateral quadrant of the PAG.

These results strongly suggest that messages conveyed by neurons in lamina I-II converge onto a restricted superficial portion of the PB area that was adequately located to contact, caudally, the PB neurons projecting to the amygdala, and rostrally, the PB neurons projecting to the hypothalamus.

The spino-parabrachio-amygdaloid pathway

An extensive electrophysiological investigation was performed on the PB region in rats under halothane anaesthesia (0.5%) in a nitrous oxide/oxygen mixture (1/2 - 2/3) [13]. Neurons were extracellularly recorded and identified by antidromic stimulation from the central nucleus of the amygdala (Ce). These neurons were located in the pontine division of the PB area (pPB), more precisely in the external lateral (pPBel) and external medial (pPBem) and dorsal lateral (pPBdl) subnuclei according to the nomenclature proposed by Fulwiler and Saper [14], (*see also* Bernard *et al.* [15]). The aim of our studies was to consider the responsiveness of PB neurons to various types of either mechanical, thermal cutaneous or visceral stimuli.

A high proportion (70%) of PB neurons backfired from the Ce (PB-Ce neurons) were exclusively excited by noxious cutaneous stimulation (nociceptive specific neurons: NS neurons), whereas other kinds of stimuli either innocuous somatic or gustatory were ineffective. The axons of these neurons exhibited a very slow conduction velocity, between 0.26m/s and 1.1 m/s, i.e. in the unmyelinated range.

The cutaneous excitatory receptive fields of these neurons were large in the majority of the cases (70%) and included several areas of the body. A more marked activation was often obtained from stimuli applied to one part of the body, denoted as the preferential receptive field. In the other cases (30%), the excitatory receptive field was relatively small and restricted to one part of the body (the tail, a paw, a hemiface, or the tongue). Both the preferential and small receptive fields were often located on the contralateral side. In addition, noxious stimuli applied outside the excitatory receptive

fields were found to strongly inhibit the responses of NS neurons. The NS neurons either exhibited absent or low spontaneous activity. They responded exclusively to mechanical (pinch or squeeze) and/or thermal (waterbath or waterjet > 44 °C) noxious stimuli with a marked and sustained activation that had a rapid onset and was generally without afterdischarge. Noxious thermal stimuli generally induced a stronger response than the noxious mechanical stimuli. These neurons exhibited a clear capacity to encode thermal stimuli in the noxious range (Figure 3 E and F):
- the stimulus-response function was always positive and monotonic;
- the slope of the curve progressively increased up to a maximum where it was very steep, then the steepness of the slope decreased close to the maximum response;
- the mean threshold was 44.1 °C ± 2 °C, and the point of steepest slope of the mean curve was around 47 °C.

All the NS neurons responded to intense transcutaneous electrical stimulation with two peaks of activation. We found that the early and the late peak were triggered by the activation of peripheral fibers with conduction velocities in the 8 - 20 m/s and 0.5 - 0.8 m/s range, i.e. A- and C- fibers, respectively (Figure 3 A - D). In numerous cases, the response due to C- fibers exhibited a wind-up phenomenon during repetitive stimulation (0.66 Hz). Intravenous morphine induced a strong depression of the response elicited by noxious thermal stimuli in a dose-related and naloxone reversible fashion, with an ED_{50} = 1.8 mg/kg [16].

In more recent studies [17], we demonstrated that a majority of PB-Ce neurons were affected by visceral stimuli (intraperitoneal injection of bradykinin and/or colorectal distension), almost exclusively in the noxious range; all of them were also affected by cutaneous noxious stimuli. Two groups of neurons were characterized:

1) those responding to intraperitoneal bradykinin and/or to strong colorectal distension with an intense and sustained increase of discharge. The response to bradykinin and to colorectal distension was often dissociated, *i.e.* the activation was often produced by only one of the stimuli, the other being ineffective or inhibitory. The viscerally activated neurons exhibited a clear capacity to encode the colorectal distension in the noxious range (Figure 4):
- the stimulus-response function was almost always positive and monotonic;
- for individual curves, the slope of the mean curve progressively increased up to the highest interval of pressure tested (100-125 mmHg);
- the threshold for neuronal response to colorectal distension was between 25 mmHg and 100 mmHg with a mean pressure threshold of 56 ± 24 (SD) mmHg ;

2) those inhibited by both strong colorectal distension and intraperitoneal bradykinin, or only by one of the stimuli, being unresponsive to the other. These neurons were either affected to a small extent, or not at all, by weak colorectal distension ≤ 25 mmHg.

These studies demonstrate that a rather high proportion of pPB neurons backfired from the Ce respond to nociceptive information. However, since Cechetto and Calaresu

[18] and Jhamandas *et al.* [19] have shown that some PB neurons responded to the activation of arterial baroreceptors, the responses observed in the PB area could be due to a blood pressure change linked to noxious stimuli. However, the possibility of such an indirect effect was improbable for the following reasons:

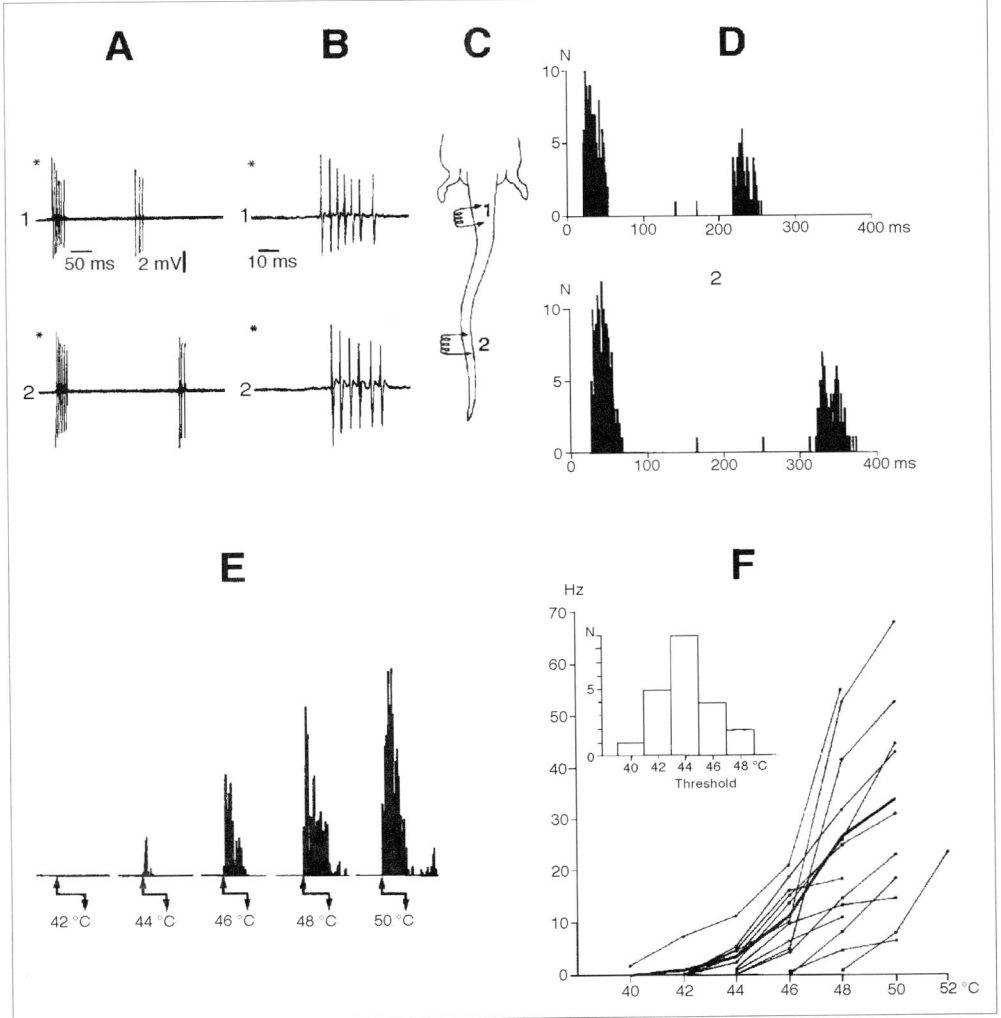

Figure 3. A1, 2: single sweep recording of the early and late peak evoked by trancutaneous electrical stimulation of the base (C1) and the tip (C2) of the tail. B1, 2: same as in A1, 2, but the scale shows detail of the early peaks. D: post-stimulus histograms (PSTH) made from responses to repetitive trancutaneous electrical stimulations (0,66 Hz, 50 trials) applied to the two sites on the tail (C 1, 2). E: Encoding properties of a nociceptive specific parabrachio-amygdaloid neuron to thermal stimulation applied to the contralateral forelimb. F: Stimulus response curve; thin lines: individual NS neurons; thick line: mean stimulus response curve. Threshold histogram is inserted in the top left. Modified from [13].

- the response of one given PB neuron was often very different according to the part of the body stimulated and/or the noxious modality used: often the stimulation of visceral and/or somatic parts of the body did not induce any response whereas an intense activation was observed in another part of the body;
- the latency of blood pressure response and the time necessary for its maximal increase was much longer than those observed when considering the electrophysiological responses, this is particularly clear when considering the response to transcutaneous electrical stimulation;
- the discharge of most of visceral nociceptive neurons was not altered by a rapid ($\approx$ 2 s) i.v. injection of ringer ($\approx$ 0.3 ml) which produced a significant increase in blood pressure (20 - 30 mmHg, see [17]). Consequently, artefactual results are improbable in most cases. However, the latter injection of ringer, that increased blood pressure, produced an activation of a few nociceptive neurons suggesting a convergence between baroreceptive and nociceptive messages.

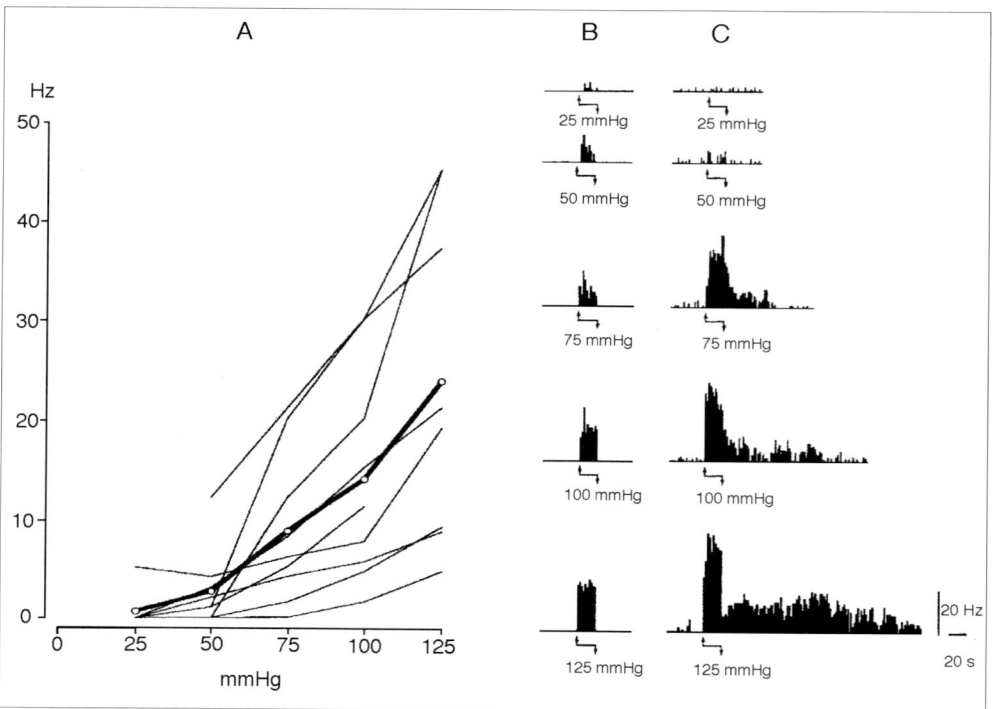

Figure 4. A: Stimulus-response curves to graded colo-rectal distension. Thin lines: individual neurons; thick line: mean stimulus response curve. B and C: Encoding properties of two individual parabrachial neurons. Increasing colo-rectal pressures (25 to 125 mmHg, 25 mmHg steps) were applied with an intracolic balloon (*see* methods). Modified from [17].

Despite numerous anatomical studies in the rat, demonstrating the efferent projection of the PB area to the Ce [8, 14, 20-24], the detailed location of terminal fibers in the Ce subregion from PB subnuclei was largely unknown to date. We therefore used the PHA-L, a very sensitive and selective anterograde axonal marker, injected into extremely restricted sites, in order to determine ascending projections from the PB with emphasis on the amygdaloid region [15, 25].

The results confirmed that the pPB area primarily and only projected onto the ipsilateral Ce, and, to a lesser extent, onto the ipsilateral posterior basolateral (BLP), anterior basomedial (BMA), and amygdaloid cortical (ACo) nuclei of the amygdala. Substantial projections were also found in the substantia innominata dorsal/ventral portion of the globus pallidus (SId/GPv), substriatal (SStr), and fondus striatal (FStr) regions which continue the amygdala rostrally. A summary diagram of these projections is illustrated in Figure 5. The results demonstrated that the projections of the pPB area onto the Ce were topically organized.

1) The region of the pPB area, mainly including the medial subnucleus (pPBm), the waist area (pPBwa), and a thin rostral lamina of the ventral lateral subnucleus (pPBvl), projects primarily to the medial portion of the Ce (CeM). Dense projections were also found in the BLP, BMA, and ACo nuclei of the amygdala. These pPB regions also diffusely project into the lateral division of the bed nucleus of the stria terminalis (BSTL) the SId/GPv, SStr and FStr rostral areas, and, to a lesser extent, to the agranular insular cortex.

2) The region of the pPB mainly including the rostral portion of the central lateral subnucleus (pPBcl) and the outer-rostral portion of the pPBel projects primarily to the lateral portion of the Ce (CeL) and the dorsal lateral subnucleus of the BST (BSTdl). Only the pPBcl subnucleus projects to the median, the anteroventral and the periventricular nuclei of the preoptic hypothalamus.

3) The region of the pPB, mainly including the pPBdl, the remaining pPBel, and the pPBem subnuclei, projects primarily to the lateral capsular portion of the Ce (CeLC) and bilaterally to its rostral portion. Dense projections were also found in the regions which extend the CeLC rostrally and, to a lesser extent, in the SId/GPv, SStr, FStr rostral areas and the nucleus of the horizontal limb of diagonal band. These pPB regions do not project onto the BST and preoptic hypothalamus.

These detailed anatomical studies, showing a dense projection of the pPB areas towards subregions of the Ce and its close vicinity, led us to perform an electrophysiological investigation at these latter levels. It must be underlined that, despite the numerous studies which have implicated the amygdala in pain processes, there was no available information on the responsiveness of Ce neurons to noxious stimuli. Thus, a systematic study was undertaken to investigate the responsiveness of Ce neurons to various types of peripheral cutaneous stimulation [26]. We used the same approach as previously described at the PB level. In these experiments, 177 neurons

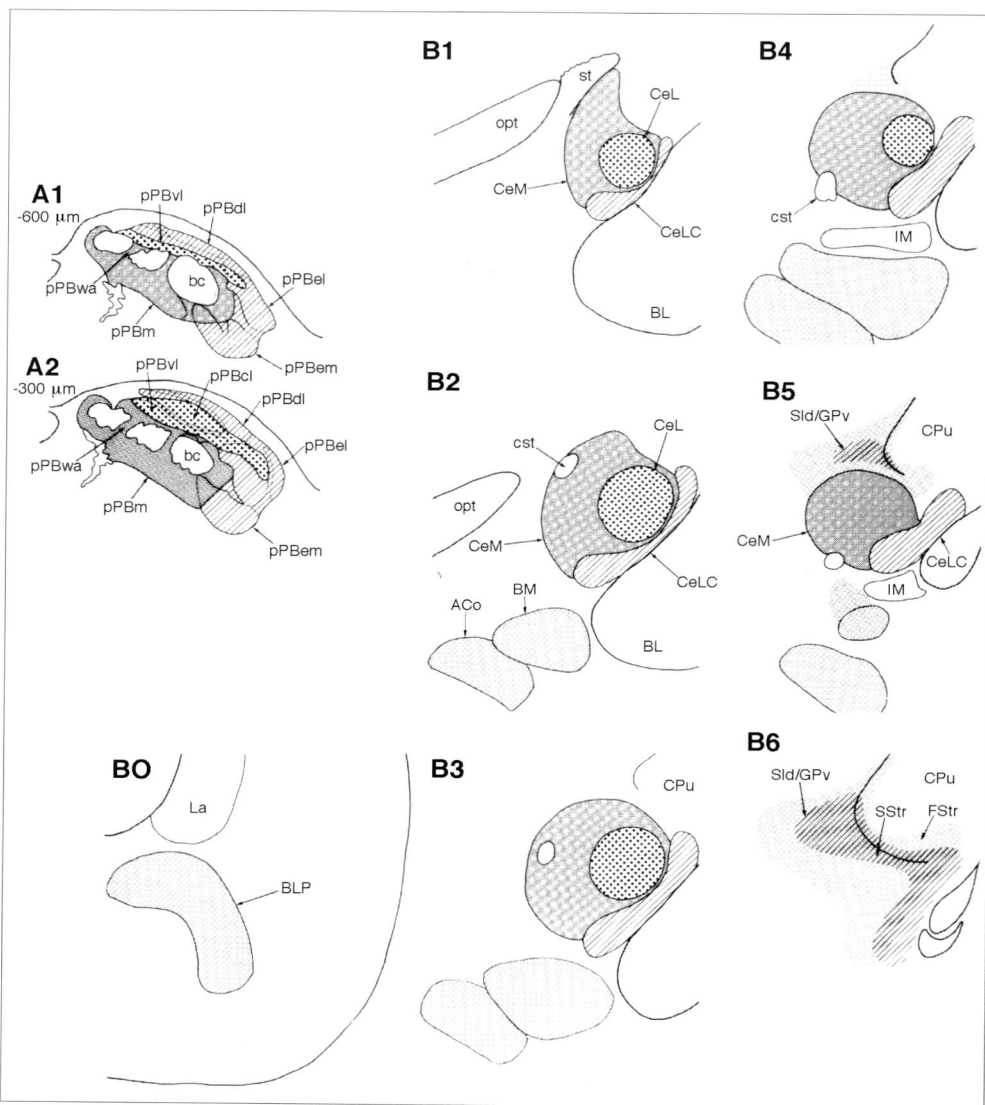

Figure 5. Summary diagram illustrating the projection pattern from the pPB area to the amygdala. The pPB grey region (A1, 2) projects very densely to the Ce grey region (CeM, B1 - 5), and densely to the other light grey regions (B0, 2 - 6). The pPB region filled with dots (A1, 2) projects very densely to the Ce region filled with dots (CeL, B1 - 4). The pPB hatched region (A1, 2) projects very densely to the Ce hatched region (CeLC, B1 - 5), and densely to the other hatched regions (B5 - 6). Scale = 500 mm. For the abbreviations, *see* the separate list of abbreviations. From [15].

were studied and the majority of them (80%) were excited or inhibited exclusively or preferentially by noxious stimuli. These units were separated into two groups: a group of neurons excited by noxious stimuli (46% of the whole population) and a group of neurons inhibited by noxious stimuli (34% of the whole population). The receptive fields of both groups of neurons were very large; in about half of the cases, the neurons responded similarly from all parts of the body.

The excited neurons were essentially located in the CeLC and in the SId/GPv. They responded to noxious mechanical (pinch or squeeze) and/or noxious thermal (water bath or water jet > 44 °C) stimuli with a marked and sustained discharge, with a clear capacity to encode thermal stimuli in the noxious range. The mean t_{50} of the stimulus response curve was around 47 °C. These neurons were clearly driven by the activation of Aδ and C fibers (nociceptive). The responses to noxious stimuli were markedly depressed by intravenous morphine in a dose-related and naloxone reversible fashion, with an ED_{50} = 1.2 mg/kg [27].

The inhibited neurons were essentially located in the remaining portion of the Ce (CeL and CeM). Their spontaneous activity was markedly decreased or suppressed by noxious stimuli. There was a clear relationship between the degree of inhibition and the intensity of peripheral stimulation in noxious range.

From these studies, it must be pointed out that the main electrophysiological characteristics of CeLC and SId/GPv excited neurons are similar to those described for pPB-Ce neurons which project densely to the former areas. Dense pPB projections have also been observed in the CeL and CeM subregions, two areas associated with inhibitory neurons, the role of which remains to be determined.

Taken together, these results demonstrate the existence of a new pain pathway, the spino-parabrachio-amygdaloid tract, the first relay being mainly the lamina I of the spinal cord (*see* introduction), the second relay, the lateral and external pPB subnuclei, the termination sites being mainly the Ce, the SId/GPv and the BSTL. A striking feature of this pathway is the high density of the projections originating from the superficial dorsal horn to the PB (*see* above). Another striking feature of this pathway is the high proportion of neurons exclusively activated by noxious stimuli at all stages of this pathway *i.e.* the superficial dorsal horn, the lateral and external PB area, the Ce and the SId/GPv areas. Additionally to this simplified view, it must be pointed out that anatomical and electrophysiological data [8, 28-31] demonstrate that another strong input, the visceral portion of the solitary tract nucleus (NTS), could relay visceral nociceptive message towards the lateral PB area. Both superficial spinal and NTS relays probably have a complementary and/or an interactive role in the transmission of visceral nociceptive messages towards the PB area.

Most of the lamina I neurons that project onto the PB area or in its vicinity ascend in the dorsolateral funiculus (DLF; *see* references in [10]). The observation that DLF section does not clearly modify the latency and the threshold in various nociceptive tests (tail-flick, paw withdrawal from heat, shock avoidance; *see* references in [32]) suggests that the spino-parabrachio-amygdaloid pathway is not primarily involved in the sensory discrimination of noxious stimuli. Because the receptive fields of PB and Ce neurons are extremely large, the involvement of such a pathway in spatial discrimination is also improbable.

Taking into account (1) the involvement of PB area in numerous autonomic processes: i.e. cardiovascular regulation [18, 19, 33-35], respiratory modulation [36-38], drinking behavior [39] and micturition [40] and (2) the involvement of Ce in fear [41-45], emotional memory and behavior [41, 46-50], autonomic regulation i.e. pupil dilatation [41, 51], cardiorespiratory regulation [52-57], adrenocortical and hormonal responses [58, 59], stomach ulcers (see references in [60]) and micturition [41], it is suggested that the spino-parabrachio-amygdaloid nociceptive pathway could be involved in the affective-emotional (fear, memory of aggression), behavioral (vocalization, flight, freezing and defense), and autonomic (pupil dilatation, cardiorespiratory, adrenocortical responses, and micturition) reactions to noxious events. In addition, the detailed anatomical studies of PB-Ce connections allow us further interpretations (see [15]). Thus, one could speculate that:

1) the pPB-CeLC pathway would be mainly implicated in affective-emotional responses to noxious aggressions and major cardio-respiratory changes. Indeed:
- the pPB region (hatched in Figure 5) receives the highest density from spinal and trigeminal lamina I afferents (nociceptive input, [7, *see* also: 61-63]) and its microstimulation induces the strongest cardiovascular changes [33],
- this pPB region and the CeLC contain a very high proportion of nociceptive neurons [13, 26] ;

2) the pPB-CeL pathway would be also implicated in affective-emotional responses to noxious agressions but in association with chemosensitive and digestive changes. Indeed:
- this area contains numerous nociceptive neurons [13] and part of this pPB region (the pPBel outer) also receives dense nociceptive inputs from spinal lamina I [7],
- the pPB region (filled with dots in Figure 5) receives the highest density of afferents from the medial NTS and the area postrema [28] ;

3) in contrast, the pPB-CeM pathway is implicated in learning taste aversion and autonomic response to feeding. Indeed:
- the pPB region (grey in Figure 5) receives the highest density of afferent from the lateral rostral (gustatory) portion of the NTS [30, 28],
- this region is well known to contain numerous gustatory neurons [64, 65] and is involved in taste aversive learning [66, 67].

4) the pPB-(SId/GPv) more diffuse pathway could play a role in memorization and arousal reactions related to noxious, autonomic and gustatory events, since the SId/GPv

that includes part of the nucleus basalis of Meynert is involved in learning and arousal processes [68].

The spino-parabrachio-hypothalamic pathway

The spino-parabrachio-amygdaloid nociceptive pathway demonstrated above deals only with the pPB division. In fact, very recent studies [7, 61-63] have shown that the terminal area of lamina I neurons is not restricted to the pPB division that sends primarily efferent projections to the Ce, but strongly spreads into the adjacent mesencephalic division of the PB area (mPB). The latter region does not project to the Ce [15] but instead, it projects densely to the hypothalamus.

In fact, despite anatomical studies demonstrating efferent projections of the PB area to the hypothalamus [14, 20, 23, 69-71, *see* also 15], the detailed location of terminal fibers into hypothalamic subregion from PB subnuclei was largely unknown to date. We therefore used the PHA-L injected into extremely restricted sites, to determine ascending projections from the PB, with emphasis on the hypothalamus.

Unpublished results demonstrated that only a restricted portion of the superior lateral (mPBsl) and the external lateral (mPBel) subnucleus projected very densely, and specifically, to the ventromedial nucleus (VMH) and retrochiasmatic area (RCh) of the hypothalamus. The remaining portion of the mPBsl and the mPBel projected, more diffusely, to the dorsomedial nucleus of the hypothalamus and also gave rise to a small but dense cluster of terminals in the dorsal aspect of the parvocellular paraventricular nucleus of the hypothalamus. In addition, a diffuse projection was observed, in the lateral hypothalamus, from most parts of the PB area. The dense projections to the VMH nucleus and the RCh area, led us to hypothetize the existence of a spino-parabrachio-hypothalamic nociceptive pathway.

Thus, a second extensive electrophysiological investigation was performed at the PB level under the same conditions as the previous studies, but only PB neurons antidromically driven from the VMH or the RCh (PB-H neurons) were selected [72]. In contrast to PB-Ce neurons that were located in the pPB area, the PB neurons projecting onto the VMH or the RCh were mainly located in the mPB division, in the mPBsl and mPBel subnuclei (Figure 6). These electrophysiological data are in good agreement with the recent anatomical investigation performed in our laboratory (*see* above). The axons of these neurons exhibited a very slow conduction velocity in the range of 0.2 - 1.4 m/s, *i.e.* corresponding to thin unmyelinated fibers.

About half (49%) of the PB-H neurons were only activated by mechanical and/or thermal (heat) cutaneous stimuli in the noxious range; most of the remaining neurons (44%) were nonresponsive.

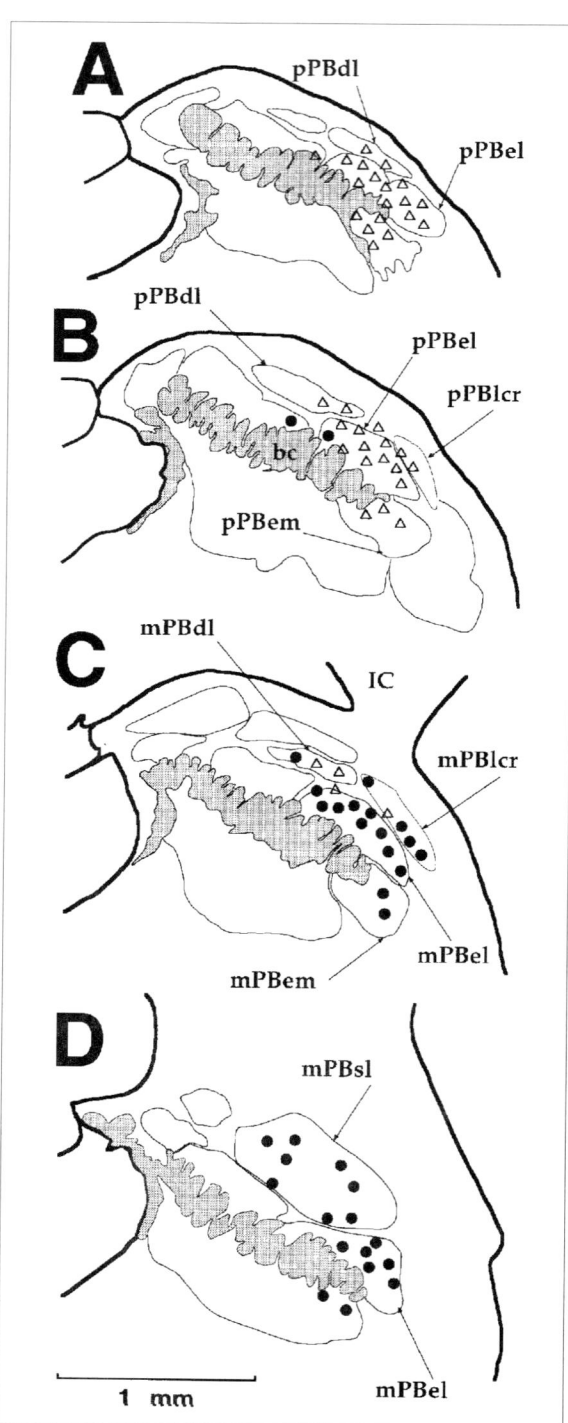

Figure 6. Location of NS neurons antidromically driven from the Ce (open triangle) and antidromically driven from the VMH (black point). A to D, camera lucida drawings of coronal section through the PB area, from caudal to rostral, 300 μm apart. A, B: pontine division of the PB area. C, D: mesencephalic division of the PB area.

The cutaneous excitatory receptive fields of the NS neurons were large in most cases (89%). In the few remaining cases (11%) they were restricted to one part of the body. In addition, in several cases, noxious stimuli applied outside the excitatory receptive field were found to strongly inhibit the discharge of NS neurons. The NS neurons exhibited very low or absent spontaneous activity, responding exclusively to mechanical (pinch or squeeze) and/or thermal (waterbath or waterjet > 44 °C) noxious stimuli with a rapid onset, a marked and sustained activation, and generally no after-discharge. These neurons exhibited a clear capacity to encode thermal stimuli in the noxious range:
- the stimulus-response function was always positive and monotonic;
- the slope of the mean curve increased up to a maximum around 48 °C then, beyond, decreased;
- the mean threshold was 44.3 ± 2.2 °C (Figure 7 B and B').

Most NS neurons responded to intense transcutaneous electrical stimulation with two peaks of activation. We found that the early and the late peaks were triggered by the activation of peripheral fibers with conduction velocities in the 5 - 17 m/s and 0.5 - 1.8 m/s range, *i.e.* Aδ- and C-fibers, respectively (Figure 7 C).

In an additional subgroup of PB-H neurons (n = 32) tested with cold stimuli (0 °C), 13% were strongly and only excited by cold stimuli (Figure 7 A), 28% responded to both cold and mechanical or hot stimuli, the remainder were nonresponsive to cooling.

It is concluded that this part of the mPB (primarily the mPBsl and mPBel) constitutes an anatomical and electrophysiological entity, which is implicated in the transmission of nociceptive messages in a spino-parabrachio-hypothalamic pathway. The role of such a pathway in pain is a matter of speculation. Since, the VMH nucleus seems to be involved not only in the regulation of food intake (*see* references in [73]) but also in (1) thermogenesis resulting from brown adipose tissue catabolism [74], (2) affective-defensive behavior [75], (3) neuroendocrine secretion of CRF [76] and (4) reproductive behavior in the female rat (see references [73]), it is suggested that this system could be involved in motivational (affective-defensive, feeding and sexual) reactions, energy (brown adipose tissues metabolism) and neuroendocrine (corticoadrenal axis) adaptations to a noxious event. A role in thermoregulative integration must also be considered.

Conclusion

The two new pain pathways described above are summarized in Figure 8. A third putative pain pathway terminating in the BSTL is also indicated. As already discussed, the anatomical data emphasized the major, extremely dense and adequately located projection that supported the physiological importance of these pathways. The electrophysiological properties of neurons recorded in some parts of this pathway (PB areas and Ce nucleus), the specific connections of the three termination sites, *i.e.* the Ce,

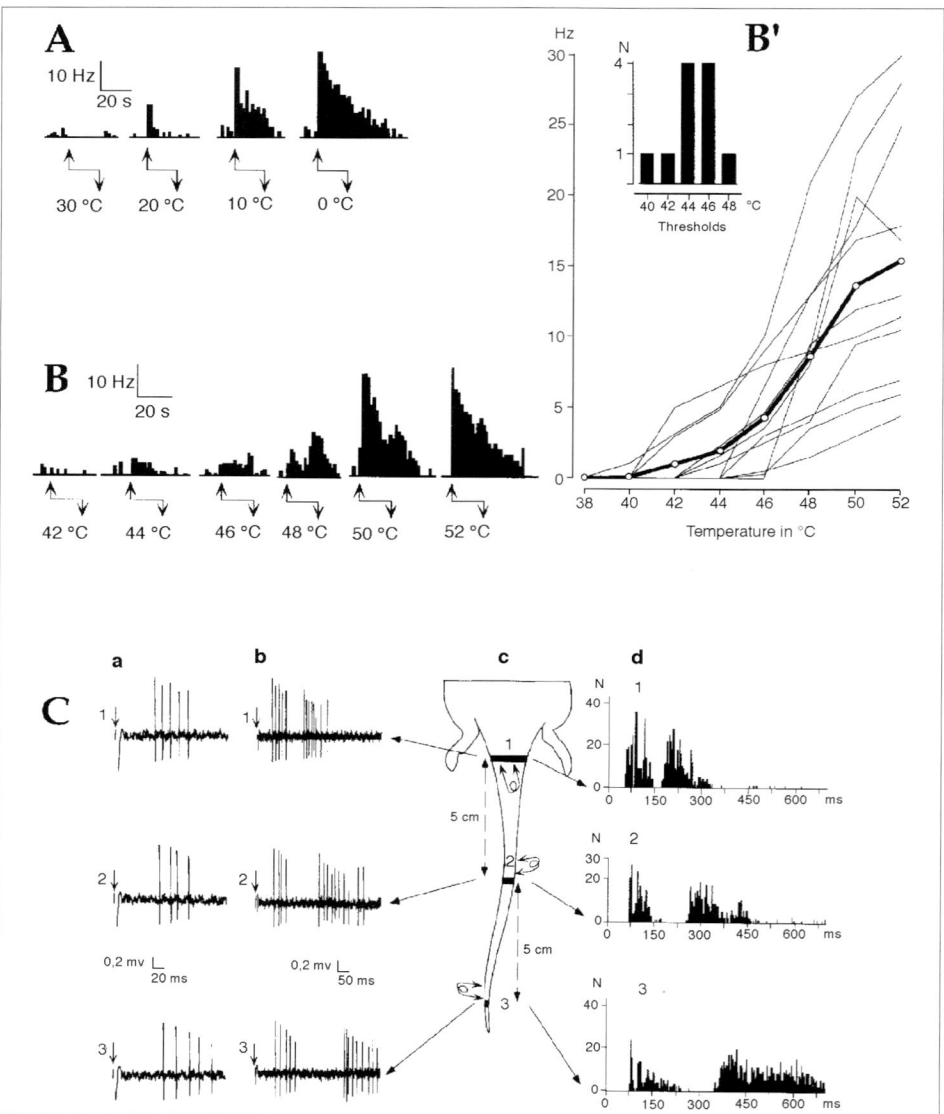

Figure 7. A: Response of a parabrachiohypothalamic neuron to cooling of the contralateral face. Graded decreasing thermal stimuli (30 - 0 °C, 10° C steps) were applied between the arrows, for 20 s. B: Response of a parabrachiohypothalamic neuron to heating of the contralateral face. Graded thermal stimuli (42 - 52 °C, 2° C steps) were applied between the arrows, for 20 s. B': Stimulus-response curves of parabrachiohypothalamic neurons to graded thermal stimuli. The response of individual neurons are represented by thin lines and the average stimulus-response curve with thick line. Temperature threshold histogram is inserted in the top left. C, a: single sweep recording of the early peak evoked by trancutaneous electrical stimulation of the base (C, a 1) the middle (C, a 2) and the tip (C, a 3) of the tail. C, b: same as in A, but the scale shows both the early and the late peaks. C, d: post-stimulus histograms (PSTH) made from responses to repetitive trancutaneous electrical stimulations (0,66 Hz, 50 trials) applied to the three sites on the tail (C, c 1 - 3). Modified from [72].

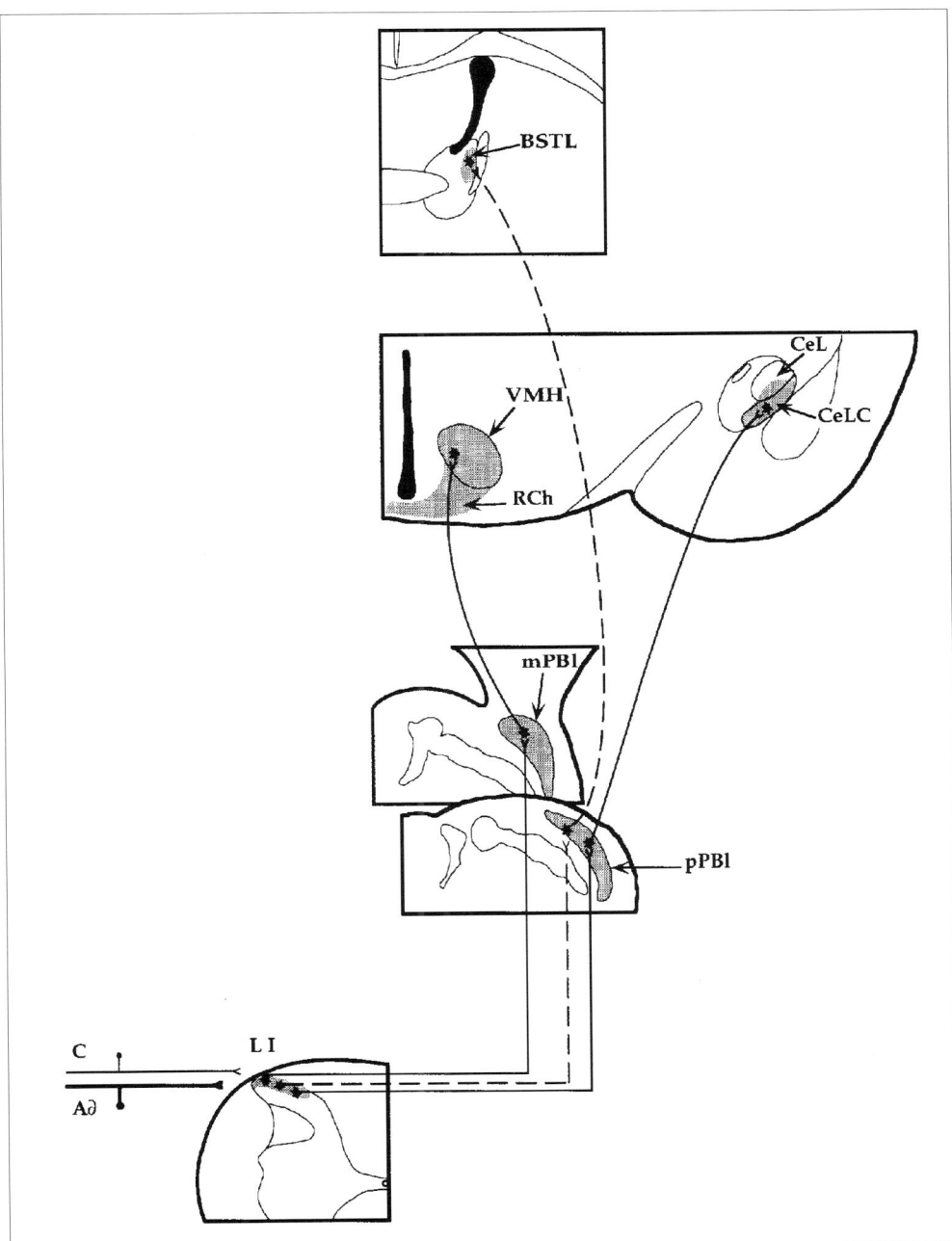

Figure 8. Summary diagram of the spino-parabrachio -amygdaloid and -hypothalamic pathways. A third putative pathway towards the bed nucleus of the stria terminalis is also represented. In grey: regions processing nociceptive messages. For the abbreviations *see* the separate list of abbreviations.

the VMH/RCh and the BSTL (the periaqueductal grey matter, the vagal motor, the ambiguous pedunculupontine tegmental nuclei) (*see* references in [77] and [73]) and their properties (*see* discussion in specific section) indicate that these pathways are strongly implicated in autonomic, affective-emotional and emotional-memory aspects of pain.

Acknowledgements

This study was supported by l'Institut National de la Santé et de la Recherche Médicale (INSERM) and by an Unrestricted Pain Research Award from Bristol-Myers Squibb Co.

Abbreviations

ACo	anterior cortical amygdaloid nucleus
bc	brachum conjunctivum
BL	basolateral amygdaloid nucleus
BLP	basolateral amygdaloid nucleus, posterior
BM	basomedial amygdaloid nucleus
BMA	basomedial amygdaloid nucleus, anterior
BST	bed nucleus of stria terminalis
BSTdl	dorsal lateral subnucleus of the BSTL
BSTL	lateral division of the BST
Ce	central nucleus of the amygdala
CeL	lateral subdivision of the Ce
CeLC	lateral capsular subdivision of the Ce
CeM	medial subdivision of the Ce
CPu	caudate putamen
cst	commissural stria terminalis
DLF	dorsolateral funiculus
FStr	fundus striati
GPv	ventral globus pallidus
IM	intercalated nucleus of the amgydala main subdivision
Kf	Kölliker-Fuse nucleus
LC	locus coeruleus
LI	lamina I
La	lateral nucleus of the amygdala
opt	optic tract
PB	parabrachial area
pPB	pontine PB area
pPBcl	central, lateral subnucleus of pPB area
pPBdl	dorsal, lateral subnucleus of pPB area
pPBel	external, lateral subnucleus of pPB area
pPBem	external, medial subnucleus of pPB area
pPBil	internal lateral subnucleus of pPB area
pPBl	lateral pPB area
pPBlcr	lateral crescent area of pPB area
pPBvl	ventral lateral pPB area
pPBm	medial subnucleus of pPB area
pPBvl	ventral, lateral subnucleus of pPB area
pPBwa	waist area of the pPB area
mPB	mesencephalic PB area
mPBel	external, lateral subnucleus of mPB area

mPBem	external, medial subnucleus of mPB area
mPBil	internal lateral subnucleus of mPB area
mPBl	lateral mPB area
mPBlcr	lateral crescent area of mPB area
mPBm	medial subnucleus of mPB area
mPBsl	superior lateral subnucleus of the mPB area
RCh	retrochiasmatic area of the hypothalamus
SId	dorsal substantia innominata
SId/GPv	transition area between the SId and the GPv
SStr	substriatal area
st	stria terminalis.
VMH	ventromedial nucleus of the hypothalamus

References

1. Cechetto DF, Standaert DG, Saper CB. Spinal and trigeminal dorsal horn projections to the parabrachial nucleus in the rat. *J Comp Neurol* 1985 ; 240 : 153-60.
2. Wiberg M, Blomqvist A. The spinomesencephalic tract in the cat: its cells of origin and termination pattern as demonstrated by the intraaxonal transport method. *Brain Res* 1984 ; 291 : 1-18.
3. Besson JM, Chaouch A. Peripheral and spinal mechanisms of nociception. *Physiol Rev* 1987 ; 67 : 67-185.
4. Hylden JLK, Hayashi H, Bennett GJ, Dubner, R. Spinal lamina I neurons projecting to the parabrachial area of the cat midbrain. *Brain Res* 1985 ; 336 : 195-8.
5. Hylden JL, Hayashi, H, Dubner R, Bennett GJ. Physiology and morphology of the lamina I spinomesencephalic projection. *J Comp Neurol* 1986 ; 247 : 505-15.
6. Light AR, Casale E, Sedivec M. The physiology and anatomy of spinal laminae I and II neurons antidromically activated by stimulation in the parabrachial region of the midbrain and pons. In : Schmidt RF, Schaible HG, Vahle-Hinz C, eds. *Fine afferent nerve fibers and pain*.Weinheim FRG: VCH 1987 : 347-56.
7. Bernard JF, Dallel R, Raboisson P, Villanueva L, Le Bars D. Organization of the efferent projections from the spinal cervical enlargement to the parabrachial area and periaqueductal grey: a PHA-L study in the rat. *J Comp Neurol* 1995 ; 353 : 480-505.
8. Bernard JF, Peschanski M, Besson JM. A possible spino(trigemino)-pontoamygdaloid pathway for pain. *Neurosci Lett* 1989 ; 100 : 83-8.
9. Ma W, Peschanski M. Spinal and trigeminal projections to the parabrachial nucleus in the rat: electron-microscopic evidence of a spino-ponto-amygdalian somatosensory pathway. *Somatosens Res* 1988 ; 5 : 247-57.
10. Hylden JLK, Anton F, Nahin RL. Spinal lamina I projection neurons in the rat: collateral innervation of parabrachial area and thalamus. *Neuroscience* 1989 ; 28 : 27-37.
11. Kitamura T, Yamada J, Sato H, Yamashita K. Cells of origin of the spinoparabrachial fibers in the rat - a study with fast blue and WGA-HRP. *J Comp Neurol* 1993 ; 328 : 449-61.
12. Menétrey D, De Pommery J. Origins of spinal ascending pathways that reach central areas involved in visceroception and visceronociception in the rat. *Eur J Neurosci* 1991 ; 3 : 249-59.
13. Bernard JF, Besson JM. The spino(trigemino)pontoamygdaloid pathway: electrophysiological evidence for an involvement in pain processes. *J Neurophysiol* 1990 ; 63 : 473-90.
14. Fulwiler CE, Saper CB. Subnuclear organization of the efferent connections of the parabrachial nucleus in the rat. *Brain Res Rev* 1984 ; 7 : 229-59.
15. Bernard JF, Aldén M, Besson JM. The organization of the efferent projections from the pontine parabrachial area to the amygdaloid complex: a *Phaseolus vulgaris* leucoagglutinin (PHA-L) study in the rat. *J Comp Neurol* 1993 ; 329 : 201-29.

16. Huang GF, Besson JM, Bernard JF. Morphine depresses the transmission of noxious messages in the spino(trigemino)-ponto-amygdaloid pathway. *Eur J Pharmacol* 1993 ; 230 : 279-84.
17. Bernard JF, Huang GF, Besson JM. The parabrachial area: electrophysiological evidence for an involvement in visceral nociceptive processes. *J Neurophysiol* 1994 ; 71 : 1646-60.
18. Cechetto DF, Calaresu FR. Parabrachial units responding to stimulation of buffer nerves and forebrain in cat. *Am J Physiol* 1983 ; 245 : R811-R819.
19. Jhamandas JH, Aippersbach SE, Harris KH. Cardiovascular influences on rat parabrachial nucleus: an electrophysiological study. *Am J Physiol* 260 (Regulatory Integrative comp Physiol 29) 1991 : R225-R231.
20. Moga MM, Herbert H, Hurley KM, Yasui Y, Gray TS, Saper CB. Organization of cortical, basal forebrain, and hypothalamic afferents to the parabrachial nucleus in the rat. *J Comp Neurol* 1990 ; 295 : 624-61.
21. Norgren R. Taste pathways to hypothalamus and amygdala. *J Comp Neurol* 1976 ; 166 : 17-30.
22. Ottersen OP. Afferent connections to the amygdaloid complex of the rat with some observations in the cat. III - Afferents from the lower brain stem. *J Comp Neurol* 1981 ; 202 : 335-56.
23. Saper CB, Loewy AD. Efferent connections of the parabrachial nucleus in the rat. *Brain Res* 1980 ; 197 : 291-317.
24. Voshart K, Van Der Kooy D. The organization of the efferent projections of the parabrachial nucleus to the forebrain in the rat: a retrograde fluorescent double-labeling study. *Brain Res* 1981 ; 212 : 271-86.
25. Aldén M, Besson JM, Bernard JF. The organization of the efferent projections from the pontine parabrachial area to the bed nucleus of the stria terminalis and neighbouring regions: a PHA-L study in the rat. *J Comp Neurol* 1994 ; 341 : 289-314.
26. Bernard JF, Huang GF, Besson JM. The nucleus centralis of the amygdala and the globus pallidus ventralis: electrophysiological evidence for an involvement in pain processes. *J Neurophysiol* 1992 ; 68 : 551-69.
27. Huang GF, Besson JM, Bernard JF. Intravenous morphine depresses the transmission of noxious messages to the nucleus centralis of the amygdala. *Eur J Pharmacol* 1993 ; 236 : 449-56.
28. Herbert H, Moga M, Saper CB. Connections of the parabrachial nucleus with the nucleus of the solitary tract and medullary reticular formation in the rat. *J Comp Neurol* 1990 ; 293 : 540-80.
29. Kobashi M, Adachi A. Projection of nucleus tractus solitarius units influenced by hepatoportal afferent signal to parabrachial nucleus. *J Auton Nerv Syst* 1986 ; 16 : 153-8.
30. Norgren R. Projections from the nucleus of the solitary tract in the rat. *Neuroscience* 1978 ; 3 : 207-18.
31. Yuan CS, Barber WD. Parabrachial nucleus: neuronal evoked responses to gastric vagal and greater splanchnic nerve stimulation. *Brain Res Bull* 1991 ; 27 : 797-803.
32. Wall PD, Bery J, Saade N. Effects of lesions to rat spinal cord lamina I cell projection pathways on reactions to acute and chronic noxious stimuli. *Pain* 1988 ; 35 : 327-39.
33. Chamberlin NL, Saper CB. Topographic organization of cardiovascular responses to electrical and glutamate microstimulation of the parabrachial nucleus in the rat. *J Comp Neurol* 1992 ; 326 : 245-62.
34. Mraovitch S, Kumada M, Reis DJ. Role of the nucleus parabrachialis in cardiovascular regulation in cat. *Brain Res* 1982 ; 232 : 57-75.
35. Ward DG. Neurons in the parabrachial nuclei respond to hemorrhage. *Brain Res* 1989 ; 491 : 80-92.
36. Bertrand F, Hugelin A. Respiratory synchronizing function of nucleus parabrachialis medialis: pneumotaxic mechanisms. *J Neurophysiol* 1971 ; 134 : 189-207.
37. Cohen MI. Switching of the respiratory phases and evoked phrenic responses produced by rostral pontine electrical stimulation. *J Physiol Lond* 1971 ; 217 : 133-58.

38. Eguchi K, Tadaki E, Simbulan D JR, Kumazawa T. Respiratory depression caused by either morphine microinjection of repetitive electrical stimulation in the region of the nucleus parabrachialis of cats. *Pfluegers Arch* 1987 ; 409 : 367-73.
39. Ohman LE, Johnson AK. Brain stem mechanisms and the inhibition of angiotensin-induced drinking. *Am J Physiol* 1989 ; 256 : 264-9.
40. Lumb BM, Morrison JFB. An excitatory influence of dorsolateral pontine structures on urinary bladder motility in the rat. *Brain Res* 1987 ; 435 : 363-6.
41. Kaada BR. Stimulation and regional ablation of the amygdaloid complex with reference to functional representations. In : Eleftheriou BE, ed. *The neurobiology of the amygdala*. New York : Plenum, 1972 : 205-82.
42. Ben-Ari Y. *The amygdaloid complex*. INSERM Symposium n°20. Amsterdam : Elsevier, 1981 : 516.
43. Hitchcock JM, Davis M. Lesions of the amygdala, but not of the cerebellum or red nucleus block conditioned fear as measured with the potentiated startle paradigm. *Behav Neurosci* 1986 ; 100 : 11-22.
44. Hitchcock JM, Davis M. Fear-potentiated startle using an auditory conditioned stimulus: effect of lesions of the amygdala. *Physiol Behav* 1987 ; 39 : 403-8.
45. Rosen JB, Davis M. Enhancement of electrically elicited startle by amygdaloid stimulation. *Physiol Behav* 1990 ; 48 : 343-9.
46. LeDoux JE. Emotional memory: in search of systems and synapses. *Brain Mechanisms* 1993 ; 702 : 149-57.
47. Lico MC, Hoffmann A, Covian MR. Influence of some limbic structures upon somatic and autonomic manifestations of pain. *Physiol Behav* 1974 ; 12 : 805-11.
48. Miczek KA, Brykczynski T, Grossman SP. Differential effects of lesions in the amygdala, periamygdaloid cortex, and stria terminalis on aggressive behaviors in rats. *J Comp Physiol Psychol* 1974 ; 87 : 760-71.
49. Pascoe JP, Kapp BS. Electrophysiological characteristics of amygdaloid central nucleus neurons during pavlovian fear conditioning in the rabbit. *Behav Brain Res* 1985 ; 16 : 117-33.
50. Shibata K, Kataoka Y, Yamashita K, Ueki S. An important role of the central amygdaloid nucleus and mamillary body in the mediation of conflict behavior in rats. *Brain Res* 1986 ; 372 : 159-62.
51. Creutzfeldt OD, Bell FR, Adey WR. The activity of neurons in the amgydala of the cat following afferent stimulation. *Prog Brain Res* 1963 ; 3 : 31-49.
52. Mogenson GJ, Calaresu FR. Cardiovascular responses to electrical stimulation of the amygdala in the rat. *Exp Neurol* 1973 ; 39 : 166-80.
53. Cechetto DF, Calaresu FR. Units in the amygdala responding to activation of carotid baro- and chemoreceptors. *Am J Physiol* 1984 ; 246 : R832-R836.
54. Pascoe JP, Kapp BS. Electrophysiological characteristics of amygdaloid central nucleus neurons in the awake rabbit. *Brain Res Bull* 1985 ; 14 : 331-8.
55. Zhang JX, Harper RM, Frysinger RC. Respiratory modulation of neuronal discharge in the central nucleus of the amygdala during sleep and waking states. *Exp Neurol* 1986 ; 91 : 193-207.
56. Cox GE, Jordan D, Paton JFR, Spyer KM, Wood LM. Cardiovascular and phrenic nerve responses to stimulation of the amygdala central nucleus in the anaesthetized rabbit. *J Physiol* 1987 ; 389 : 541-56.
57. Iwata J, Chida K, LeDoux JE. Cardiovascular responses elicited by stimulations of neurons in the central amygdaloid nucleus in awake but not anaesthetized rats resemble conditioned emotional responses. *Brain Res* 1987 ; 418 : 183-8.
58. Beaulieu S, Di Paolo T, Côté J, Barden N. Participation of the central amygdaloid nucleus in the response of adrenocorticotropin secretion to immobilization stress: opposing roles of the noradrenergic and dopaminergic systems. *Neuroendocrinology* 1987 ; 45 : 37-46.

59. Roozendaal B, Koolhaas JM, Bohus B. Attenuated cardiovascular, neuroendocrine and behavioral responses after a single footshock in central amygdala lesioned male rats. *Physiol Behav* 1991 ; 50 : 771-5.
60. Henke PG, Ray, A, Sullivan RM. The amygdala: emotions and gut functions. *Dig Dis Sci* 1991 ; 36 : 1633-43.
61. Slugg RM, Light AR. Spinal cord and trigeminal projections to the pontine parabrachial region in the rat as demonstrated with *Phaseolus vulgaris* leucoagglutinin. *J Comp Neurol* 1994 ; 339 : 49-61.
62. Feil F, Herbert H. Topographic organization of spinal and trigeminal somatosensory pathways to the rat parabrachial and Kölliker-Fuse nuclei. *J Comp Neurol* 1995 ; 353 : 506-28.
63. Panneton WM, Johnson SN, Christensen ND. Trigeminal projections to the peribrachial region in the muskrat. *Neuroscience* 1994 ; 58 : 605-25.
64. Norgren R., Leonard CM. Taste pathways in rat brainstem. *Science* 1971 ; 173 : 1136-9.
65. Ogawa H, Hayama T, Ito S. Response properties of the parabrachio-thalamic taste and mechanoreceptive neurons in rats. *Exp Brain Res* 1987 ; 68 : 449-57.
66. Reilly S, Grigson PS, Norgren R. Parabrachial nucleus lesions and conditioned taste aversion: evidence supporting an associative deficit. *Behav Neurosci* 1993 ; 107 : 1005-17.
67. Spector AC, Norgren R, Gill HJ. Parabrachial gustatory lesions impair taste aversion learning in the rats. *Behav Neurosci* 1992 ; 106 : 147-61.
68. Everitt BJ, Robbins TW, Evenden JL, Marston HM, Jones GH, Sirkia TE. The effects of excitotoxic lesions of the substantia innominata, ventral and dorsal globus pallidus on the acquisition and retention of a conditional visual discrimination: implications for cholinergic hypotheses of learning and memory. *Neuroscience* 1987 ; 22 : 441-69.
69. Fulwiler CE, Saper CB. Cholecystokinin-immunoreactive innervation of the ventromedial hypothalamus in the rat: possible substrate for autonomic regulation of feeding. *Neurosci Lett* 1985 ; 53 : 289-96.
70. Krukoff T L, Harris KH, Jhamandas JH. Efferent projections from the parabrachial nucleus demonstrated with the anterograde tracer *Phaseolus vulgaris* leucoagglutinin. *Brain Res Bull* 1993 ; 30 : 163-72.
71. Mcbride RL, Sutin J. Amygdaloid and pontine projections to the ventromedial nucleus of the hypothalamus. *J Comp Neurol* 1977 ; 174 : 377-96.
72. Bester H, Menendez L, Besson JM, Bernard JF. The spino(trigemino)-parabrachiohypothalamic pathway: electrophysiological evidence for an involvement in pain processes. *J Neurophysiol* 1995 ; 73 : 569-85.
73. Swanson LW. The hypothalamus. In : Hökfelt T, Swanson LW, eds. *Hanbook of chemical neuroanatomy*, vol 5, integrated systems of the CNS, part I. Amsterdam, Oxford : Elsevier, 1987 : 1-124.
74. Preston E, Triandafillou J, Haas N. Colchicine lesions of ventromedial hypothalamus: effects on regulatory thermogenesis in the rat. *Pharmacol Biochem Behav* 1989 ; 32 : 301-7.
75. Yardley CP, Hilton SM. The hypothalamic and brainstem areas from which the cardiovascular and behavioural components of the defence reaction are elicited in the rat. *J Auton Nerv Syst* 1986 ; 15 : 227-44.
76. Filaretov AA, Filaretova LP. Role of the paraventricular and ventromedial hypothalamic nuclear areas in the regulation of the pituitary-adrenocortical system. *Brain Res* 1985 ; 342 : 135-40.
77. De Olmos J, Alheid GF, Beltramino CA. Amygdala. In : Paxinos G, ed. *The rat nervous system*, Volume 1. Academic Press Australia, 1985 : 223-334.

4

The spino-hypothalamic tract

G.J. GIESLER Jr

Department of Cell Biology and Neuroanatomy, University of Minnesota, Minneapolis, USA.

In 1928, Wallenberg [1] reported that lesions of the sacral spinal cord in monkeys caused degeneration of fibers that could be followed through the medial lemniscus into the mammillary nuclei and the hypothalamus. This was the first indication that spinal cord neurons project directly to the hypothalamus. The possibility of such a projection is of interest, because it is likely that the hypothalamus contributes of a number of types of responses to noxious stimuli. The hypothalamus probably contributes to autonomic responses to noxious stimulation such as increased blood pressure, increased blood flow to the heart and skeletal muscles, decreased blood flow to skin and viscera, decreased gastrointestinal motility, piloerection and sweat secretion [2]. The hypothalamus also contributes to neuroendocrine responses to noxious stimuli such as cause the release of ACTH from the anterior pituitary and vasopressin from the posterior pituitary [2]. In addition, since the hypothalamus is strongly interconnected with other areas in the limbic system including the amygdala, septal nuclei, frontal cortex and the cingulate gyrus [3], it is likely that nociceptive neurons in the hypothalamus contribute to affective and motivational responses to pain.

In 1949, Chang and Ruch [4] confirmed and extended Wallenberg's observations. They reported that, following lesions in the spinal cord white matter in monkeys, a bundle of degenerating axons could be followed across the ipsilateral internal capsule in the posterior thalamus and into the supraoptic decussation (SOD), a small area of white matter located medially adjacent to the optic tract. These axons coursed anteriorly, ventrally and medially within the SOD. At the level of the posterior optic chiasm in the anterior hypothalamus, the degenerating axons crossed the midline. The fibers were also followed within the contralateral diencephalon as they turned posteriorly and descended in the mirror image location to that in which they had ascended in the SOD. These axons were followed posteriorly to the level of the medial geniculate where their numbers decreased and the projection appeared to disappear. In 1951, Morin *et al.* [5] confirmed virtually every aspect of the results of Chang and Ruch [4], again using the degeneration methods in monkeys. Thus, using methods that are less sensitive than those in use today, a prominent projection was described from spinal neurons in primates that ascended to the hypothalamus, then made a "U turn" and descended through the hypothalamus and thalamus on the opposite side. Several studies have since confirmed various aspects of these original descriptions of the spinohypothalamic tract (SHT) in several species [6-9]. Nonetheless, the possible existence of direct spinal projections to the hypothalamus received almost no attention until relatively recently.

In 1987, Burstein *et al.* [10] reported that neurons in the lumbar spinal cord of rats could be antidromically activated using small current pulses from the lateral and ventral hypothalamus, in or near the SOD. In these studies, antidromic stimulating pulses were systematically delivered throughout the diencephalon and the antidromic thresholds were determined at 200 µm intervals. Axons were initially activated antidromically in the posterior thalamus and attempts were made to follow them anteriorly using antidromic activation techniques. The axons did not appear to terminate within the thalamus. They were followed ventrally and medially, out of the thalamus and into the hypothalamus. Several of the lowest threshold points located anteriorly in the hypothalamus were surrounded medially, laterally, ventrally, dorsally and anteriorly by tracks in which the antidromic threshold increased markedly, or the axon could not be activated with 500 µA pulses, suggesting that the examined axons ended within the hypothalamus. Each of the seven neurons that were tested responded differentially to noxious stimuli, suggesting that they were capable of carrying nociceptive information to the hypothalamus.

The cells of origin of the spinohypothalamic tract have been determined using retrograde tracers in rats [10-13] and cats [14]. Injections that were restricted to the hypothalamus and did not spread into the overlying zona incerta or thalamus consistently labeled many numbers of neurons in all segments that were examined in the spinal cord of rats [11] (Figure 1). Based on cell courting in 18 segments and application of correction factors to reduce the effect of double-counting split neurons, it was estimated that a total of roughly 9000 neurons were labeled in the most effective case. Therefore, the total of numbers of spinothalamic [15] and spinohypothalamic tract neurons are similar in rats, suggesting that the spinohypothalamic tract is large and it may also make important contributions to nociceptive processing. Note in Figure 1 that many SHT neurons were located in the marginal zone, the lateral reticulated area and the area around the central canal [11], areas that each receive direct input from primary afferent nociceptors, contain many nociceptive neurons, and contribute large numbers of neurons to other ascending nociceptive tracts [16]. This finding reinforces the idea that the SHT may be involved in transmission of nociceptive information.

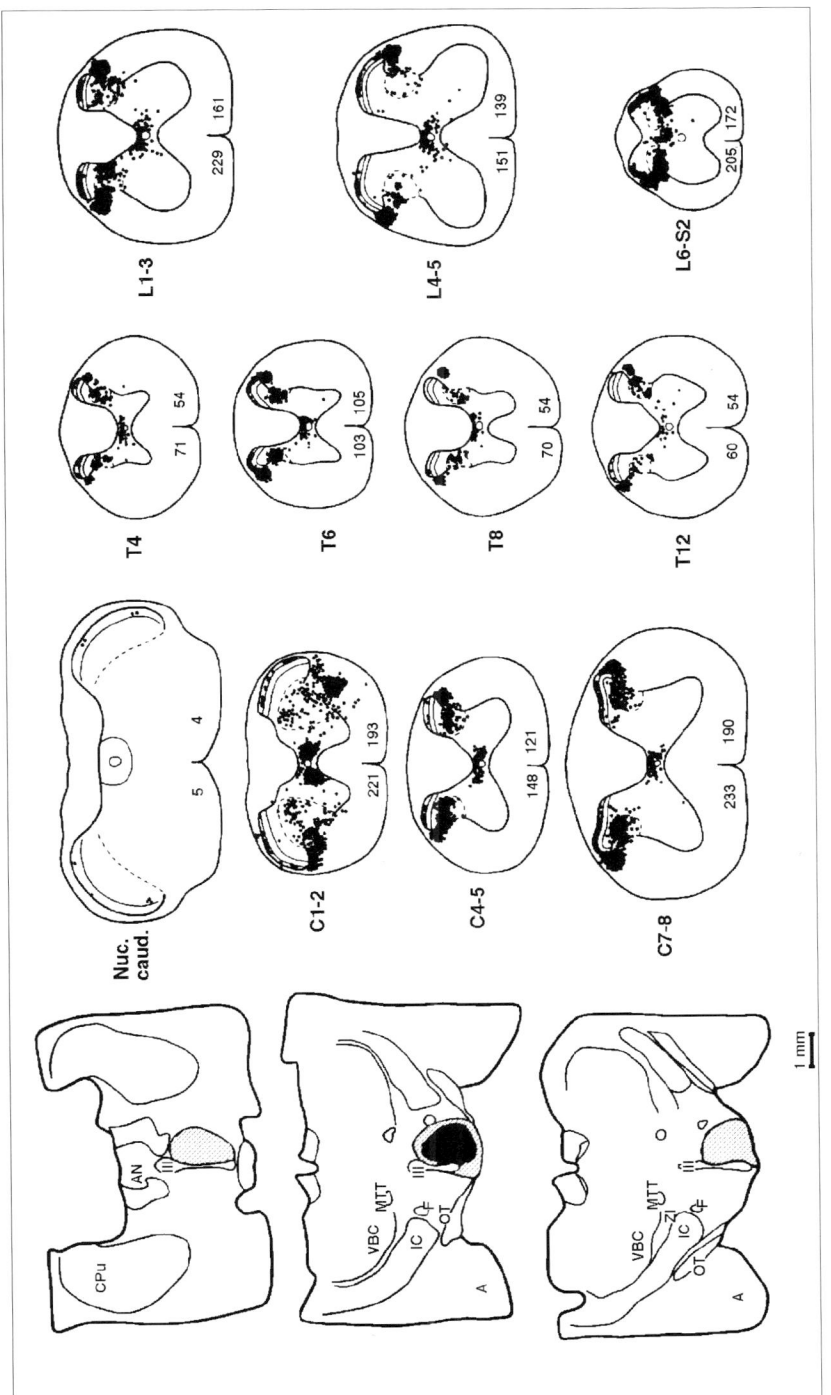

Figure 1. Drawings of injection of FG into medial and lateral hypothalamus (left) and the labeling it produced in the spinal cord (right). Black area indicates the core of the injection, and cross-hatching the diffuse halo of FG. The drawing at top left depicts the most anterior spread of the injection. The drawing at center depicts the center of the injection site. The drawing at bottom depicts the most caudal spread of injection. Locations of 4127 labeled neurons plotted in alternate sections are indicated by black dots. The right side of all segments is ipsilateral to the injected area. The total number of labeled neurons found in each side of the indicated segments is shown. Note the high concentrations of labeled neurons in the marginal zone, lateral reticulated area, the area around the central canal and the lateral spinal nucleus. Scale bar, 1mm. Reprinted from [11].

The course and termination of the spinohypothalamic tract has also been examined using modern anterograde tracing techniques. Cliffer et al. [17] injected PHAL into the spinal cord gray matter and reported labeled axons in several areas of the hypothalamus (Figure 2). Many labeled axons were located in the SOD bilaterally. A number appeared to cross the midline in the SOD and posterior part of the optic chiasm, confirming earlier observations in monkeys [4, 5]. In addition, labeled axons and varicosities were found throughout the hypothalamus including the lateral hypothalamus, posterior hypothalamic area, dorsal hypothalamic area, the dorsomedial nucleus, the paraventricular nucleus, the periventricular nucleus, the suprachiasmatic nucleus and the lateral and medial preoptic areas [17]. Recently, Newman et al. [18] injected biotin-dextran into the upper cervical segments or cervical enlargements of rats and monkeys. In both species, injections into either area labeled large numbers of axons and terminals in several areas of the hypothalamus including the medial, lateral, dorsal and posterior hypothalamus, and the lateral preoptic area. Many labeled axons were also observed in the SOD and some of these gave off branches that appeared to terminate within the hypothalamus (Apkarian, personal communication). These findings indicated that the SHT projects to a large number of nuclei that are located throughout much of the hypothalamus.

Spinohypothalamic tract neurons have now been examined physiologically at several levels of the spinal cord [10, 19-22] and in nucleus caudalis of the trigeminal system [23] in rats. Burstein et al. [19] recorded from 79 neurons in the lumbar enlargement that were initially antidromically activated with low amplitude current pulses delivered in the contralateral hypothalamus. Eighty-seven percent responded preferentially or specifically to noxious mechanical stimulation of receptive fields on the hindlimbs.

Figure 2. Locations of labeled fibers in transverse sections through the diencephalon and telencephalon following injections of PHAL into the cervical enlargement of a rat. Each thick line represents the location and extent of a labeled axon. The approximate distance rostrocaudally from the anterior commissure is indicated at lower right of each drawing. Ipsilateral is at left; contralateral at right. Abbreviations: AC: anterior commissure; Am: amygdala; AM: anteromedial thalamic nucleus; APT: anterior pretectal nucleus; Ar: arcuate hypothalamic nucleus; AV: anteroventral thalamic nucleus; B: basal nucleus of Meynert; BST: bed nucleus of stria terminalis; CAm: central nucleus of amygdala; CC: corpus callosum; CL: central lateral thalamic nucleus; CM: central medial thalamic nucleus; CPd: cerebral peduncle; CPu: caudate-putamen; DA: dorsal hypothalamic area; DLG: dorsal lateral geniculate nucleus; DM: dorsomedial hypothalamic nucleus; EC: external capsule; F: fornix; .FR: fasciculus retroflexus; GP: globus pallidus; H: habenula; HDB: diagonal band of Broca: horizontal limb; IC: internal capsule; IL: infralimbic cortex; LD: laterodorsal thalamic nucleus; LH: lateral hypothalamus; LO: lateral olfactory tract; LPO: lateral preoptic area; LV: lateral ventricle; MD: mediodorsal thalamic nucleus; MG: medial geniculate nucleus; ML: medial lemniscus; MPO: medial preoptic area; MS: medial septal nucleus; MT: mammillothalamic tract; NA: nucleus accumbens; OC: optic chiasm; OT: optic tract; PAG: periaqueductal gray; PC: paracentral thalamic nucleus; PCm: posterior commissure; PF: parafascicular thalamic nucleus; PH: posterior hypothalamic area; Po: posterior thalamic nuclear group; PV: paraventricular thalamic nucleus; PVA: paraventricular thalamic nucleus, anterior; PVH: paraventricular hypothalamic nucleus; SC: suprachiasmatic nucleus; SCo: superior colliculus; Sm: nucleus submedius; SM: stria medullaris thalami; SN: substantia nigra; SOD: supraoptic decussation; ST: stria terminalis; STh: subthalamic nucleus; VB: ventrobasal thalamic complex; VDB: diagonal band of Broca, vertical limb; VL: ventrolateral thalamic nucleus; VLG: ventral lateral geniculate nucleus; VM: ventromedial thalamic nucleus; VMH: ventromedial hypothalamic nucleus; VP: ventral pallidum; VTA: ventral tegmental area; ZI: zona incerta; 3V: third ventricle. Adapted from [17].

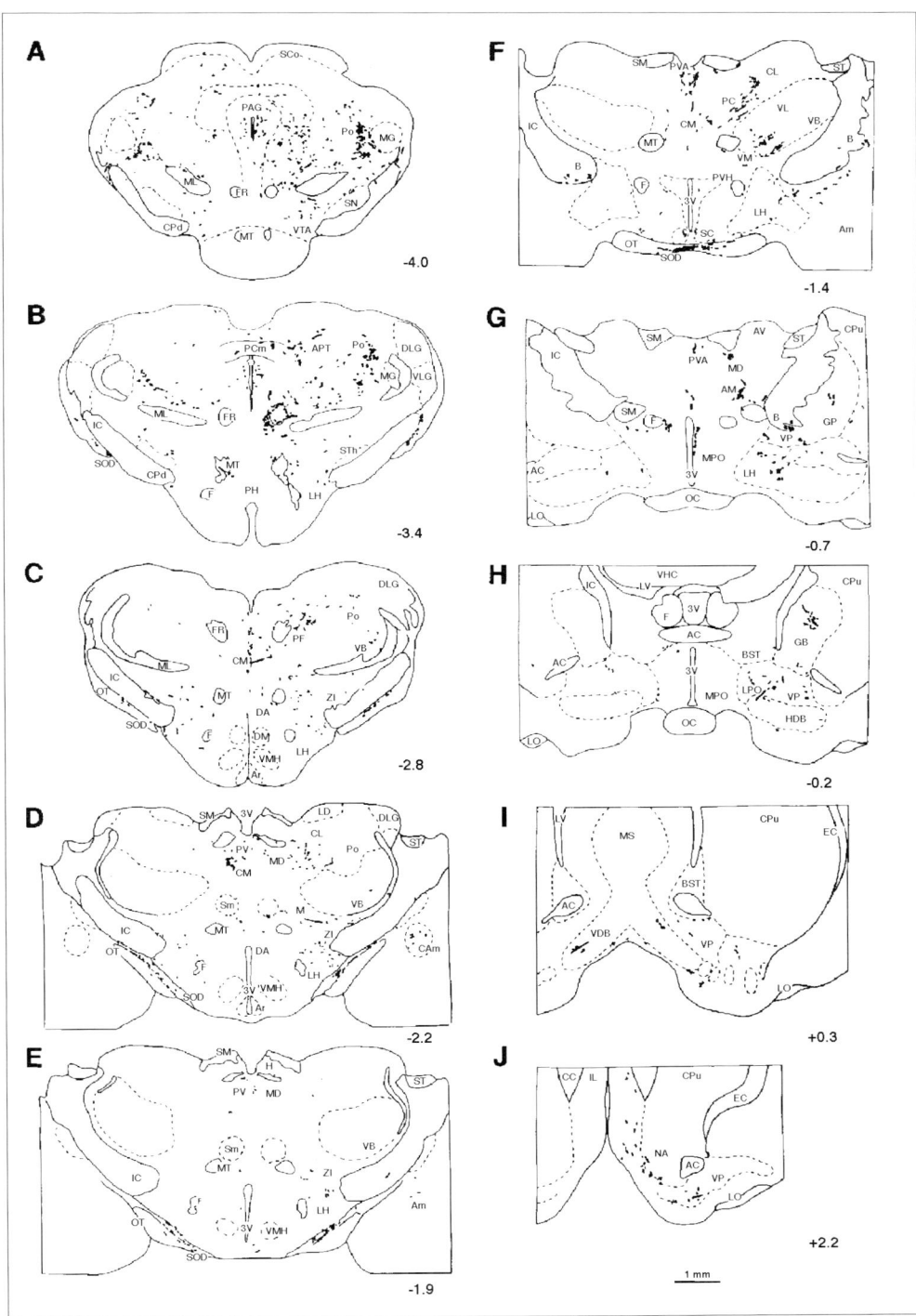

Fifty-six percent of the examined neurons responded incrementally to increasing intensities of noxious heat. An example of one such neuron is presented in Figure 3. This SHT neuron was recorded in the superficial dorsal horn (3B) and was antidromically activated using 5 µA in the SOD (3A). It responded to innocuous mechanical stimuli (brushing, 3D) but was more powerfully activated by noxious

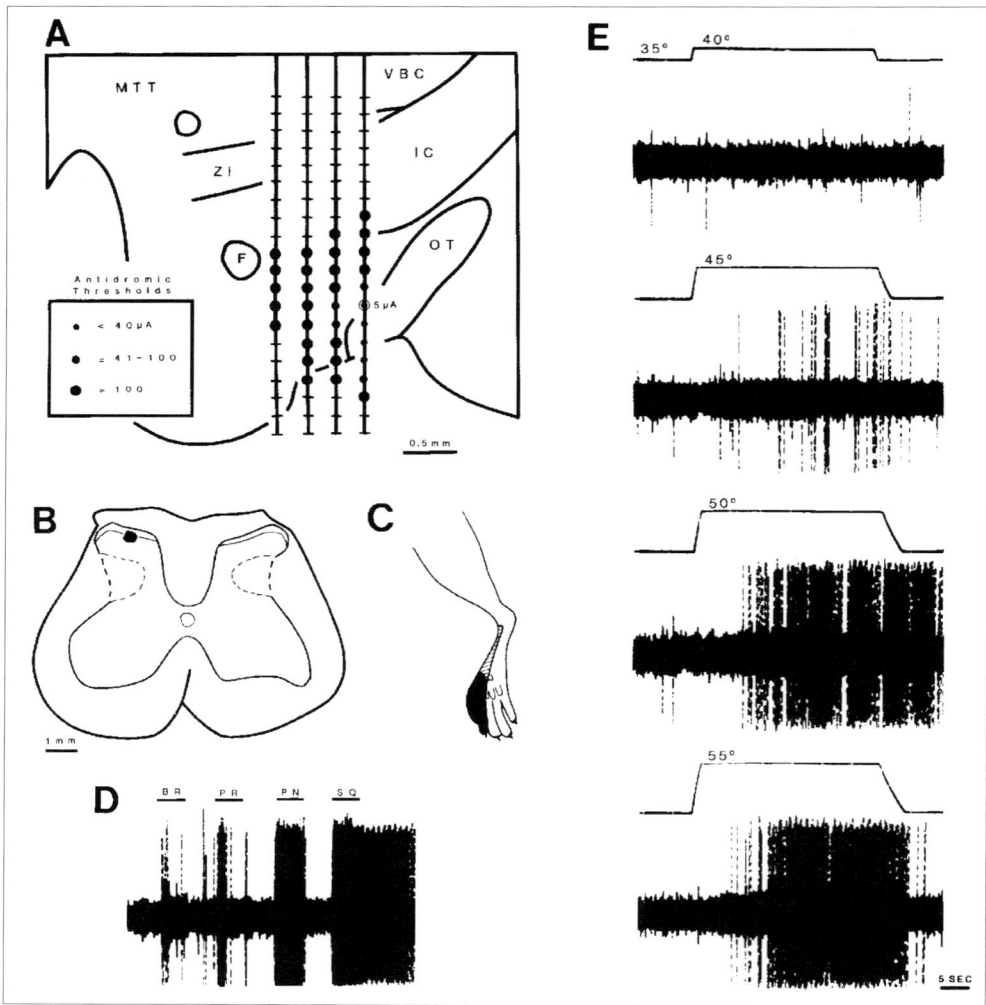

Figure 3. Characterization of a SHT neuron recorded in the superficial dorsal horn that was classified as a wide dynamic range neuron. A. Locations of tracks of a stimulating electrode in the hypothalamus, showing thresholds for antidromic activation, and a low-threshold point in the supraoptic decussation (circled). B. Drawing of lesion marking the recording location. C. Receptive field. D. Oscillographic tracing of responses to brushing (BR), pressure (PR), pinch (PN), and squeeze (SQ) of the receptive field. E. Responses to noxious heat. Temperature tracings are presented above responses. Scale bar, 0.5 mm for A and B. Reprinted from [19].

mechanical stimuli (pinch and squeeze, 3D). Therefore, this unit was classified as a wide dynamic range neuron. It also responded to noxious heating (3E) of its receptive field (3C). In 8 cases, attempts were made to examine the course of the examined SHT axons using antidromic activation [19]. The axons were activated frequently from low threshold points in the SOD and several axons were followed at increasing latencies as they apparently crossed the midline in the posterior part of the optic chiasm.

Dado et al. [20] examined neurons in the cervical enlargement of rats that were initially antidromically activated from the level of the posterior thalamus. In 38 cases, attempts were made to determine whether the axons of the examined cells ascended to other areas in the diencephalon such as the ventrobasal complex, the central lateral nucleus or the hypothalamus. In 80% of the cases, the examined neurons that were initially antidromically activated in the posterior thalamus could not be antidromically activated from low threshold points in more anteriorly located thalamic nuclei. However, they were activated at longer latencies from points in the contralateral hypothalamus. These axons appeared to leave the posterior thalamus laterally, enter the SOD, course anteriorally and medially within the SOD and enter the hypothalamus. The points from which SHT neurons could be antidromically activated in this study are presented in Figure 4. It was also found that in 83% of the cases, the axons crossed the midline in the posterior optic chiasm and entered the ipsilateral hypothalamus (top, Figure 4). Several examined axons were followed using antidromic activation as they descended in the ipsilateral brain. Such axons descended within the SOD (upper left, Figure 4). In two cases, axons were followed into the midbrain. These data and those of Burstein et al. [19] confirmed earlier anatomical findings that indicated that spinal axons cross the midline in the SOD, turn posteriorly, descend in the SOD and reach levels at least as far posterior as the thalamus.

Dado et al. [21] also examined the responses of the same neurons to noxious and innocuous cutaneous stimuli. Virtually all of the examined neurons (94%) responded preferentially or exclusively to noxious stimulation of the ipsilateral forelimb. These receptive fields were often restricted to several toes. Responses to noxious thermal stimuli were also examined. Figure 5 illustrates the responses of wide dynamic range and high threshold SHT neurons in the cervical enlargement to noxious heating of their receptive fields. Roughly 80% of the examined neurons responded incrementally to increased levels of noxious heat. The natural logs of the mean responses of the activated SHT neurons are plotted in Figure 6. These responses were highly accelerating functions; the exponent of the power function was 3.5. Therefore, SHT neurons are capable of producing clear increases in their firing rates in response to small changes in the intensity of the noxious heat stimulus. Human psychophysical studies indicate that the stimulus-response functions that describe the human sensory experience of noxious heat have slopes of from 2.0 to 3.0 [24]. The thresholds of the SHT neurons for responses to noxious heat was extrapolated from the stimulus-response function. It was determined to be 43.2 °C, a temperature that is near the human pain threshold for heat stimuli delivered on the hand. Thus, it appears that SHT neurons are capable of

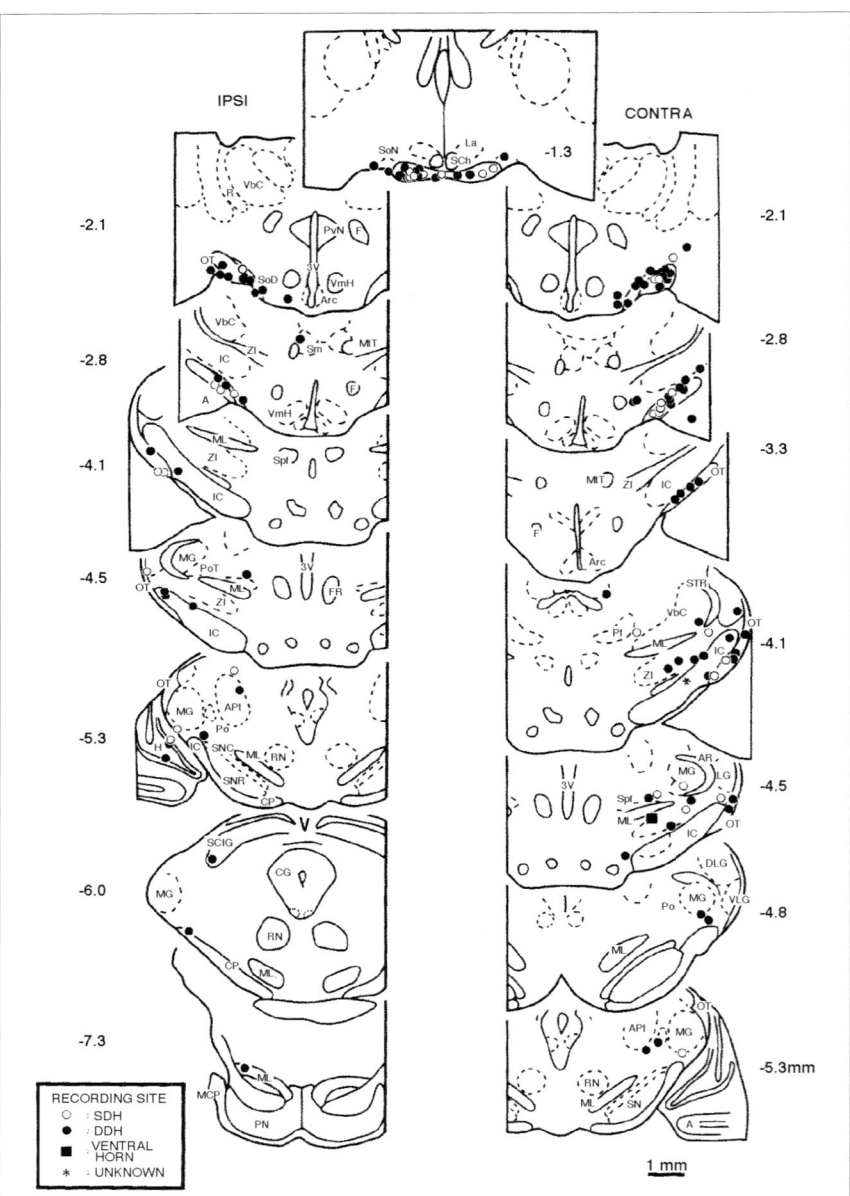

Figure 4. Summary of the locations of lesions marking 125 lowest threshold points for antidromic activation of 27 spinal neurons that were antidromically activated in the thalamus and hypothalamus. The position of each symbol indicates the location of a lowest threshold point; the type of symbol indicates the location of the recording site (lower left). Lesions on the right were located contralateral to the recording site. Numbers indicate the posterior distance from bregma. Antidromic latencies increased for all neurons at each progressively more anterior point on the contralateral side (right side of the figure) and at each progressively more posterior point on the ipsilateral side (left side of the figure). Reprinted from [20].

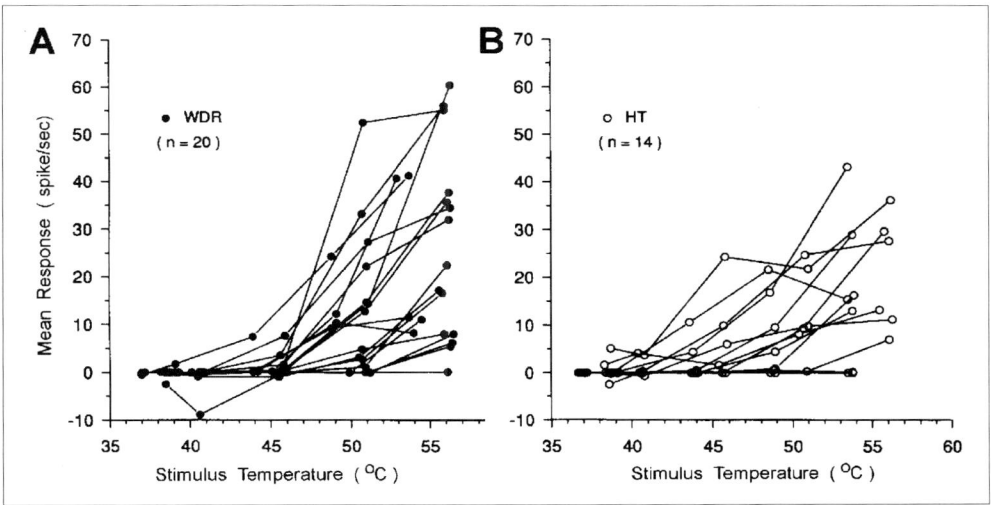

Figure 5. Mean responses to innocuous and noxious heat stimuli of neurons classified as wide dynamic range (WDR, A) or as high threshold (HT, B). The majority of cells of each type responded clearly to noxious heat. The mean responses of WDR and HT neurons were not significantly different. Adapted from [21].

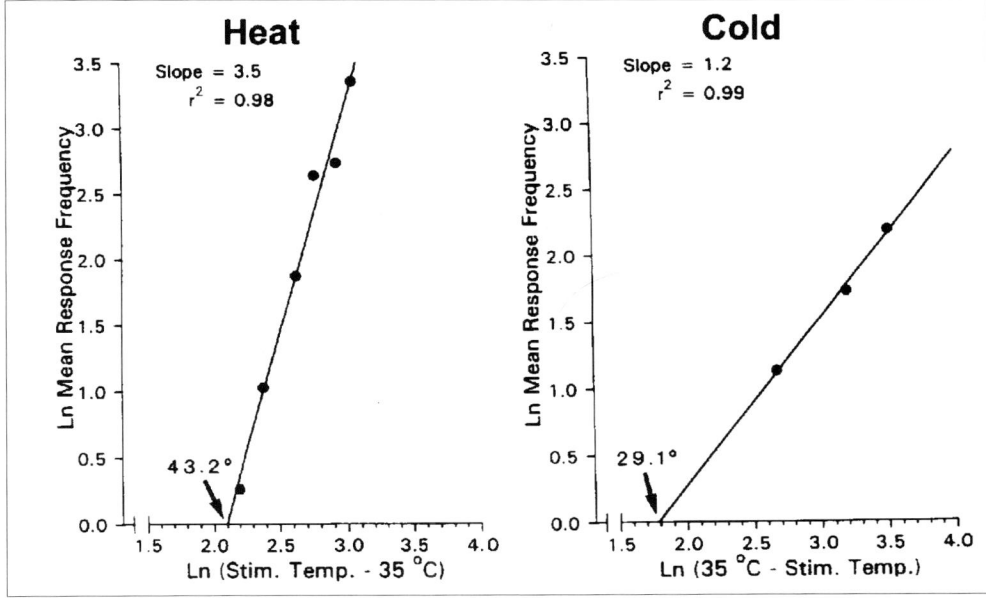

Figure 6. Ln-Ln plot of responses to innocuous and noxious heat (left) and cold (right). The difference between stimulus temperatures and baseline temperature are plotted *versus* the mean frequency of the responses. The relationship for responses to heat was described by a power function with an exponent of 3.5 ($r^2 = 0.98$); The relationship for responses to cold was described by a power function with an exponent of 1.2 ($r^2=0.99$). The arrows indicate the calculated response thresholds. Adapted from [21].

providing information that could be involved in the production of sensory responses to noxious heat.

Responses of noxious cold stimuli were also determined [21]. Ten neurons (29%) responded incrementally to increasingly intense noxious cold. Examples of the responses of one neuron are shown in Figure 7A and the responses of each of the ten are depicted in the graph in Figure 7B. The stimulus-response function of these neurons is illustrated in double natural log plots in Figure 6B. The exponent of this power function was 1.2, indicating the responses to noxious cold differ from those of the same

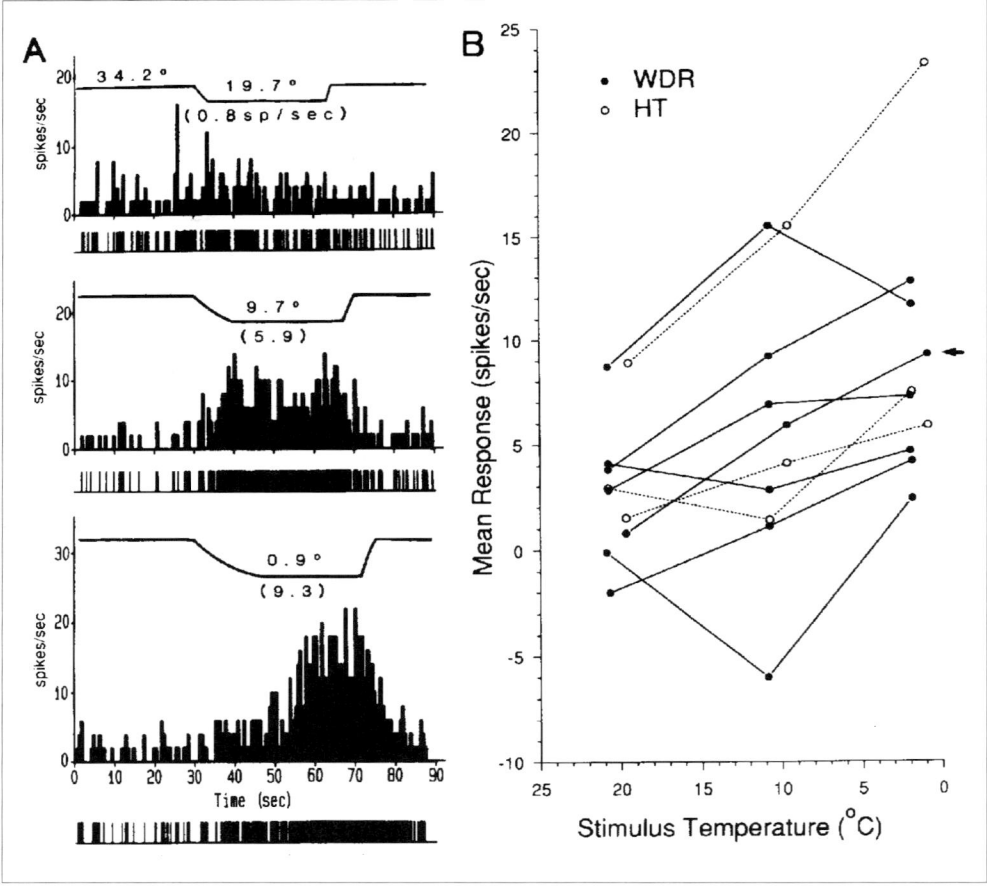

Figure 7. Responses to innocuous and noxious cold stimuli. A: example of the response of an individual neuron (indicated by the arrow in B) to increasingly intense cooling. The baseline temperature was 34.2 °C for each trial. Stimulus temperatures are indicated above each temperature trace. Numbers in parentheses indicate the mean frequency (spikes/sec) of the response to each stimulus temperature. This neuron responded at higher frequencies as the temperature decreased into the noxious range. B: Individual mean response frequencies for 10 neurons that responded to cooling. Note that the responses of over half of the neurons incremented to increasingly intense cooling. Reprinted from [21]

cells to noxious heat. Responses to cold were less robust and accelerated at a slower rate. Thus, decreases of skin temperature by several degrees typically produced modest increases in firing rates in SHT neurons. Human psychophysical responses are characterized by stimulus-responses functions with slopes of approximately 1.0 [25]. Thus, the responses of SHT neurons to both noxious heat and cold parallel human sensory responses, suggesting that SHT neurons could provide information to the production of the sensation of either type of stimulus.

The extrapolated threshold for the responses to cold stimuli was determined to be 29.3 °C, a temperature that is considerably warmer than the threshold for cold pain in humans. Therefore, it appears that SHT neuron may be capable of providing information about innocuous as well as noxious reductions in skin temperature. The hypothalamus is known to play an important role in thermoregulation, and it is known that many neurons within it respond to innocuous cooling [26]. Our findings raise the possibility that SHT neurons may provide information regarding skin temperature to hypothalamic neurons that are involved in thermoregulation.

Recently, Zhang et al. [27] attempted to examine in greater detail the course and termination of SHT axons after they decussate in the hypothalamus and travel posteriorly in the ipsilateral brain. SHT neurons in the cervical enlargement of rats were initially antidromically activated in the contralateral SOD. Antidromic tracking was then performed at multiple levels of the ipsilateral thalamus and brainstem. In these studies more than half of the 44 axons that were examined traveled crossed the midline in the hypothalamus and then descended as far posteriorly as the ipsilateral midbrain. Several such axons were surrounded dorsally, ventrally, medially, laterally and posteriorly. This indicated that the examined axon probably terminated in the surrounded area. Roughly one-quarter of the axons that were surrounded in the ipsilateral midbrain, appeared to terminate in the intermediate and deep layers of the superior colliculus. Many neurons in these layers of the superior colliculus are nociceptive and some have bilateral receptive fields [28]. It is possible that descending SHT axons provide nociceptive information originating in the ipsilateral body to neurons in the superior colliculus and other areas of the brainstem that have ipsilateral or bilateral receptive fields. In addition, Zhang et al. [27] found that the cuneiform nucleus and the midbrain reticular formation also receive prominent inputs from descending SHT axons. A number of axons were found that descended even farther in the ipsilateral brainstem. These descended in the ventral and medial pontine reticular formation. A small number of axons was also followed into the ventral medial medulla near the raphe magnus, at the level of the rostral inferior olive. It is interesting to note that the parent axons of these descending SHT axons ascend only a few millimeters away in the contralateral medulla (*see* below). Yet, these descending axons ascend as much as 18 mm to the posterior part of the optic chiasm and then descend the same distance to reach an area in the ipsilateral medulla that is within 2 to 4 mm of the ascending parent axon. For technical reasons, none of these axons in the pons and medulla could be surrounded posteriorly. Thus, their site of termination is unknown. These findings indicate that SHT axons may provide nociceptive information bilaterally to a large number of areas in the diencephalon, midbrain, pons, and medulla that are involved in nociceptive processing.

Kostarczyk et al. [29] have recently used the same methods of antidromic activation to examine the course of ascending SHT axons in the brainstem contralateral to the recording site. Eighty-eight neurons in the cervical enlargement of rats were initially antidromically activated from the contralateral hypothalamus. A second electrode was then lowered into the contralateral brainstem, and tracks were made across the mediolateral extent of the brainstem at multiple anterior-posterior planes. The antidromically activated spikes at each low threshold point were collided with those elicited from the electrode in the hypothalamus to insure that the action potentials evoked from the two sites traveled in the same axon. In the medulla, SHT axons appeared to ascend within or surrounding the lateral reticular nucleus. What appeared to be branches from these axons, based on the presence of multiple low threshold points at multiple latencies at one anterior-posterior level, were found within the reticular formation, the cuneate nucleus, and the solitary nucleus. Thus, it appears that branches from SHT axons contribute to postsynaptic projections to the cuneate nucleus and also to the spinosolitary and spinoreticular tracts. In the pons, most ascending SHT axons were located near the facial nucleus. Several apparent branches were also seen at this level in nucleus gigantocellularis, in the lateral reticular formation and near the raphe magnus. In the caudal midbrain, SHT axons were located near the lateral lemniscus. These axons travelled dorsally at this level, leaving an area near the ventral surface of the brainstem and assumed a more dorsal position. Several low threshold points located in the cuneiform nucleus. Therefore, it appears that the cuneiform nucleus may receive inputs from both ascending and descending SHT axons. In the rostral midbrain, most SHT axons ascended near the brachium of the inferior colliculus. As SHT axons entered the posterior thalamus, they assumed a position medial to the medial geniculate. These findings indicate that SHT axons ascend in a ventral and lateral position within the medulla and pons, then course dorsally and enter the diencephalon through the posterior nucleus of thalamus.

The results described here indicate that a large number of neurons throughout the length of the spinal cord in rats project directly to the hypothalamus. These SHT axons ascend through the ventral and lateral brainstem where they appear to give rise to large numbers of collateral branches that supply several nociceptive areas with sensory input. Many of these axons ascend through the lateral midbrain and pass through the area of the posterior nucleus of thalamus as they enter the diencephalon. SHT axons then pass laterally through the internal capsule and enter the supraoptic decussation. In the SOD, SHT axons course anteriorly and medially in the ventral and lateral hypothalamus. Collateral branches appear to leave the SOD and supply a number of areas in the hypothalamus. The parent SHT axons frequently ascend to the posterior part of the optic chiasm where the decussate and enter the ipsilateral hypothalamus. The majority of SHT axons turn posteriorly and descend within the SOD on the side ipsilateral to the cell bodies of origin. Descending SHT axons terminate in several regions of the midbrain including, most prominently, the superior colliculus and the cuneiform nucleus. The remaining SHT axons course medially and ventrally, and descend into the caudal pons and even the rostral medulla. Ascending and descending SHT axons appear to be capable of providing nociceptive input to a large number of nociceptive areas in the brainstem and diencephalon bilaterally.

Acknowledgements

I am grateful to Drs R Burstein, KD Cliffer, RJ Dado and JT Katter, E Kostarczyk and X Zhang who participated in many of the studies described here. This work was supported by NS25932.

References

1. Wallenberg A. Anatomie, Physiologie und Pathologie des sensiblen Systems. *Deutsch Zeitsch Nervenh* 1928 ; 101 : 111-55.
2. Janig W. The sympathetic nervous system in pain: physiology and pathophysiology. In : Stanton-Hicks M, ed. *Pain and the sympathetic nervous system.* Boston : Kluwer, 1990 : 17-89.
3. Swanson LW. The hypothalamus. In : Björklund A, Hökfelt T, Swanson LW, eds. *Handbook of chemical neuroanatomy.* Amsterdam : Elsevier, 1987 : 1-124.
4. Chang HT, Ruch TC. Spinal origin of the ventral supraoptic decussation (Gudden's commissure) in the spider monkey. *J Anat* 1949 ; 83 : 1-9.
5. Morin F, Schwartz HG, O'Leary JL. Experimental study of the spinothalamic and related tracts. *Acta Psychiat Neurol* 1951 ; 16 : 371-96.
6. Anderson FD, Berry CM. Degeneration studies of long ascending fiber systems in the cat brain stem. *J Comp Neurol* 1959 ; 111 : 195-230.
7. Minderhoud JM. Observations on the supra-optic decussations in the albino rat. *J Comp Neurol* 1967 ; 129 : 297-312.
8. Kerr FWL. The ventral spinothalamic tract and other ascending systems of the ventral funiculus of the spinal cord. *J Comp Neurol* 1975 ; 159 : 335-55.
9. Ring G, Ganchrow D. Projections of nucleus caudalis and spinal cord to brainstem and diencephalon in the hedgehog (*Erinaceus europaeus* and *paraechinus aethiopicus*): a degeneration study. *J Comp Neurol* 1983 ; 216 : 132-51.
10. Burstein R, Cliffer KD, Giesler GJ Jr. Direct somatosensory projections from the spinal cord to the hypothalamus and telencephalon. *J Neurosci* 1987 ; 7 : 4159-64.
11. Burstein R, Cliffer KD, Giesler GJ Jr. The cells of origin of the spinohypothalamic tract in the rat. *J Comp Neurol* 1990 ; 291 : 329-44.
12. Carstens E, Leah J, Lechner J, Zimmerman M. Demonstration of extensive brainstem projections to medial and lateral thalamus and hypothalamus in the rat. *Neurosci* 1990 ; 35 : 609-26.
13. Menetrey D, de Pommery J. Origins of spinal ascending pathways that reach central areas involved in visceroception and visceronociception in the rat. *Eur J Neurosci* 1991 ; 3 : 249-59.
14. Katter JT, Burstein R, Giesler GJ Jr. The cells of origin of the spinohypothalamic tract in cats. *J Comp Neurol* 1990 ; 303 : 101-12.
15. Burstein R, Dado RJ, Giesler GJ Jr. The cells of origin of the spinothalamic tract of the rat: a quantitative reexamination. *Brain Res* 1990 ; 511 : 329-37.
16. Willis WD Jr, Coggeshall RE. *Sensory mechanisms of the spinal cord.* New York : Plenum, 1991

17. Cliffer KD, Burstein R, Giesler GJ Jr. Distributions of spinothalamic, spinohypothalamic and spinotelencephalic fibers revealed by anterograde transport of PHA-L in rats. *J Neurosci* 1991 ; 11 : 852-68.
18. Newman HM, Stevens RT, Pover CM, Apkarian AV. Spinal-suprathalamic projections from the upper cervical and the cervical enlargement in rat and squirrel monkey. *Neurosci Abs* 1994 ; 20 : 118.
19. Burstein R, Dado RJ, Cliffer KD, Giesler GJ Jr. Physiological characterization of spinohypothalamic tract neurons in the lumbar enlargement of rats. *J Neurophysiol* 1991 ; 66 : 261-84.
20. Dado RJ, Katter JT, Giesler GJ Jr. Spinothalamic and spinohypothalamic tract neurons in the cervical enlargement of rats. I. locations of antidromically identified axons in the thalamus and hypothalamus. *J Neurophysiol* 1994 ; 71 : 959-80.
21. Dado RJ, Katter JT, Giesler GJ Jr. Spinothalamic and spinohypothalamic tract neurons in the cervical enlargement in rats. II. responses to innocuous and noxious mechanical and thermal stimuli. *J Neurophysiol* 1994 ; 71 : 981-1002.
22. Katter JT, Dado RJ, Giesler GJ Jr. Response properties and locations of axons of lumbosacral spinothalamic (STT) and spinohypothalamic (SHT) tract neurons in rats. *Neurosci Abs* 1992 ; 18 : 498.
23. Burstein R, Strassman AM, Maciewicz RJ. Anatomical and physiological studies of the trigeminohypothalamic tract. *Neurosci Abstr* 17 ; 1991 : 1009.
24. Price DD. *Psychological and neural mechanisms of pain.* New York : Raven, 1988.
25. Chery-Croze S. Relationship between noxious cold stimuli and the magnitude of pain sensation in man. *Pain* 1983 ; 15 : 265-9.
26. Hensel H. *Thermoreception and temperature regulation.* London : Academic Press, 1981 : 77-142.
27. Zhang X, Kostarczyk E, Giesler GJ Jr. Spinohypothalamic tract neurons in the cervical enlargement of rats: location of antidromically identified axons in the ipsilateral brain. *Neurosci Abs* 1994 ; 20 : 547.
28. Stein, BE, Dixon JP. Superior colliculus cells respond to noxious stimuli. *Brain Res* 1978 ; 158 : 65-73.
29. Kostarczyk E, Zhang X, Giesler GJ Jr. Spinohypothalamic tract (SHT) neurons in the cervical enlargement of rats: location of antidromically identified axons in the contralateral brain. *Neurosci Abs* 1995 (in press).

5

Thalamic processing of sensory-discriminative and affective-motivational dimensions of pain

M.C. BUSHNELL

Département de Stomatologie and Centre de recherche en sciences neurologiques, Université de Montréal, Montréal, Québec, Canada.

Much evidence now indicates that the thalamus is not just a passive synaptic relay site along sensory pathways, but, in fact, plays an important role in sensory gating and analysis. For example, state-dependent high-frequency bursting activity patterns in thalamic relay neurons are observed during slow-wave sleep, but not during wakefulness and REM sleep, when thalamocortical systems are activated [1]. Additionally, levels of arousal have been shown to alter the responsiveness of thalamic nociceptive neurons [2, 3], so that cells are generally most responsive when the monkey is in a quiet waking state.

Nociceptive information is transmitted to the thalamus directly by the trigemino- and spinothalamic tracts, and indirectly by other pathways, including the spinoreticular and spinomesencephalic tracts. Although fibers in these tracts terminate in a variety of thalamic areas, several nuclei in particular have been shown to receive dense projections from laminae I and V of the dorsal horn, where most spinal nociceptive and thermoreceptive neurons are located. These nuclei include the ventroposterior lateral and medial nuclei (VPL and VPM), VMpo of the posterior thalamus, and the ventrocaudal portion of the medial dorsal (MDvc) and parafascicular (Pf) nuclei of the medial thalamus [4-13]. These nuclei show differential connections with the cortical regions most often shown in human brain imaging studies to be activated by painful stimuli, i.e., primary and secondary somatosensory cortices (SI and SII), anterior cingulate cortex and insular cortex [14-17].

My colleagues and I have examined response characteristics of nociceptive and thermoreceptive neurons in medial, lateral and posterior thalamic regions, in order to assess the role of these various areas in the processing of nociceptive information [18-21]. Since pain is a complex experience, encompassing discriminative, emotional and motivational components, the variety of thalamocortical nociceptive pathways may well represent different components of the pain experience. Because of the state-dependent responsiveness of nociceptive neurons, for most of our studies we have used an awake, trained monkey model to determine receptive field and stimulus-response characteristics of thalamic neurons during an alert waking state. We have also examined modulation of such neuronal activity related to differences in behavioral state, which could contribute to the emotional and/or behavioral responses to painful stimuli.

This chapter will describe how neurons located in medial, lateral and posterior thalamic regions might contribute to sensory-discriminative and affective-motivational aspects of pain processing. Using an awake trained monkey model, we have recorded in VPM of the lateral thalamus [18, 20], and throughout the medial thalamus, including the central lateral (CL), central median (CM), medial dorsal (MD) and parafascicular (Pf) nuclei [19]. In the barbiturate anaesthetized monkey, we have recorded in VMpo of the posterior thalamus [21]. Figure 1 shows the locations of nociceptive and/or thermoreceptive neurons recorded in VPM and medial thalamus (Figure 1A) and VMpo (Figure 1B). Whereas tactile neurons were distributed throughout VPM (not shown), neurons sensitive to thermal and noxious stimuli were preferentially located at the dorsomedial and ventroposterior borders of VPM. Medial thalamic neurons responsive to noxious heat and/or pinch were found almost exclusively in Pf and MDvc.

Some monkeys used for the awake recording experiments received reward for sitting quietly while the experimenter mapped receptive fields and examined response properties to mechanical stimuli [18], whereas others were trained to perform a variety of detection tasks involving heat, cold, airpuff and visual stimuli. In these tasks, a 1-cm diameter feedback-controlled thermode with attached airpuff stimulator was placed in the receptive field of the neuron (*see* Figure 2). By pressing a lever, the monkey initiated trials in which stimuli were presented. The monkey received juice reward for releasing the lever in response to changes in the intensity of the heat, cold, airpuff or visual stimuli, with the basic task being the same for all stimulus modalities. For heat trials, when the monkey depressed the lever, the temperature of the thermode increased from the neutral range (34 °C - 37 °C) to some temperature between 45 °C and 49 °C (T1). After 3 - 9s, the temperature increased another small step of 0.1 °C to 2.0 °C (T2), and the monkey received a reward for releasing the lever within 1 sec of T2 onset. The monkeys also performed a comparable cooling task (T1's = 33 °C to 25 °C; T2's = 0.4 °C to 2.0 °C), as well as airpuff and visual tasks (Figure 2). In all the experiments, single unit extracellular activity was recorded using insulated tungsten microelectrodes.

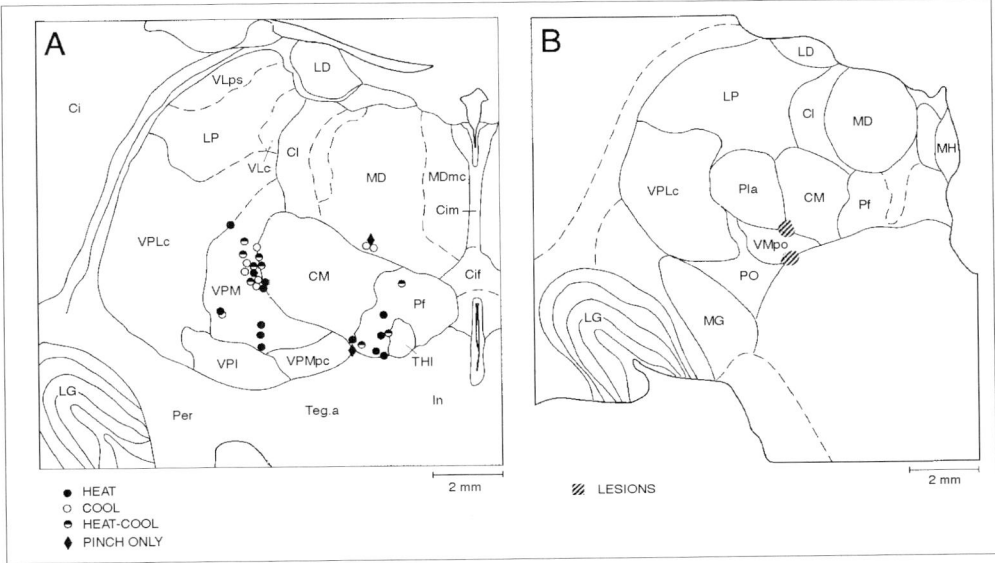

Figure 1. Part A shows the approximate locations of recording sites of thermosensitive and nociceptive neurons in the medial and lateral thalamus of the awake monkey. The data from four monkeys are combined onto a drawing from Olszewski [22] at A5.1. Part B is a camera lucida drawing from one monkey of cytoarchitectonic boundries and lesions deliniating the top and bottom of the region in posterior thalamus in which nociceptive and thermoreceptive neurons were isolated. Ci: internal capsule; Cif: central inferior nucleus; Cim: central intermediate nucleus; Cl: central lateral nucleus; CM: central medial nucleus; In: interstitial nucleus; LD: lateral dorsal nucleus; LG: lateral geniculate nucleus; LP: lateral posterior nucleus; MD: medial dorsal nucleus; Per: peripeduncular nucleus; Pf: parafascicular nucleus; Pla: anterior pulvinar; Teg.a: anterior tegmental nucleus; THI: habenulo-interpeduncular tract; VMpo: posterior division of ventromedial nucleus; VPLc: caudal ventroposterior lateral nucleus; VPI: ventroposterior inferior nucleus; VPM: ventroposterior medial nucleus; VPM: parvocellular division of VPM.

Sensory-discriminative properties of thalamic neurons

Humans can precisely localize cutaneous painful or thermal stimuli [23] and can detect changes of less than 1 °C in the intensity of noxious heat or innocuous cool [24-26]. We also perceive qualitative differences in the pain associated with noxious heat, cold or mechanical stimulation [27]. Thus, there must be some differential thalamocortical representation to subserve these varied perceptions. Our studies suggest that pain localization, modality identification and intensity discrimination are not all processed by the same neurons, but in fact different regions of thalamus may subserve each of these features.

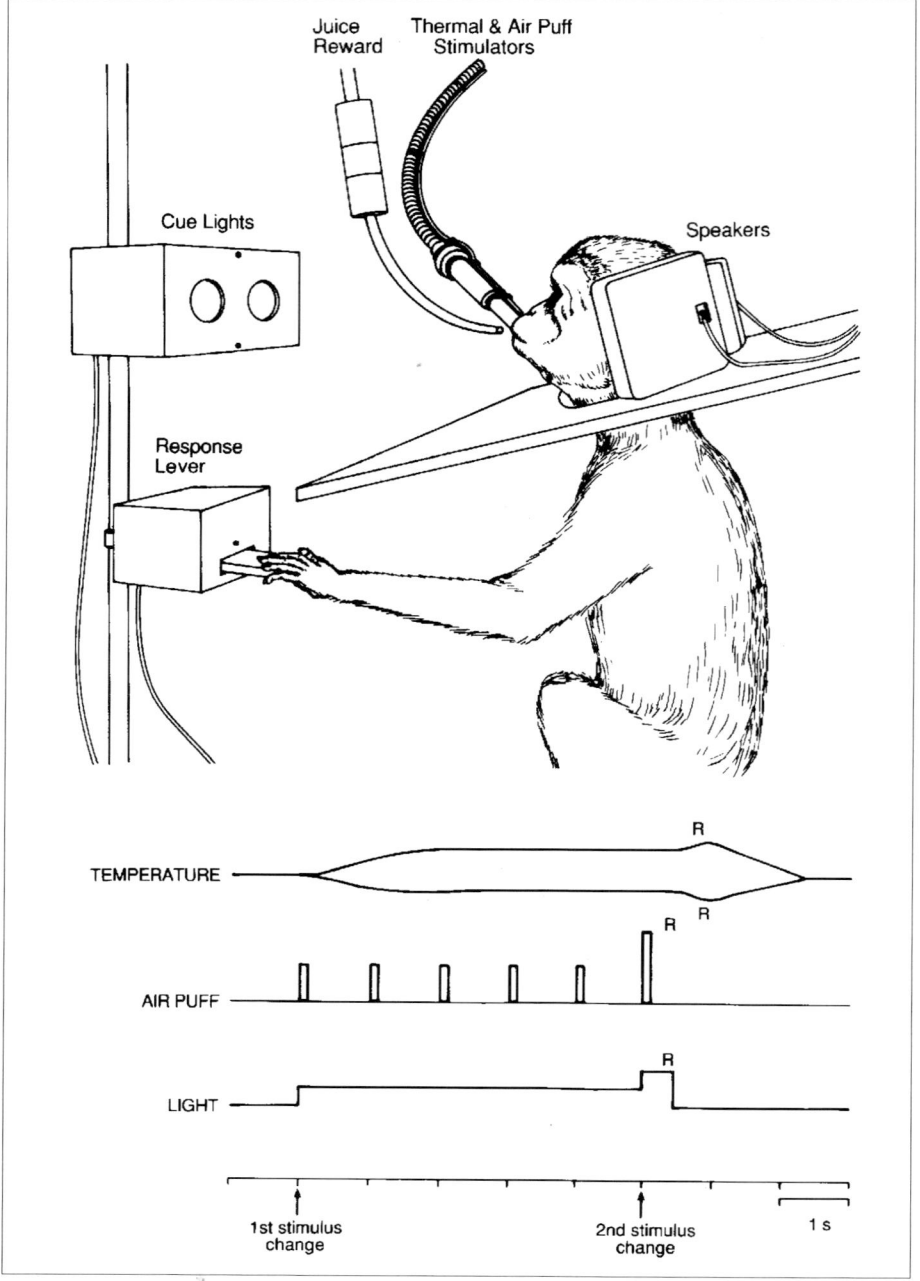

Figure 2. Representation of the experimental procedures. The drawing at the top shows the location of the thermal, airpuff and visual stimuli, response lever, speakers for presentation of a white noise masking stimulus, and juice reward delivery system. The diagrams at the bottom depict the temporal sequence of events for thermal, airpuff, and visual trials. From [20].

Pain localization

Receptive field sizes of nociceptive or thermoreceptive neurons in lateral, medial and posterior thalamus differed considerably (*see* Table I). Neurons in VPM all had restricted receptive fields, whereas those in Pf/MDvc had large, often bilateral fields. There was a larger variation in receptive field size of neurons in VMpo than in the other regions, with half the neurons having small receptive fields, and a fourth having large or bilateral fields. Receptive field size in VPM did not appear to vary according to the monkey's behavioral state or after repeated stimulation. In contrast, receptive fields were extremely difficult to characterize in medial thalamus, because their boundries changed as the monkey became agitated or excited. Since receptive fields in VMpo were characterized in anaesthetized monkeys, the effect of behavioral state could not be determined. However, receptive fields sometimes expanded with repeated noxious stimulation. These findings indicate that activity in VPM is sufficient to account for pain and temperature localization. Activity in VMpo could also be important for such localization, but further studies in awake monkeys are needed to examine the stability of receptive field size across behavioral states.

Table I. Comparison of receptive field size in medial, lateral, and posterior thalamus.

Nucleus	Small[1]	Medium	Large[2]	Bilteral
VPM (n = 19)	89%	11%	0%	0%
VMpo (n = 73)	48%	26%	15%	11%
Pf/MDvd (n = 6)	0%	17%	50%	33%

1: Less than 3-cm diameter
2: Most of contralateral face or limb

Modality specificity

Humans are able to distinguish pain evoked by noxious heat, noxious cold and noxious mechanical stimuli. Whereas noxious heat is felt as primarily superficial and burning, noxious cold is perceived as a deep, aching, diffuse pain, even when presented cutaneously using a small contact thermode [27]. Although there are a number of ways in which the nervous system could code these perceptual differences, modality specific neuronal activity would probably constitute a primary contributor to such specific percepts. Among the thalamic nuclei we studied, the region showing the most modality specificity was VMpo. In this region, more than 80% of the neurons showed specific nociceptive or thermal responses. Only 7% had wide dynamic range (WDR) characteristics, in which the neurons responded to both innocuous touch and noxious pinch, with the response frequency being proportional to the stimulus intensity. In Pf/MDvc, of eight neurons responding to noxious and/or thermal stimuli, only one showed WDR characteristics; the others responded either to skin cooling or to noxious heat or pinch. Nevertheless, the response characteristics of these cells were highly variable, depending upon the monkey's behavioral state (*see* below). In VPM, few neurons responding to noxious or thermal stimuli were modality specific. Seventy-seven percent of the neurons in VPM activated by noxious stimuli were WDR. Similarly, 100% of the neurons responding to skin cooling also responded to tactile stimuli. Many neurons in VPM responded to touch, pressure, pinch, noxious heat and innocuous cool. Figure 3 shows an example of such a neuron. It can be seen that a weak airpuff generated instantaneous response frequencies higher than those produced by noxious heat stimuli (48 °C). Further, the response pattern evoked by a 1 °C increase from 47 °C to 48 °C (Figure 3B) is similar to that produced by a 3 °C cooling shift from 31 °C to 28 °C. These findings show that although the activity of single neurons in VPM can account for spatial discrimination of pain and temperature, it cannot easily account for modality discrimination. The responsiveness of neurons in VMpo, MDvc and Pf appears to be better suited to distinguish noxious and innocuous temperatures, and it may be activity in these regions that is important to identify a stimulus as potentially harmful.

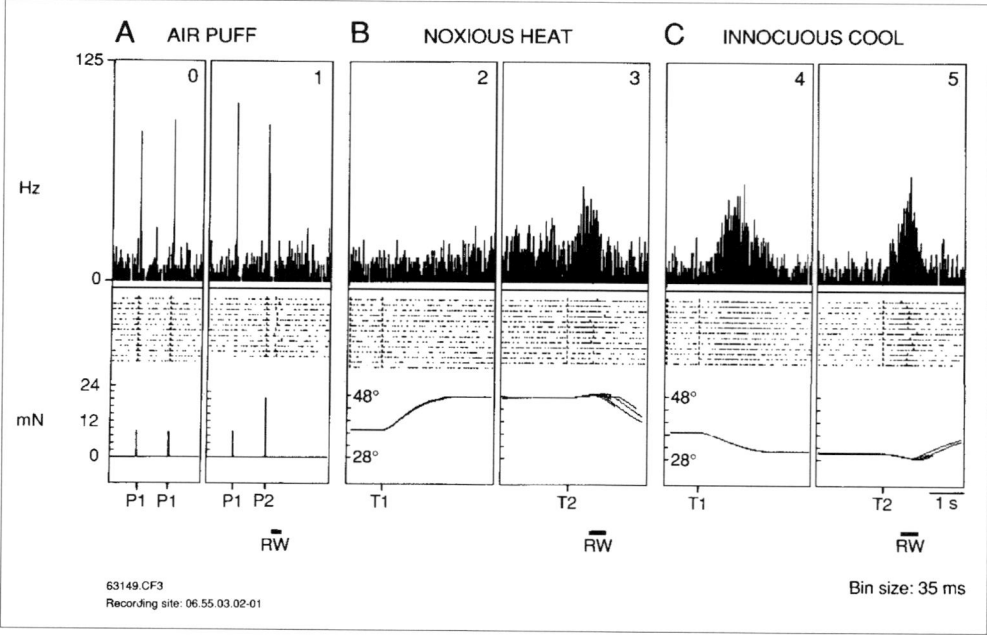

Figure 3. Histograms and associated dot rasters showing the responses of a single VPM neuron that responded to airpuff (A), noxious heat (B) and innocuous cool (C) applied above the maxillary lip. From [20].

Intensity discrimination

The intensity of a noxious stimulus is not only a sensory-discriminative feature in itself, but is one of the most important contributors to pain-related emotional feelings and behavioral reactions. Thus, it would not be surprising to find that nociceptive neurons involved in either sensory-discriminative or affective-motivational components of pain respond differentially to various intensities of a noxious stimulus. This, in fact, appears to be the case both within thalamus [19-21, 28, 29], and in many other regions of the brain, including the spinal cord [30-32], parabrachial region [33], amygdala [34], SI cortex [35, 36], area 7b cortex [37], and anterior cingulate cortex [38].

Figure 4 shows examples of neuronal responses in VPM, VMpo and Pf to noxious heat stimuli. Neurons in each region respond differentially to noxious temperatures between 43 °C and 50 °C, a temperature range usually described by humans as painful but tolerable [39-41]. For neurons in VPM and MDvc/Pf, we also examined their ability to respond to small changes in the intensity of noxious heat [19, 20]. In both regions, neurons responded to the smallest temperature change detectable by the monkey. Figure 5 shows the responses of a single neuron in VPM to temperature changes ranging from 1.0 °C to 0.2 °C from a baseline of 48 °C. Although the neuron discharged more vigorously to the large temperature changes, it also responded consistently to 0.2 °C, which is only detectable about 50% of the time by both monkeys and humans [20, 25].

Despite the finding that neurons throughout thalamus discriminate the intensity of noxious heat stimuli, activity in ventroposterior thalamus may be particularly important to maximize discriminative ability. For neurons in VPM, there is a significant correlation between the neuronal response to a small change in noxious heat intensity and the monkey's ability to detect the temperature step. Figure 6 shows the positive

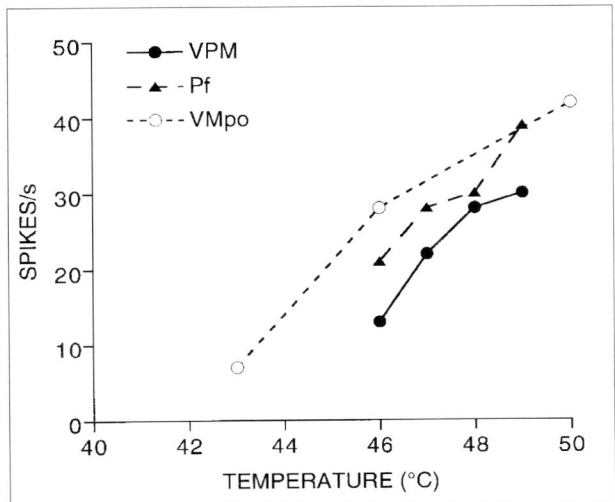

Figure 4. Mean neuronal response frequency to temperature pulses between 43 °C and 50 °C for single neurons in VPM (filled circles), Pf (filled triangles), and VMpo (open circles).

relationship in VPM between neuronal activity and the percentage of stimuli detected for temperature steps between 0.2 °C and 1.0 °C at a 47 °C baseline. An even stronger indication that VPM is necessary for the finest discriminative performance comes from our studies of reversible inactivation of VPM activity by lidocaine microinjection [42]. Figure 7 shows that, when small amounts of lidocaine were injected into locations within VPM in which nociceptive neurons were identified, the monkey's detection of small noxious temperature changes dropped to chance levels.

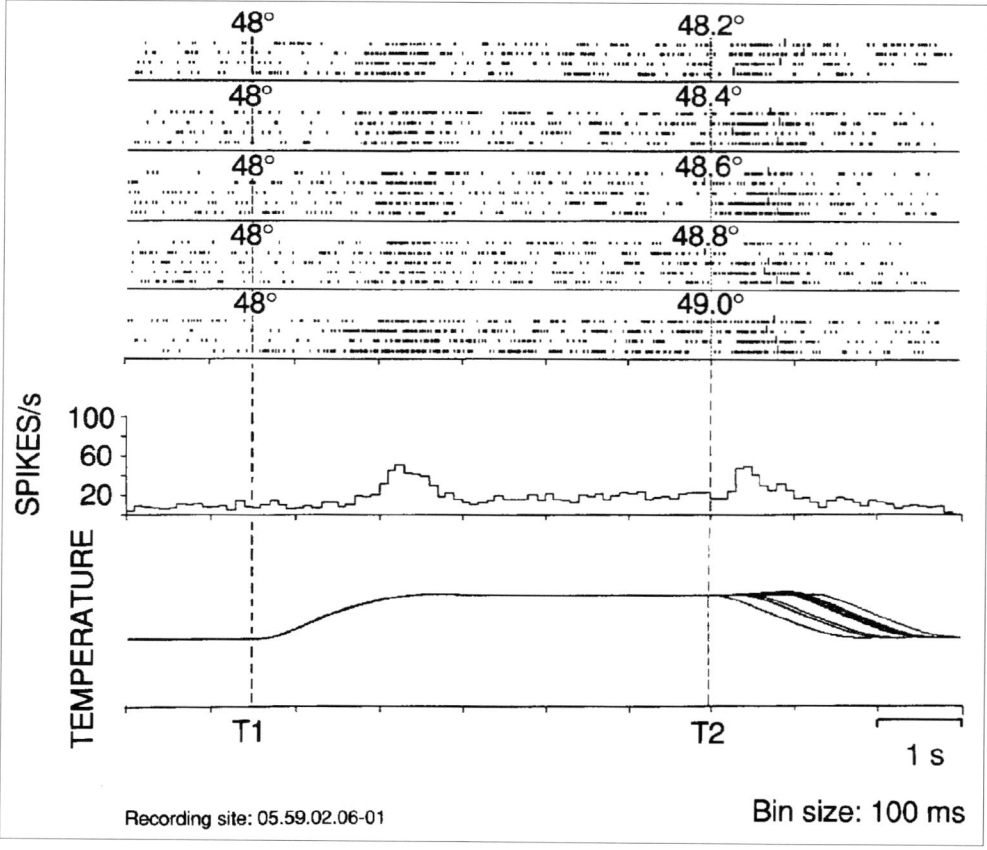

Figure 5. Top: Dot rasters showing the response of a singe VPM neuron to T1 shifts from 37 °C to 48 °C and T2 shifts from 48 °C to 48.2 °C-49.0 °C. Middle: mean response frequency for all trials depicted above. Bottom: Representation of the temperature changes associated with the neuronal activity.

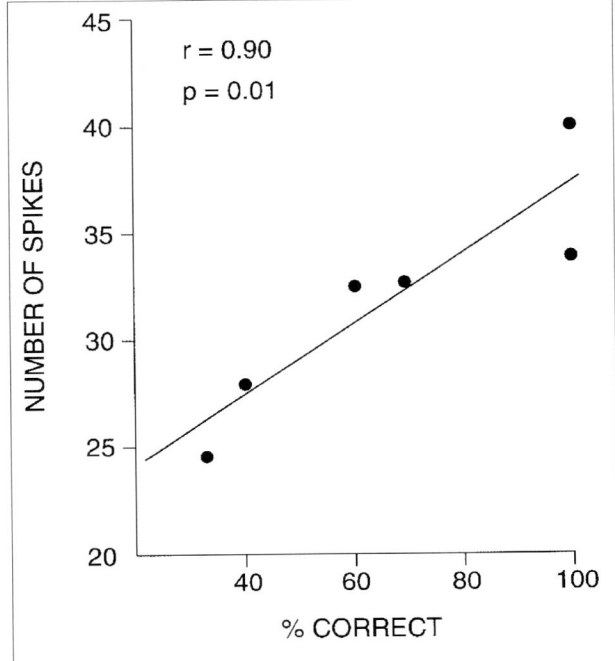

Figure 6. Neuronal response (number of spikes) plotted as a function of the monkey's accuracy (% correct) in detecting the stimulus change that evoked the neuronal response. There was a signficant correlation between the behavioral and neuronal response in VPM (Pearson's correlation coefficient: r = 0.90, p = 0.01).

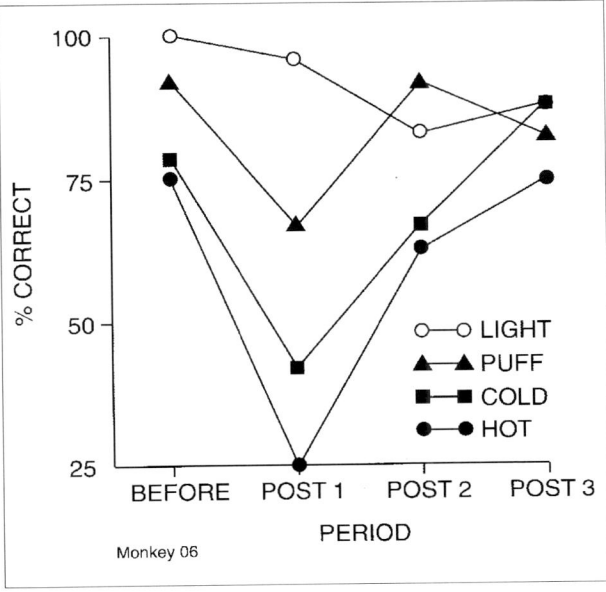

Figure 7. Percent correct detection of heat, cold, airpuff and visual stimuli before and after a double injection of 2% lidocaine (2.8µl and 1.8µl, 1 mm apart) into mid- and caudal VPM. There was a significant decrease in perception of hot, cold, and airpuff stimuli detected, but visual discrimination was unaltered (from [42]).

Affective-motivational properties of thalamic neurons

To understand which thalamic regions may be important for emotional and behavioral reactions to pain, we need to consider both the characteristics of the neurons in the region and the cortical connections of these neurons. Reactions to painful stimuli are highly modulated by the meaning of the stimulus, the context in which it is presented and the attentional and/or emotional state of the individual at the time of pain onset. Whereas pain threshold is relatively invariant across experimental conditions, pain tolerance depends on many factors, including the rewarding value of tolerating the stimulus [43]. People will submit to surgical procedures which produce extreme post-operative pain if the procedure is thought to be life-saving, but would clearly refuse to be subjected to the same pain if there was no perceived gain. Similarly, most adults are able to inhibit pain-evoked escape behavior while in the dentist's office. Thus, thalamic regions important for our affective and/or motivational reactions to pain might well contain neurons whose activity varies according to the behavioral context. Further, it would be reasonable for these neurons to project to motor and limbic regions of the cerebral cortex.

Cortical connectivity

Based on connectivity to cortical regions implicated in pain processing, MDvc/Pf and VMpo are more likely than VPL/VPM to be important for emotional or behavioral reactions to pain. The cortical regions most often identified in human brain imaging studies to be activated by pain are SI, SII, area 24 of the anterior cingulate cortex, and rostral insular cortex [14-17]. Of these regions, it is the anterior cingulate and insular cortices that most probably subserve emotional and behavioral reactions to pain (*see* [15] for review). Most evidence indicates that nociceptive regions of VPL/VPM do not project to cingulate or insular cortex, but, instead, project to primary somatosensory cortex (SI) [44, 45]. In contrast, cortical connectivity of MDvc/Pf and VMpo suggests that activity in these thalamic nuclei may be particularly important for the affective-motivational component of pain. Evidence is now accumulating that MDvc and Pf project to area 24 of the anterior cingulate cortex [46-48] and that VMpo projects to the rostral insular cortex (*see* chapter by A.D. Craig).

Modulation by behavioral state

We have examined the effect of behavioral state on nociceptive neuronal activity in VPM and MDvc/Pf [19, 20], but not on activity in VMpo. A striking contrast was found in behavioral modulation of nociceptive activity between medial and lateral thalamic regions. Whereas, in medial thalamus, the activity of almost all neurons was modulated by the behavioral state, no such change was observed in VPM. Two types of modulation were examined:

THALAMIC PROCESSING

- neuronal activation present when the monkey was performing a task and absent when the monkey sat quietly (i.e., task-related responses),
- differential stimulation-evoked activity when the monkey was rewarded for attending and responding to a noxious stimulus and when the noxious stimulus was presented while the monkey performed a visual task (i.e., attentional modulation).

Figure 8 shows the activity of a neuron recorded from Pf which demonstrated both task-related responses and attentional modulation. As shown at the beginning of each

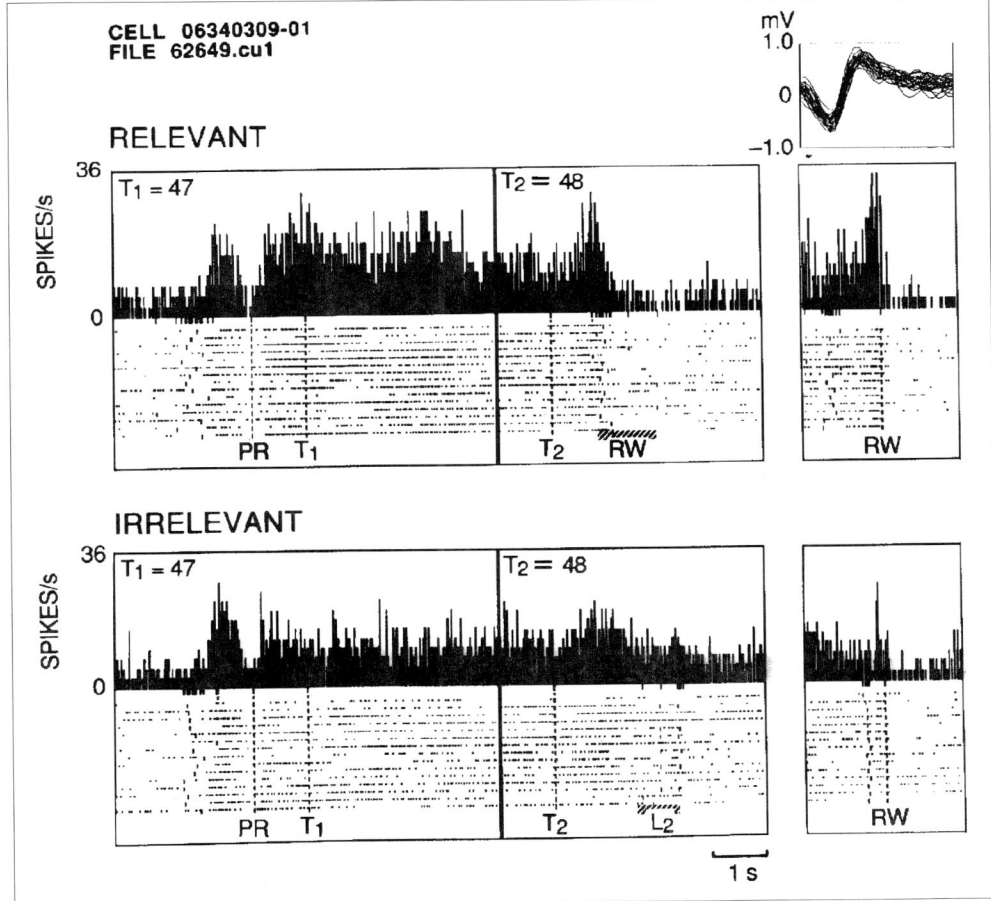

Figure 8. Top: histograms and associated dot rasters showing the response of a single neuron in Pf during trials in which the monkey received reward for responding to 1 °C changes from a T1 of 47 °C to a T2 of 48 °C (RELEVANT). Bottom: response of the same neuron during trials in which the monkey was rewarded for detecting changes in the intensity of a visual stimulus (L1 to L2). During these trials, irrelevant thermal stimuli were presented (T1 = 47 °C, T2 = 48 °C), but the monkey was never rewarded for responding to temperature changes. PR represents the lever press and RW shows time of rewarded lever release.

trace, the baseline activity of the cell was low (approximately 5 Hz), when the monkey was not performing the task. However, the cell's activity increased dramatically when the red light indicating trial availability was illuminated (hash marks before PR). When the monkey pressed the lever to begin the trial (PR), there was a transient decrease in response rate, followed by a tonic activation of the cell until the end of the trial (RW). In addition, the cell responded to the temperature change from 47 °C to 48 °C (T2), independent of the monkey's response to this change. By contrast, there was no such activation to L2 when the monkey performed the visual task.

Both the task-related responses and the T2-evoked thermal response were more pronounced when the temperature was the relevant stimulus for reward (RELEVANT) than when the light was the relevant stimulus (IRRELEVANT). In both cases the same temperatures (T1 = 47 °C, T2 = 48 °C) were presented, but the neuronal response to T2 was much greater when the monkey received reward for detecting the temperature (Figure 8, top) than for detecting the light (L2 in Figure 8, bottom).

The enhanced neuronal activation when the monkey is performing a task involving noxious stimulation may reflect a heightened readiness for behavioral reaction. The ubiquitous nature of such modulation in medial thalamus strongly implicates this region in the affective-motivational dimension of pain. The relative absense of such task-related activity and attentional modulation of nociceptive responses in lateral thalamus suggests that it is part of a less variable sensory detection pathway. Nevertheless, lateral thalamic activity is not totally insensitive to behavioral state. Activity in both medial and lateral thalamus is modulated by changes in state of arousal, with neurons being most active during a quiet waking state similar to that of the monkeys in our experiments [2, 3]. Attentional manipulations may also alter lateral thalamic activity in tasks involving detection of the absence of stimulation [49]. The finding that lateral thalamus is influenced somewhat, but to a lesser degree than medial thalamus, by changes in behavioral state is consistent with psychophysical observations that similar manipulations have a small but consistent effect on perceived stimulus intensity [50]. Nociceptive activity in posterior thalamus has not been investigated in the awake monkey, so that state-related modulation of these neurons in unknown. However, the strong connectivity of VMpo to limbic cortex suggests that activity in this part of thalamus might well be influenced by behavioral state.

In summary, the fully elaborated experience of pain may require co-activation within a number of neural pathways. Various regions of thalamus appear to process noxious stimuli in distinct fashions, and thus are likely to be involved in different aspects of pain processing. The multiplicity of thalamocortical circuits involved in nociception might explain why infarcts involving the thalamus produce such variable effects on pain perception, and why post-stroke pain syndromes involving thalamocortical pathways are so difficult to treat [51].

References

1. Steriade M, McCormick DA, Sejnowski TJ. Thalamocortical oscillations in the sleeping and aroused brain. *Science* 1993 ; 262 : 679-85.
2. Casey KL. Unit analysis of nociceptive mechanisms in the thalamus of the awake squirrel monkey. *J Neurophysiol* 1966 ; 29 : 727-50.
3. Morrow TJ, Casey KL. State-related modulation of thalamic somatosensory responses in the awake monkey. *J Neurophysiol* 1992 ; 67 : 305-17.
4. Apkarian AV, Hodge CJ. Primate spinothalamic pathways: III. Thalamic terminations of the dorsolateral and ventral spinothalamic pathways. *J Comp Neurol* 1989 ; 288 : 493-511.
5. Applebaum AE, Leonard RB, Kenshalo DR Jr, Martin RF, Willis WD. Nuclei in which functionally identified spinothalamic tract neurons terminate. *J Comp Neurol* 1979 ; 188 : 575-86.
6. Berkley KJ. Spatial relationships between the terminations of somatic sensory and motor pathways in the rostral brainstem of cat and monkeys I. Ascending somatic sensory inputs to lateral diencephalon. *J Comp Neurol* 1980 ; 193 : 283-317.
7. Boivie J. An anatomical reinvestigation of the termination of the spinothalamic tract in the monkey. *J Comp Neurol* 1979 ; 186 : 343-70.
8. Burton H, Craig AD. Distribution of trigeminothalamic projection cells in cat and monkey. *Brain Res* 1979 ; 161 : 515-21.
9. Ganchrow D. Intratrigeminal and thalamic projections of nucleus caudalis in the squirrel monkey (*Saimiri sciureus*): a degeneration and autoradiographic study. *J Comp Neurol* 1978 ; 178 : 281-312.
10. Mehler WR, Federman ME, Nauta WJH. Ascending axon degeneration following antero-lateral cordotomy. An experimental study in the monkey. *Brain* 1960 ; 83 : 718-50.
11. Craig AD. Lamina I trigeminothalamic projections in the monkey. *Soc Neurosci Abstr* 1990 ; 16 : 1144.
12. Craig AD. Organization of lamina I terminations in the posterior thalamus of the cynomolgus monkey. *Soc Neurosci Abstr* 1992 ; 18 : 385.
13. Ralston HJ,III, Ralston DD. The primate dorsal spinothalamic tract: evidence for a specific termination in the posterior nuclei (Po/SG) of the thalamus. *Pain* 1992 ; 48 : 107-18.
14. Talbot JD, Marrett S, Evans AC, Meyer E, Bushnell MC, Duncan GH. Multiple representations of pain in human cerebral cortex. *Science* 1991 ; 251 : 1355-8.
15. Coghill RC, Talbot JD, Evans AC, Meyer E, Gjedde A, Bushnell MC, Duncan GH. Distributed processing of pain and vibration by the human brain. *J Neurosci* 1994 ; 14 : 4095-108.
16. Casey KL, Minoshima S, Berger KL, Koeppe RA, Morrow TJ, Frey KA. Positron emission tomographic analysis of cerebral structures activated specifically by repetitive noxious heat stimuli. *J Neurophysiol* 1994 ; 71 : 802-7.
17. Jones AKP, Brown WD, Friston KJ, Qi LY, Frackowiak RSJ. Cortical and subcortical localization of response to pain in man using positron emission tomography. *Proc R Soc Lond (Biol)* 1991 ; 244 : 39-44.
18. Bushnell MC, Duncan GH. Mechanical response properties of ventroposterior medial thalamic neurons in the alert monkey. *Exp Brain Res* 1987 ; 67 : 603-14.
19. Bushnell MC, Duncan GH. Sensory and affective aspects of pain perception: is medial thalamus restricted to emotional issues ? *Exp Brain Res* 1989 ; 78 : 415-8.
20. Bushnell MC, Duncan GH, Tremblay N. Thalamic VPM nucleus in the behaving monkey. I. Multimodal and discriminative properties of thermosensitive neurons. *J Neurophysiol* 1993 ; 69 : 739-52.

21. Craig AD, Bushnell MC, Zhang E-T, Blomqvist A. A thalamic nucleus specific for pain and temperature sensation. *Nature* 1994 ; 372 : 770-3.
22. Olszewski J. *The thalamus of the* Macaca mulatta: *an atlas for use with the stereotaxic instrument.* Basel : S. Karger, 1952.
23. Morin C, Bushnell MC, Lamarre Y. Temperature localization without tactile information in a deafferented patient. *Soc Neurosci Abstr* 1995 ; 25.
24. Bushnell MC, Duncan GH, Dubner R, Jones RL, Maixner W. Attentional influences on noxious and innocuous cutaneous heat detection in humans and monkeys. *J Neurosci* 1985 ; 5 : 1103-10.
25. Bushnell MC, Taylor MB, Duncan GH, Dubner R. Discrimination of noxious and innocuous thermal stimuli in human and monkey. *Somatosen Res* 1983 ; 1 : 119-29.
26. Chen CC, Rainville P, Bushnell MC. Noxious and innocuous cold discrimination in humans. *Soc Neurosci Abstr* 1994 ; 20 : 127.
27. Morin C, TenBokum L, Bushnell MC. Temporal and qualitative differences in heat and cold pain. *Soc Neurosci Abstr* 1994 ; 20 : 127.
28. Apkarian AV, Shi T. Squirrel monkey lateral thalamus. I. Somatic nocirespnsive neurons and their relation to spinothalamic terminals. *J Neurosci* 1994 ; 14 : 6779-95.
29. Kenshalo DR,Jr., Giesler GJ, Leonard RB, Willis WD. Responses of neurons in primate ventral posterior lateral nucleus to noxious stimuli. *J Neurophysiol* 1980 ; 43 : 1594-614.
30. Ferrington DG, Sorkin LS, Willis WD. Responses of spinothalamic tract cells in the superficial dorsal horn of the primate lumbar spinal cord. *J Physiol* 1987 ; 388 : 681-703.
31. Surmeier DJ, Honda CN, Willis WD. Natural groupings of primate spinothalamic neurons based on cutaneous stimulation. Physiological and anatomical features. *J Neurophysiol* 1988 ; 59 : 833-60.
32. Price DD, Dubner R, Hu JW. Trigeminothalamic neurons in nucleus caudalis responsive to tactile, thermal, and nociceptive stimulation of monkey's face. *J Neurophysiol* 1976 ; 39 : 936-53.
33. Bernard JF, Besson JM. The spino(trigemino)pontoamygdaloid pathway: electrophysiological evidence for an involvement in pain processes. *J Neurophysiol* 1990 ; 63 : 473-90.
34. Bernard JF, Huang GF, Besson JM. Effect of noxious somesthetic stimulation on the activity of neurons of the nucleus centralis of the amygdala. *Brain Res* 1990 ; 523 : 347-50.
35. Kenshalo DR Jr, Isensee O. Responses of primate SI cortical neurons to noxious stimuli. *J Neurophysiol* 1983 ; 50 : 1479-96.
36. Kenshalo DR Jr, Chudler EH, Anton F, Dubner R. SI nociceptive neurons participate in the encoding process by which monkeys perceive the intensity of noxious thermal stimulation. *Brain Res* 1988 ; 454 : 378-82.
37. Dong WK, Chudler EH, Sugiyama K, Roberts VJ, Hayashi T. Somatosensory, multisensory, and task-related neurons in cortical area 7b (PF) of unanaesthetized monkeys. *J Neurophysiol* 1994 ; 72 : 542-64.
38. Sikes RW, Vogt BA. Nociceptive neurons in area 24 of rabbit cingulate cortex. *J Neurophysiol* 1992 ; 68 : 1720-32.
39. Price DD, McGrath P, Rafii A, Buckingham B. The validation of visual analogue scales as ratio scale measures for chronic and experimental pain. *Pain* 1983 ; 17 : 45-56.
40. Rainville P, Feine JS, Bushnell MC, Duncan GH. A psychophysical comparison of sensory and affective responses to four modalities of experimental pain. *Somatosens Mot Res* 1992 ; 9 : 265-77.
41. Feine JS, Bushnell MC, Miron D, Duncan GH. Sex differences in the perception of noxious heat stimuli. *Pain* 1991 ; 44 : 255-62.
42. Duncan GH, Bushnell MC, Oliveras J-L, Bastrash N, Tremblay N. Thalamic VPM nucleus in the behaving monkey. III. Effects of reversible inactivation by lidocaine on thermal and mechanical discrimination. *J Neurophysiol* 1993 ; 70 : 2086-96.

43. Rollman GB, Harris G. The detectability, discriminability, and perceived magnitude of painful electrical shock. *Perception and Psychophysics* 1987 ; 42 (3) : 257-68.
44. Rausell E, Jones EG. Chemically distinct compartments of the thalamic VPM nucleus in monkeys relay principal and spinal trigeminal pathways to different layers of the somatosensory cortex. *J Neurosci* 1991 ; 11 : 226-37.
45. Rausell E, Bae CS, Viñuela A, Huntley GW, Jones EG. Calbindin and parvalbumin cells in monkey VPL thalamic nucleus: distribution, laminar cortical projections, and relations to spinothalamic terminations. *J Neurosci* 1992 ; 12 : 4088-111.
46. Musil SY, Olson CR. Organization of cortical and subcortical projections to anterior cingulate cortex in the cat. *J Comp Neurol* 1988 ; 272 : 203-18.
47. Vogt BA, Pandya DN, Rosene DL. Cingulate cortex of the rhesus monkey: I. Cytoarchitecture and thalamic afferents. *J Comp Neurol* 1987 ; 262 : 256-70.
48. Vogt BA, Sikes RW, Vogt LJ. Anterior cingulate cortex and the medial pain system. In : Vogt BA, Gabriel M, eds. *Neurobiology of cingulate cortex and limbic thalamus: a comprehensive handbook*. Boston : Birkhauser, 1993.
49. Morrow TJ, Casey KL. Effects of attention on VP thalamic neuronal responses in awake monkey. *Soc Neurosci Abstr* 1990 ; 16 : 225.
50. Miron D, Duncan GH, Bushnell MC. Effects of attention on the intensity and unpleasantness of thermal pain. *Pain* 1989 ; 39 : 345-352.
51. Boivie J, Leijon G. Clinical findings in patients with central poststroke pain. In : Casey KL, ed. *Pain and central nervous system disease: the central pain syndromes*. New York : Raven Press, 1991 : 65-75.

6

Thalamic and cortical processing in rat models of clinical pain

G. GUILBAUD, J.M. BENOIST

Unité de Recherches de Physiopharmacologie du Système Nerveux, INSERM U161, Paris, France

The electrophysiological approach to demonstrate the role of supraspinal structures, particularly the thalamus and cortex, in pain processing is used by relatively few groups, as compared to the numerous teams studying pain mechanisms at the periphery and spinal cord levels [1].

On the basis of anatomical data, we have systematically explored the thalamic ventrobasal complex (VB) of the rat, which receives terminals of the spinothalamic tract and thus, nociceptive messages. Subsequently, the primary somatosensory cortex (SM1) where most, if not all, VB neurons project in this species, was systematically studied. A few other groups have studied similar structures in the monkey and obtained roughly comparable data [1].

In the initial experiments, it was necessary to record reliable neuronal responses in these structures, which can account for nociceptive responses in normal rats. In fact, these 2 structures contain neurons which can be activated, sometimes exclusively, by noxious stimuli. Multiple experimental series performed under similar conditions (anaesthesia, age, weight, stimulus...) have clearly emphasized the reproducibility of neuronal ventrobasal thalamic responses elicited by thermal and mechanical noxious stimuli (Table I). Activation thresholds of those neurons were similar to those of nociceptive behavioural reactions; for example, noxious heat threshold of 44 °C - 45 °C. These neurones are able to encode the stimulus charateristics, in the sense that the intensity of the response was dependent on the stimulus intensity, surface and duration. In addition, the responses are suppressed by anterolateral cordotomy and strongly depressed by morphine, or other opioid agonists and inhibitors of enkephalin degrading enzymes. Although less studies have focused on the somatosensory cortex, SM1 neuronal responses to noxious stimuli such as pinch and heat are also reproducible (Table I).

Table I. Neuronal responses to pinch stimulus (15 sec) in normal rats.

	vb	sm1
Mean number of spikes	504 ± 42	162 ± 38
Duration (seconds)	42 ± 2	14 ± 2
n	174	8

The ultimate purpose of these studies is a better understanding of pain in humans, our latter studies have thus been performed in rat models of clinical pain. The first aim was to search for neuronal responses accounting for the pain behaviours seen in the awake, unrestrained rats. The second aim was to study whether, and to what extent central mechanisms contribute to the persistence of pain and evolution towards chronic pain.

Inflammatory and neuropathic pain models

Models of inflammatory pain consisted of rats rendered polyarthritic by Freund's adjuvant injection into the tail, and rats with a localized inflammatory process induced by intraplantar carrageenin injection in one hindpaw. These models have been widely used by many laboratories with several approaches [2, 3].

Among the various neuropathic pain models recently proposed, and based on the chronic injury of one sciatic nerve [4, 5], we chose the moderate chronic constriction (CCI) of one sciatic nerve, as proposed by Bennett and Xie [5], that we have extensively investigated in our group [3, 6, 7]. More recently, following the initial description of Vos et al. [8, 9], we started to study another model of nerve injury, consisting of a chronic constriction of one infraorbital nerve (ION). Contrasting with the sciatic nerve, this branch of the Vth nerve is purely sensory and supplies, alone, a well-defined facial area of great functional importance in the rat, without any functional overlap with the other trigeminal branches. The rats with such a nerve constriction exhibit some reactions reminiscent of some aspects of trigeminal pain [8, 9]. Lesions of this nerve has already been used to study cortical plasticity in general [10], but without considering the "pain" aspect. In fact, rats with a ION injury developed abnormal pain-related behaviours reminiscent of some aspects of trigeminal pain, currently encountered in clinical situations [8].

Carrageenin injection induces an inflammatory pain lasting between 60 minutes and several days. It is thus an ideal model to study the development of acute inflammatory pain, since it is possible to study changes in activities of a single neurone during several hours. In addition, neuronal recordings in rats still hyperalgesic 1-4 days after the beginning of the inflammation, can also be used to study sub-acute inflammatory pain.

The polyarthritic and mononeuropathic rats are considered as models of persistent pain, since the pain-related behaviours were maximum between 3-4 weeks after injection of Freund's adjuvant, with a recovery at week 11. Whereas, with mononeuropathic rats, maximum pain-related was between the 2nd and 3rd week after the nerve ligature, with a recovery at week 8-10. In these models, electrophysiological recordings were performed at time of the maximum pain-related behaviours, and tested with several behavioural tests beforehand.

Changes in the neuronal responsivity and responses to somatic stimulus usually ineffective

Electrophysiological neuronal recordings in the ventrobasal thalamic complex (VB) (or in the ventro-postero-median thalamus, VPM for rats with ION constriction) and in the primary somatosensory cortex (SM1) have emphasized the existence of changes in the neuronal activities which can account for hyperalgesia or allodynia to mechanical and thermal stimuli observed in the awake unrestrained animals [2, 4, 8].

Pinch responses

- Changes in pinch responses of a single neuron recorded before and after an intraplantar injection of carrageenin into the hindpaw were observed (Figure 1).
- Twenty four hours -post carrageenin, and 2-3 weeks after a CCI of one sciatic nerve, neuronal pinch responses from the injured limb were also increased as compared to responses corresponding to the non-injured paw. These changes included a decrease in the activation thresholds to thermal and/or mechanical stimulus, discharges of a long duration, (often beyond 1 minute) which was termed "spontaneous" since such activity occurs without an intentional stimulus (Figure 2).
- Studies performed in the ventro-postero-median (VPM) thalamus in rats with a ION constriction (Figure 3) [9] have also emphasized changes in the neuronal activities which might account for some of the pain-related behaviours observed in these rats.

Changes in classical neuronal responses to light touch

At the level of the VB, responses to light touch were apparently stable under the different situations of inflammatory pain (acute, subacute, chronic) but the responses were strongly modified at the level of the SM1 neurons in acute and subacute

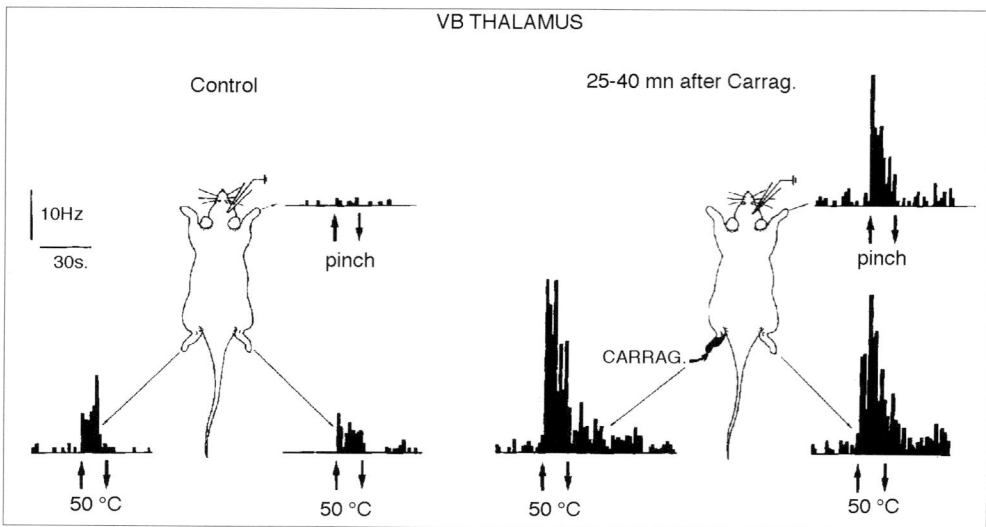

Figure 1. Responses of one right VB neuron to a pinch stimulus applied to the right forepaw, and to a 50 °C water bath applied alternately to each hind paw before and after carageenin injection in the left plantar hindpaw. Note the increase responses to 50°C for both injected and non-injected hindpaw, and the occurence of a pinch response for the forepaw 25-40 minutes after the carrageenin injection.

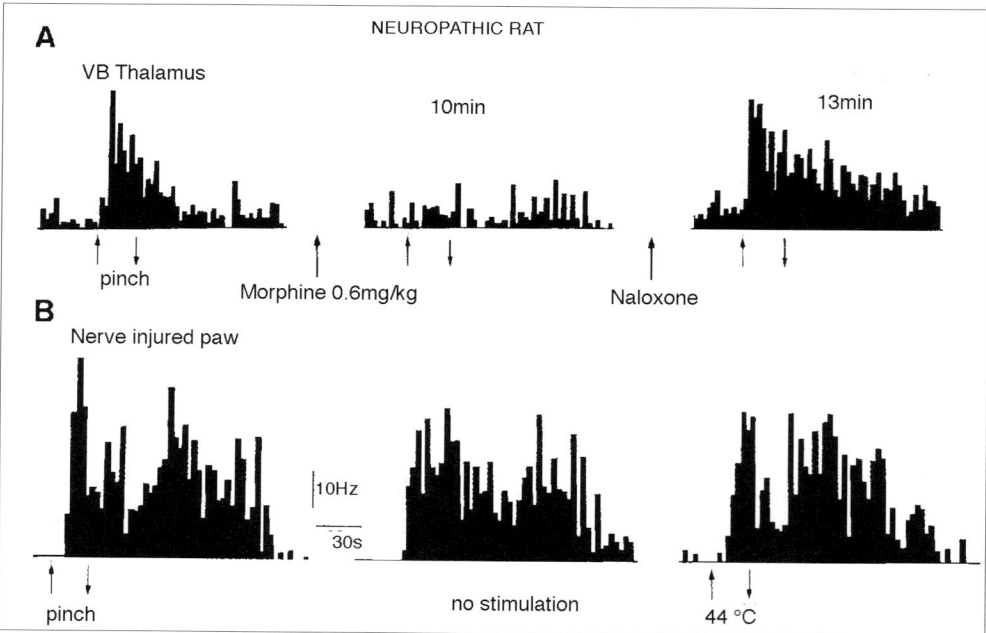

Figure 2. Two VB neurons recorded in 2 neuropathic rats and excited by a pinch stimulus applied to the nerve injured paw. The response of neuron A was supressed by 0.6 mg/kg i.v.morphine, the effect being reversed by the antagonist naloxone; neuron B was also excited when the nerve injured paw was immersed in a 44 °C water bath, and exhibited a discharge without any stimulus.

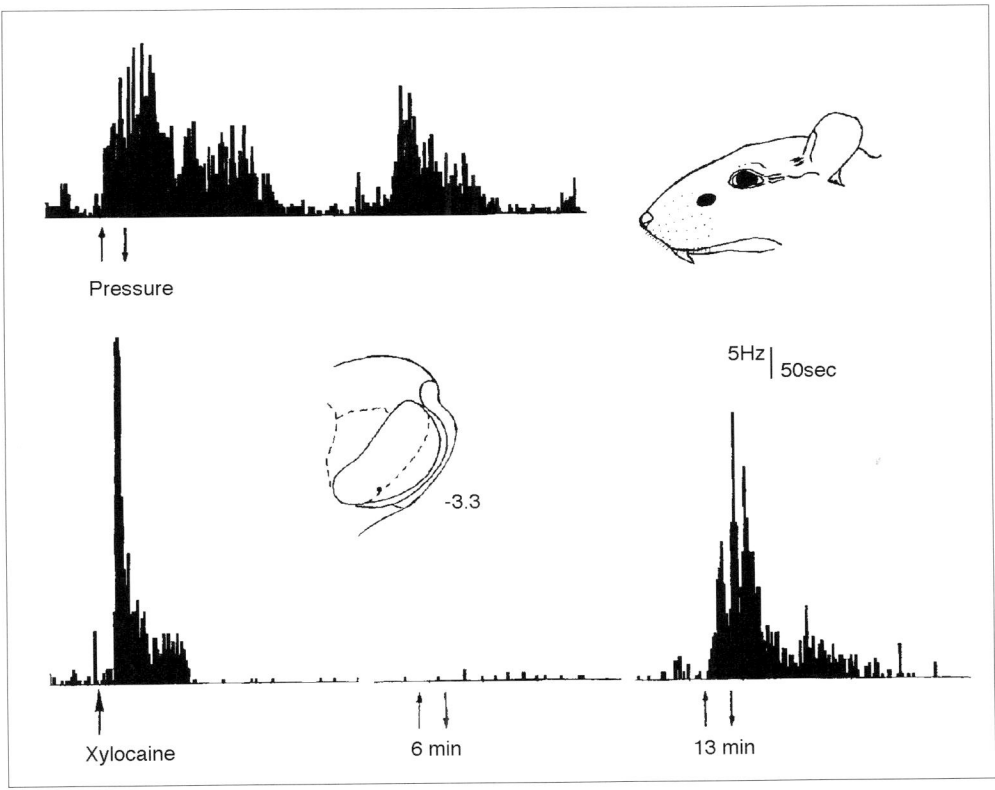

Figure 3. Responses of one VPM neuron to mild pressure applied to the RF indicated on the figure. Note the discharge occuring "spontaneously" a few minutes after the first stimulus, the response induced by the needle when xylocaine was injected, resulting in the total suppression of the response, followed by a recovery of the pressure response (6 and 13 minutes after the nerve block respectively).

inflammation due the carrageenin injection in one hindpaw: these modifications consisted of changes in the background activity, an increase in responses, and an enlargement of the receptive fields (RFs) (Figures 4, 5).

Occurence of responses to some stimulus modalities normally not effective
(Figures 6, 7)

For instance, there was a dramatic increase in neurons responding to the stimulation of the inflamed joints in arthritic animals, and also to a lesser extent in 24h-post-carrageenin injected rats. These differences were usually more marked at cortical than at thalamic level.

Surprisingly, such an increase of joint inputs was also noted in the SM1 cortex of neuropathic rats, possibly partly due to the sensitization of the peripheral joint afferent fibers (Figure 7). From the preliminary study in rats with ION constriction, such a reorganization has not been observed in the cortical area corresponding to the vibrissae so far.

Functional relevance of these changes: pharmacological studies

Since the neuronal responses were highly reproducible (Table II), pharmacological studies could be performed. Such studies demonstrated the functional relevance of the altered neuronal responses in the VB and SM1 cortex. Indeed, the neuronal responses

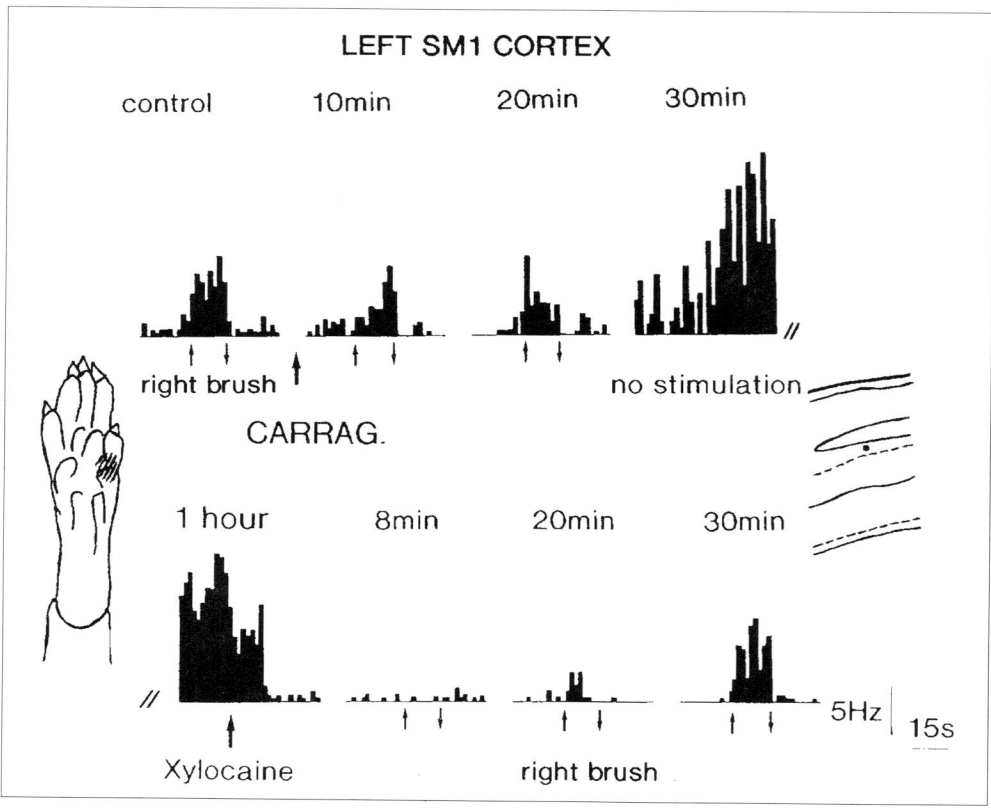

Figure 4. Responses of a SM1 cortex neuron responding to brushing applied to the small receptive field indicated on the right hindpaw before, and after the carrageenin injection in the medial plantar region of this paw. Note the unchanged responses at 10 or 20 minutes after carrageenin, then the sudden increase of the background activity occuring at 30 minutes. This activity was still maintained 1 hour after carrageenin injection, but suppressed by xylocaine injected locally at this time. The evoked neuronal response to brush was absent for 8 minutes following the anaesthetic injection; recovery was then progressive.

Table II. Neuronal responses to joint stimulus (15 sec.) in polyarthritic rats

	VB	SM1
Mean number of spikes	469 ± 41	230 ± 38
Duration (seconds)	43 ± 3	27 ± 5
n	98	37

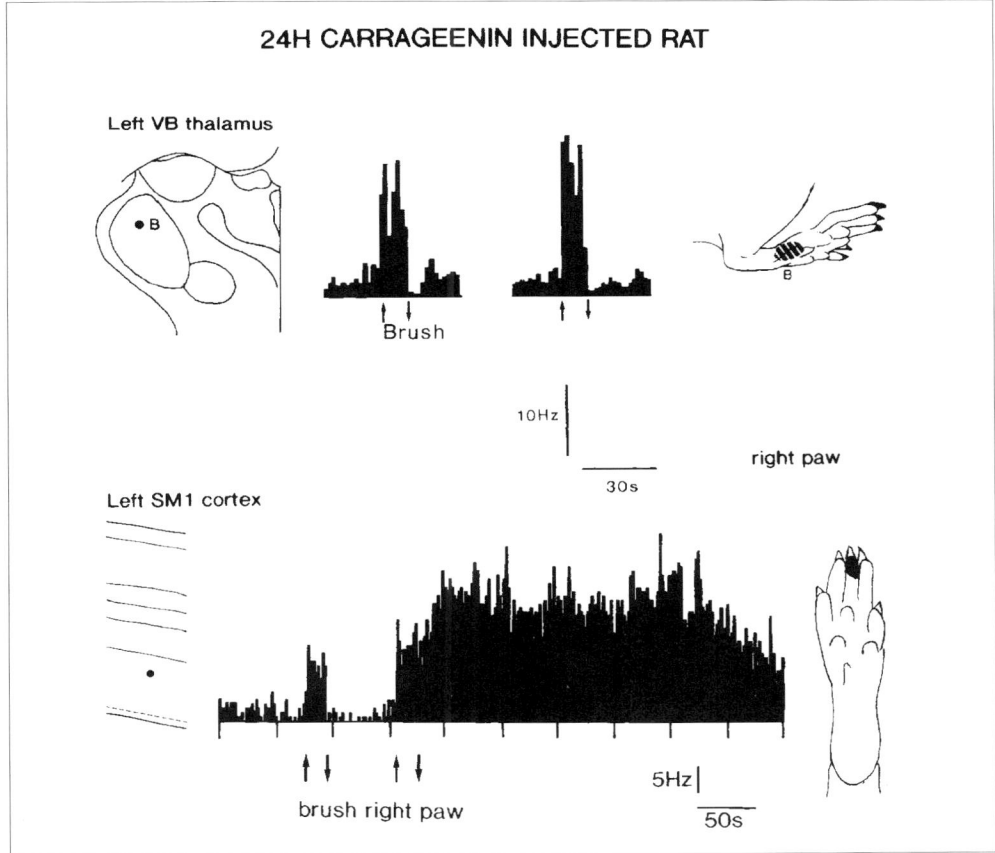

Figure 5. Responses of one ventrobasal (VB) thalamic and one SM1 cortex neuron to brushing applied to their small contralateral field in 24-hours post-carrageenin injected rats. While VB responses remained normal, a SM1 neuronal discharge was triggered by the second stimulus, this discharge persited up to 30 minutes and was depressed by local xylocaine [adapted from 19].

were depressed, suppressed or prevented by low doses of pharmacological analgesic substances (opioids and non-opioids), which are antinociceptive when tested in the awake animals (Figures 2, 4, 6). In rats with a ION constriction, some responses reflecting an excess in peripheral inputs could also be suppressed by a xylocaine nerve block (Figure 3).

Beside these different alterations in the neuronal responsiveness which seem to be directly linked to the peripheral injury, other modifications were also apparent.

Secondary distant hyperalgesia and neuronal counterpart

In rat models of unilateral inflammatory or neuropathic pain, distant secondary hyperalgesia, remote to the initial injury has been emphasized: such a distant secondary hyperalgesia was evident by the significant decrease in the vocalization threshold to paw pressure, and a decrease in the struggle latency to thermal stimuli, from the opposite non-lesionned hindpaw (even from the forepaws in some cases) [3, 7, 11, 12].

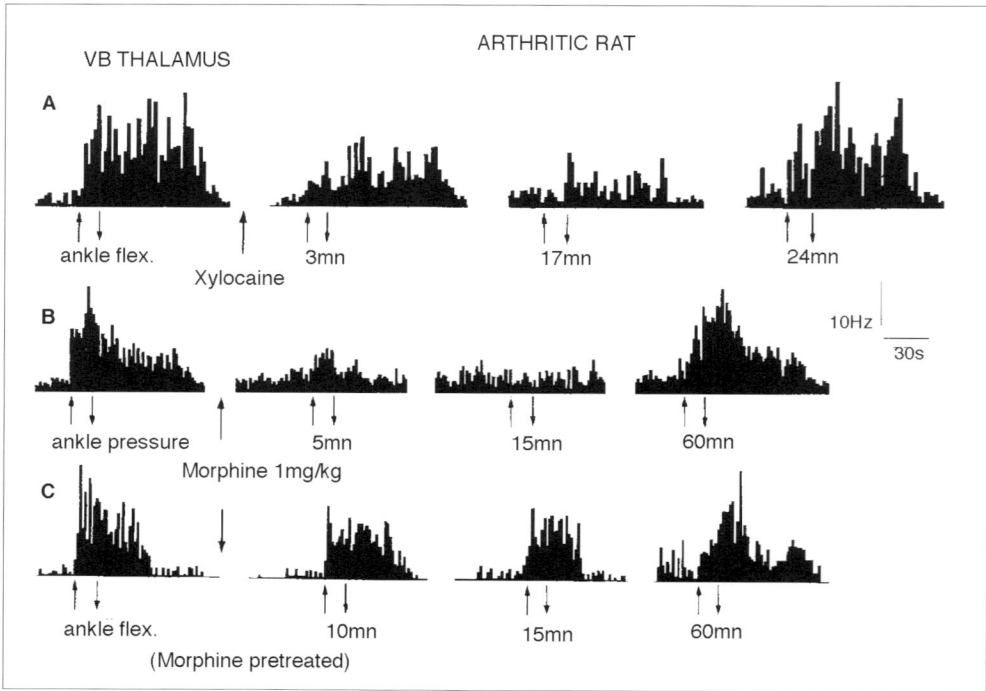

Figure 6. Responses to ankle flexion or mild pressure of 3 VB thalamic neurons, in 3 arthritic rats, were strongly depressed by local xylocaine (A), or morphine which is effective in naive (B) but not in morphine pretreated (C) animals.

In fact, there is electrophysiological evidence for a distant hyperalgesia since thalamic and cortical neuronal responses, obtained from part of the non-injured-body, were also increased as compared to the pre-injury values. In addition, it was possible to influence these neuronal changes (as also seen for behaviour) by treating the peripheral process itself. Indeed, several compounds, such as local anaesthetics, or antagonists of inflammatory substances, could prevent, depress or even suppress the VB or SM1 neuronal responses obtained not only from the injury, but also from the non-injured limb (Figure 1) [3, 11, 12].

Thus, although most of the data strongly emphasized a major role of the peripheral process, it also seems clearly that the peripheral abnormalities can trigger additional central mechanisms. These phenomena, seen in animal models of pain, are especially helpful for our understanding of mirror pain occuring in clinical situations of inflammatory and neuropathic pain.

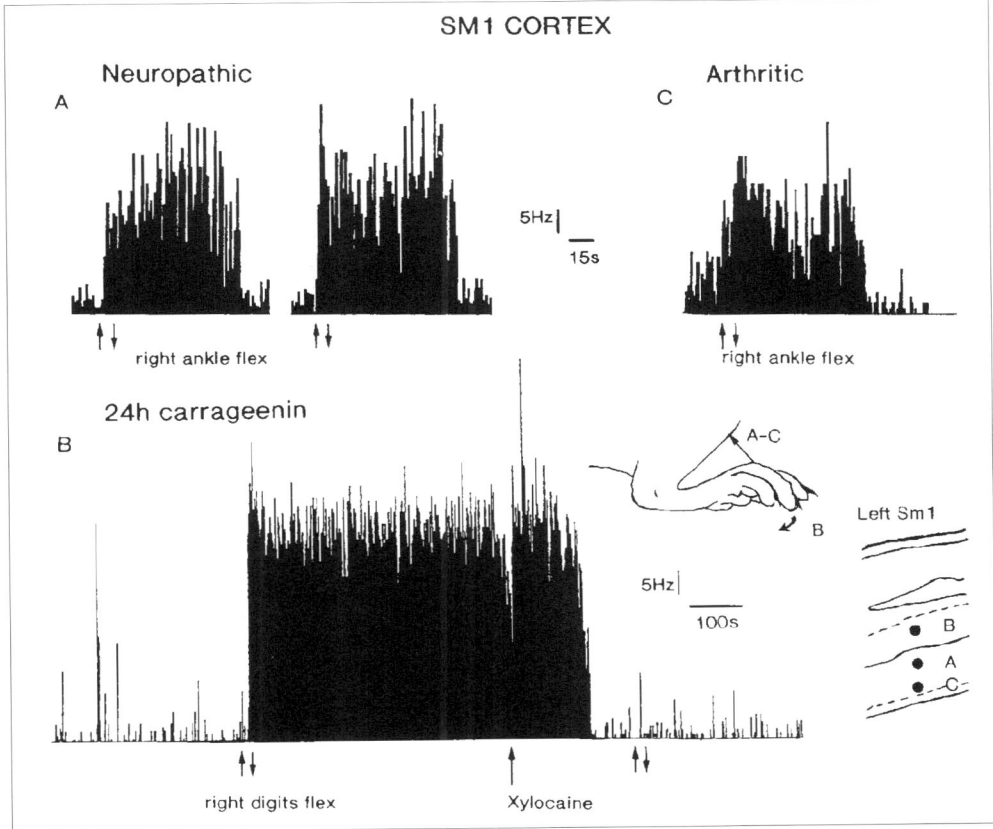

Figure 7. Responses to ankle or digit flexion of 3 SM1 cortical neurons recorded in 3 different models of clinical pain. The example obtained in 24 h-carrageenin injected rats also illustrates the depressive effect of local xylocaine.

Reorganization of the somatic inputs in SM1 cortical area in models of inflammatory and neuropathic pain: homeostatic processes

Comparison of our successive investigations performed, under similar experimental conditions, in various experimental models of pain led us to note some intriguing data concerning the SM1 cortex.

The occurrence of "new" neuronal responses to some specific inputs, mentioned above, was often concomitant to a simultaneous decrease in the number of neurons driven by other inputs (Figure 8).

In polyarthritic rats

Despite the increase in responsivity of VB and SM1 neurons to joint stimuli which can account for the pain behaviours, there was no modification of the total number of neurons excited by somatic inputs, since the number of neurons responding to light touch and pinch was dramatically decreased [3, 11]. This reduction was possibly due to an increase in descending inhibitory controls observed in chronic inflammation [13, 14, 15], in addition to specific cortical control [16].

In neuropathic rats

There was a decrease in the number of neurons responding to light touch from the sciatic nerve territory. This may be accounted for by a major drop in the number of large myelinated fibers in this nerve. In contrast, an increase in saphenous nerve inputs was observed, partly due to an unmasking phenomenon and disinhibition of initially silent synapses [16-18]. There was also an increase in the number of neurons driven by joint inputs (Figures 7, 8), suggested to be linked to the sensitization of peripheral joint fibers as a consequence of the abnormal position of the nerve-injured paw. Finally, in this model of neuropathic pain, the number of SM1 cortical neurons driven by somatic stimuli was comparable to that observed in normal rats (Figure 8) [3, 7].

This rearrangement of cortical inputs, which maintains a fixed number of somatosensory neurons in the cortical hindpaw area, has previously been described after sciatic nerve section, and was suggested to be linked to some homeostatic processes [16-18]. Interestingly, such a rearrangement occurs here, in two different models of pain, both of which have a component of persistent pain which lasts over a 1-2 week period. These phenomena thus appear to be able to attenuate an excess, or to replace a lack of, inputs either in arthritic or neuropathic rats, respectively.

It is not known whether these phenomena have some functional implication, but, since they appear linked to the persistence of pain-related behaviours, we wondered whether they are specific of this pain type, or if they also exist at an earlier stage of an hyperalgesic state.

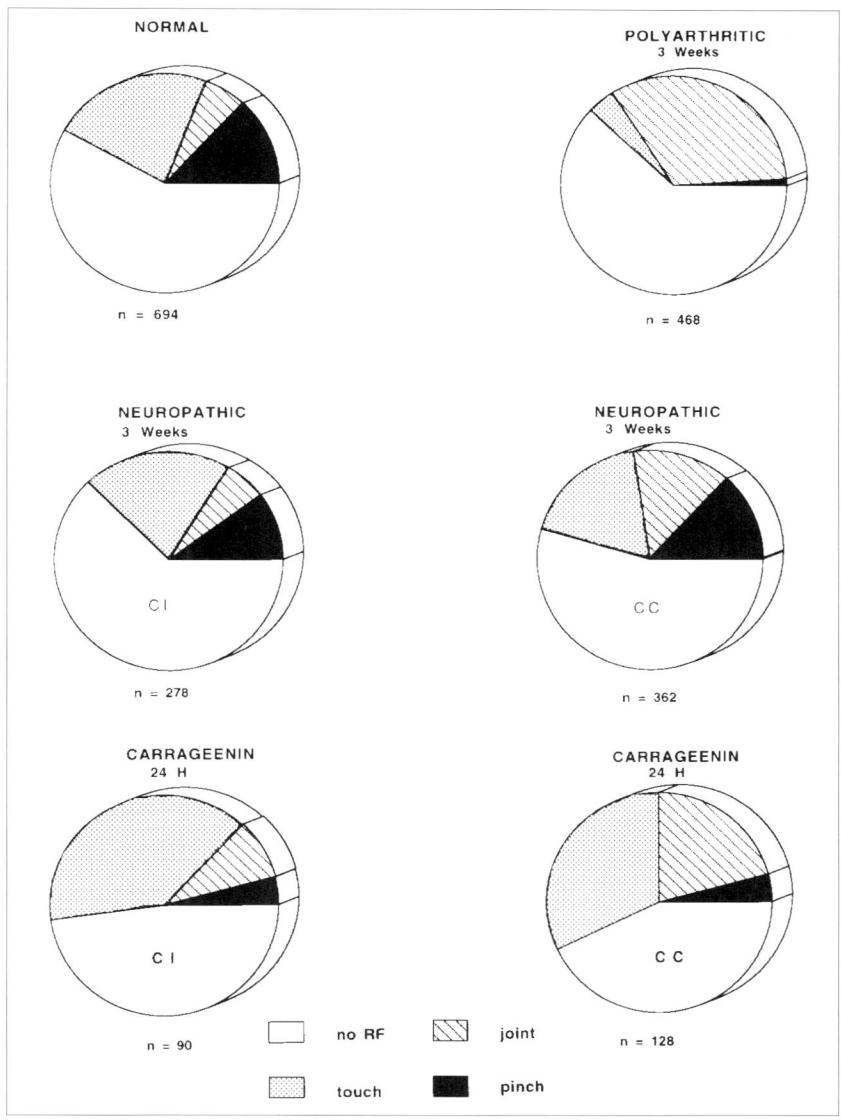

Figure 8. The proportion of cortical SM1 neurons without receptive fields (RF) or driven by touch, pinch, or joint movement in: normal and polyarthritic rats (upper line); in the SM1 cortex ipsilateral (CI) or contralateral (CC) to the nerve-injured paw in neuropathic rats (middle line); in the SM1 cortex ipsilateral (CI) or contralateral (CC) of 24 hour post-carrageenin-injected rats (bottom line). The CI is contralateral to the paw without injury.
The number of neurons with RFs is higher in the SM1 cortices of 24 h-carrageenin-injected rats, difference being significant for the CC $0.1 > P > 0.01$, 2 test.

In the 24 h-carrageenin injected rats

In this model of sub-acute inflammatory pain, the proportion of SM1 neurons driven by somatic inputs in the hindpaw cortical area was significantly enhanced, as compared to the normal state (Figure 8) [7, 11]. In fact, although the number of neurons driven by pinch were less numerous than in normal rats, there were significantly more somatosensory neurons as a result of the increase in the number of neurons driven by light touch, and stimulation of the inflamed joints (*see* above) (Figure 8).

This observation in the subacute inflammatory state and the changes in neuronal responsivity observed in the acute phase (Figures 4, 5), suggest that it may be of interest to determine other time points of the cortical re-organization of the somatic inputs over the whole time course of an hyperalgesia.

Since these homeostatic processes occured in 2 models of persistent pain which, in our hands, recovered totally a few weeks later, the possible link between the occurence of homeostatic processes and some characteristics of the pain behaviours, including their recovery may also be questioned.

Finally, whether these phenomena observed for the model of pain concerning the limbs and essentially one or both hindpaws also exist for other body regions is another question.

In rats with ION constriction

In addition to the excess of inputs mentioned above, other observations from the VPM of such rats, seem to reflect major signs of deafferentation, which are likely to be due to the dramatic decrease in large myelinated fibers innervating the vibrissae, as a consequence of the nerve constriction. Indeed, there was a major decrease in the number of neurons driven by vibrissae ($< 5\%$ *versus* 35%), or guard hairs of the muzzle (0 *versus* 20%) [9] in the VPM corresponding to the nerve injury, as compared to the opposite side.

Similarly, from preliminary neuronal recordings in rats with ION constriction, in the cortical area corresponding to the vibrissae pad, major signs of deafferentation have been noted. These changes included a dramatic decrease of responsive neurons to vibrissae stimulation, but no obvious new "responses" to other somatic inputs which could balance the massive lack of vibrissae inputs in this cortical area. This observation greatly contrasts with the data obtained from recordings in the cortical hindpaw representation of rats with a chronic constriction of one sciatic nerve. Further experiments could examine whether this lack of reorganization is limited to the vibrissae pad area, or extends to the other cortical face representation. In any case, the present data suggest that the infraorbital nerve constriction could be more suitable as compared to the sciatic nerve constriction for the study of the deafferentation component of neuropathic pain.

Conclusion

The systematic electrophysiological neuronal recordings of the VB thalamus and of the SM1 cortex in different rat models of clinical pain address, almost exclusively, the sensory discriminative component of pain, and are surely not sufficient to answer the different questions arisen by pain in humans. However, their interest is enhanced by the reproducibility of the data obtained from a consistent number of successive experimental series over 15 years, and the relation between neuronal responses and pain-related, or antinociceptive behaviours observed in unrestrained, awake animals. In fact, many data have emphasized that such studies could represent a useful tool for pharmacological approaches, in particular for the study of analgesic drugs. With these studies it has been possible to detect not only differences, but also similarities, in basic mechanisms involved in either inflammatory or neuropathic pain; in particular there is a major role of the peripheral process in all of these models, which is able to trigger additional central mechanisms. Finally, these studies have pointed out some data apparently more specific to the cortical pain processing, suggesting the interest of further studies of other cortical areas.

References

1. Guilbaud G, Bernard JF, Besson JM. Brain areas involved in nociception and pain. In : Wall PD, Melzack R, eds. *Textbook of pain*, 3rd ed. Edinburgh : Churchill Livingstone, 1994 : 113-28.
2. Besson JM, Guilbaud G. *The arthritic rat as a model of clinical pain* ? Amsterdam : Excerpta Medica, Elsevier, 1988.
3. Besson JM, Guilbaud G. *Lesions of primary afferent fibers as a tool for the study of clinical pain* ? Amsterdam : Excerpta Medica, Elsevier, 1991.
4. Bennett GJ. Animal models of neuropathic pain. In : Gebhart GF, Hammond DL, Jensen TS, eds. *Proceedings of the 7th world congress on pain, progress in pain research and management*, Vol.2. Seattle : IASP Press, 1994 : 495-510.
5. Bennett GJ, Xie YK. A peripheral mononeuropathy in rat that produces disorders of pain sensation like those seen in man. *Pain* 1988 ; 33 : 87-107.
6. Attal N, Jazat F, Kayser V, Guilbaud G. Further evidence for "pain-related" behaviours in a model of unilateral peripheral mononeuropathy. *Pain* 1990 ; 41 : 235-51.
7. Guilbaud G, Benoist JM. Central transmission of somatosensory inputs in the thalamic ventrobasal complex and somatosensory cortex in rat models of clinical pain. In : Boivie J, Hansson P, Lindblom U, eds. *Touch, temperature and pain in health and disease: mechanisms and assessments; progress in pain research and management*, Vol.3. Seattle : IASP Press, 1994 : 339-54.
8. Vos B, Strassman AM, Maciewicz R. Behavioral evidence of trigeminal neuropathic pain following chronic constriction injury to the rat's infraorbital nerve. *J Neurosci* 1994 ; 14 : 2708-23.
9. Vos B, Gautron M, Benoist JM, Guilbaud G. Responses of ventral posteromedial thalamic nucleus neurons after chronic constriction injury to the rat's infraorbital nerve. *Soc Neurosci Abstr* 1994 ; 2 : 1572, 644.1

10. Welker E, Soriano E, Van der Loos H. Plasticity in the barrel cortex of the adult mouse: effects of peripheral deprivation on GAD-immunoreactivity. *Exp Brain Research* 1989 ; 74 : 441-52.
11. Guilbaud G. 15 years of explorations in some supraspinal structures in rat inflammatory pain models. Some informations, but further questions. *APS Journal* 1994 ; 3 : 168-79.
12. Guilbaud G, Kayser V, Attal N, Benoist JM. Evidence for a central contribution to secondary hyperalgesia. In : Willis W, ed. *Hyperalgesia and allodynia: the Bristol-Myers Squibb symposium on pain research* . New York : Raven Press, 1992 : 187-201.
13. Calvino B, Villanueva L, Le Bars D. Dorsal horn (convergent) neurons in the intact anaesthetized arthritic rats. II. Heterotopic inhibitory influences. *Pain* 1987 ; 31 : 359-79.
14. Ferrell WR, Wood L, Baxendale RH. The effect of acute joint inflammation on flexion reflex excitability in the decerebrate, low-spinal cat. *QJ Exp Psychol* 1988 ; 73 : 95-102.
15. Schaible H, Grubb BD. Afferent and spinal mechanisms of joint pain. *Pain* 1993 ; 55 : 5-54.
16. Clark SA, Terry A, Jenkins WM, Merzenich MM. Receptive fields in the body-surface map in adult cortex defined temporally correlated inputs. *Nature* 1988 ; 332 : 444-5.
17. Dykes RW, Lamour Y. An electrophysiological laminar analysis of single somatosensory neurons in partially deafferented rat hindlimb granular cortex subsequent to transection of the sciatic nerve. *Brain Res* 1988 ; 449 : 1-17.
18. Wall JT, Cusick CG. The representation of peripheral nerve inputs in the S-I hindpaw cortex of rats raised with incompletely innervated hindpaws. *J Neurosci* 1986 ; 6 : 1129-47.
19. Vin-Christian K, Benoist JM, Gautron M, Levante A, Guilbaud G. Further evidence for the involvement of SM1 cortical neurons in nociception: modifications of their responsiveness over the early stage of a carrageenin-induced inflammation in the rat. *Somatosens Motor Res* 1992 ; 9 : 245-61.

7

Thalamic anatomy and physiology of pain perception: connectivity, somato-visceral convergence and spatio-temporal dynamics of nociceptive information coding

A.V. APKARIAN

Department of Neurosurgery, SUNY Health Science Center, Syracuse, New York, USA.

Central processing of nociceptive information remains for the most part to be studied. Very little is known about the properties of the neurons involved in this process, especially above the spinal cord. We have been studying the anatomy and physiology of nociceptive inputs to the thalamus for a number of years. Some of this work is reviewed here, emphasizing new ideas and hypotheses that emerge from the data. At the end of the chapter, very preliminary results are described based on a number of new techniques we recently started using to untangle the dynamics of information processing from a temporal viewpoint, *i.e.* taking into consideration information embedded in the serial ordering of spike trains, and a spatial viewpoint, *i.e.* exploring the interactions of nearby neurons. These new approaches should enable answering questions regarding nociceptive, somatic and visceral, information processing at the level of networks of thalamic neurons.

Nociceptive inputs to the thalamus: organization of the dorsal and ventral spinothalamic pathways

The spinothalamic pathway is still assumed to be the major route for nociceptive information access to the cortex, as a result it is also the best studied. Existence of other direct spinal-forebrain and spinal-brainstem-forebrain pathways have recently been demonstrated mainly in the rat (*see* other chapters in the book). We recently established the existence of direct spinostriatal and spinolimbic pathways in the squirrel monkey and the rat [1], in close agreement to the results shown earlier in the rat [2-4]. It should be emphasized that these alternate pathways may provide nociceptive inputs to forebrain sites and these inputs may be critical in at least assessing the affective significance of noxious stimuli. Although the specific contribution of these alternative pathways to pain perception remains to be studied.

It has long been known that axons of projecting spinal cord neurons are widely distributed in the contralateral white matter of the spinal cord. The axons of the spinothalamic tract, although concentrated in the anterolateral spinal cord white matter, have now been shown to contain a portion which extends dorsally into the dorsolateral funiculus [5-8]. This dorsally segregated, lamina I spinothalamic tract has been termed the DSTT, while the remaining ventrally located tract, originating from deeper spinal laminae is termed the VSTT. Retrograde transport studies using HRP or fluorescent dyes, in the cat and the squirrel and macaque monkeys, combined with selective spinal cord white matter lesions show differential effects on labeling of STT cell populations depending on the funicular location of the lesion. It was shown that a dorsolateral funiculus lesion abolishes more than 90% of the spinothalamic cells located in the marginal layer of the spinal cord at all segments below the lesion, leaving the label in the deeper layers intact, and leaving the labeled cells in all layers intact at segments above the lesion [5]. In contrast, when the spinal cord lesion is limited to the ventral quadrant of the white matter, at segments below the lesion, labeled spinothalamic cells are located mainly in the marginal layer of the spinal cord. These studies do not point to the exact position of these two pathways but certainly provide positive and negative results indicating an anatomical segregation along the dorsoventral axis of the spinal cord white matter for axons of marginal layer STT neurons and those of deeper spinal laminae.

Evidence for a dual organization for the spinothalamic projection has existed from early clinical studies in humans. Pain and temperature conducting fibers were known to cross locally within one or two segments of the spinal cord to the anterolateral portion of the contralateral white matter. However, the location of these fibers was seen to shift dorsally at more rostral levels as additional fibers contribute to the tract [9]. Stookey described distinct spinal pathways for temperature and pain conduction since cordotomy results using very small lesions of the lateral spinothalamic tract located just ventral to the dentate ligament and extending to the region lateral to the ventral horn could relieve pain while preserving temperature sensation [10]. His assumption was that temperature sense coursed immediately ventral to this small lesion. It is, however, now clear that cells of the superficial dorsal horn project more dorsally. Foerster and Gagel suggested from their cordotomy results that the fibers transmitting temperature sensibility were preferentially shifted dorsally (spared) following anterolateral lesions [11]. Kuru also demonstrated in humans that, although the location of the STT is mainly within the anterolateral spinal cord white matter, a portion extends to the dorsolateral regions, especially at more rostral spinal levels [12]. Additionally, Kuru extended these observations, pointing out that the dorsal-most fibers were selectively the finest caliber fibers, that they originate from posteromarginal cells, and were primarily nociceptive and thermoceptive in nature. Additionally, the most recent reports of human cordotomy cases have suggested that a DSTT exists in humans, which conveys primarily temperature sensation while pain sensation is conveyed more ventrally [13]. These clinical findings support experimental studies which have shown that lamina I, the primary component of the DSTT, is the main region conveying thermal nociceptive information cephalad [14, 15].

There is considerable evidence from recent animal studies to support the view that the lamina I portion of the contralateral, ascending projection is dorsally segregated. Early studies by McMahon and Wall [16] demonstrated in rat that projecting lamina I neurons were antidromically activated by electrical stimulation within the contralateral dorsolateral funiculus (DLF) while anterolateral stimulation activated neurons in deeper gray matter. A similar dorsal segregation of ascending lamina I fibers was demonstrated in cat by retrograde [17] and anterograde [18] tracing techniques. Further studies in cat and monkey showed that this dorsally segregated lamina I projection extends to the thalamus [5-8, 19, 20]. More recently, Dado *et al.* demonstrated that a DSTT exists in rat when they mapped lowest threshold points for axons of projecting neurons and determined that axons of superficial dorsal horn neurons are preferentially (69%) located in the contralateral DLF [21]. At the most rostral spinal levels, 74% of all projecting axons, from both superficial and deep dorsal horn, had shifted dorsally into the DLF.

Although the results of Craig indicate the existence of lamina I STT axons in the DLF, he concludes that lamina I STT axons are found widely spread in the lateral funiculus, with a main concentration in the lateral funiculus [18]. His emphasis is that these fibers are located neither dorsally nor ventrally, but intermediate to both, just at the level of the dentate ligament, an area where lesions in the cat result in temperature discrimination deficits [22]. We have examined the location of the STT fibers in the cat and squirrel monkey white matter (Figure 1), and their locations in the squirrel monkey generally correspond to that described by Craig in the cat [18]. We found a large discrepancy between the number of labeled cells and the number of axons observed in the white matter, implying that a significant number of the axons were not seen. It was also noted that the dorsally located fibers were of fine caliber approaching the limit of resolution at the level of the light microscope [8]. In another study where the STT cells were labeled retrogradely in combination with white matter lesions impinging just on the lateral funiculus, sparing most of the DLF, the results showed preservation of most of the lamina I STT label below the level of the lesion [6]. Thus, we conclude that the STT axons observed by retrograde or anterograde transport studies are most likely the largest sized STT fibers, and that the portion of DSTT traveling in the more dorsal portions of the DLF are too thin to be adequately labeled and observed by current

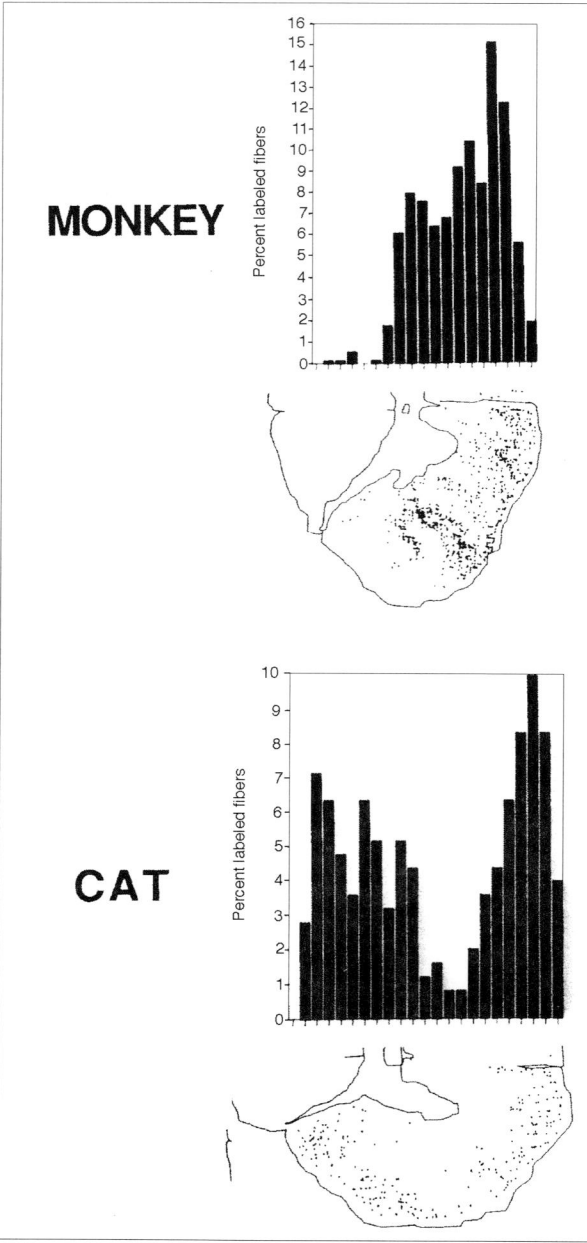

Figure 1. Plots of the locations of spinothalamic fibers, retrogradely labeled with WGA-HRP, from sample spinal cord sections in one cat and one squirrel monkey. The histograms illustrate the percentage of contralaterally labeled spinothalamic fibers in horizontal bins, dorsoventrally. Thalamic injections of WGA-HRP were combined with intraspinal colchicine injections. From [8].

techniques, even though the cell bodies of these cells are properly filled by anterograde tracers injected in the thalamus.

In the lateral thalamus, our physiologic studies (*see* below) strongly imply that the DSTT terminates in the VPI region of the lateral thalamus of the monkey but not in VP proper [23]. On the other hand the VSTT seems to terminate in both VP and VPI in the squirrel monkey. Since the cortical projections of VP (mainly to SI, [24]) are, for the most part, distinct from those of VPI (mainly to SII, [25]), the distinct parallel information flow through the DSTT and VSTT seems, at least partially, preserved up to the cortex. The nociceptive and thermal responsive cells recently described by Craig *et al.* in the posterior part of the ventral medial nucleus (VMpo) of the macaque may be yet another component of the DSTT projecting to the insular cortex [26].

Connectivity between STT terminations and thalamocortical cells

Since STT terminates in VPL, VPI, POa, Pulo, CL and MD and the cortical targets of these thalamic nuclei include SI, SII, posterior parietal cortex, cingulate cortex as well as SMA, these cortical areas are candidate targets to receive STT inputs. So far only the distributions of STT inputs in SI and SII have been studied anatomically. Ralston and his coworkers studied STT terminals anterogradely labeled with HRP within VPL of the cat, rat, and monkey at the electron microscopic level [27]. They showed that the STT terminals synapsed on dendrites of VPL neurons that were regarded thalamocortical since these neurons were not interneurons or GABAergic neurons [28]. In our laboratory, Gingold *et al.* used both anterograde and retrograde tracers to anterogradely label STT terminals from the spinal cord, and retrogradely label thalamocortical cells from SI in the squirrel monkey [24]. Ralston *et al.* [27, 29] and Ma *et al.* [30] have shown that most STT terminations are usually located on dendritic profiles within 100 μm of the soma of thalamic neurons. Therefore, the putative connections between STT terminals and thalamocortical cells were estimated by counting the thalamocortical cells located within 100 um of STT terminals [24]. These overlapped cells were presumed to be capable of receiving STT inputs and hence conveying nociceptive information into SI. This study showed that VPL, VPI and CL contain 90% of the overlapping cells, concluding that these three thalamic nuclei must be the major pathways through which STT nociceptive information is conveyed to SI. The results of the study are consistent with the prediction that SI receives STT inputs [31, 32]. Using a similar method as Gingold *et al.*, Shi *et al.* [33] found that the percentages of the overlapping cells among all thalamocortical cells retrogradely labeled selectively from the superficial layers of SI were almost the same as those percentages shown by Gingold *et al.* in VPL, VPI and CL [24]. This suggests that STT inputs innervate both superficial and deep layers.

In a more recent study, we directly visualized the connectivity of the STT terminals on cortically projecting cells at the light microscopic level. Shi and Apkarian used anterograde and retrograde tracing techniques were combined with intracellular Lucifer yellow (LY) injections in fixed tissue of the squirrel monkey [34]. In this study, BD was used to label STT terminals, LY used to further label SI-projecting cells and a dual immunocytochemical staining method for LY-filled thalamocortical cells and for biotin-dextran labeled STT terminals was applied. It was found that many STT boutons were near the filled SI-projecting cells and their dendrites. The SI-projecting cells with STT contacts were observed in VPL (Figure 2), VPI, CL and anterior PO. This is the first study to show STT terminals contacting the identified SI-projecting thalamic neurons in the primate at the light microscopic level. This finding is consistent with the electron microscopic study by Ralston *et al.*, and further supports the idea that STT inputs are directly relayed to SI not only through VPL but also through VPI, CL and PO [27]. Furthermore, the results of Shi and Apkarian show that the neurons in VPL, VPI and PO had few STT terminal-dendritic contacts, implying that the STT input is highly divergent in these nuclei [34]. The SI-projecting neurons in CL seemed to have more STT contacts than the VPL or VPI neurons, which suggests that CL is an important nucleus in relaying STT inputs to SI.

Physiologically, somatic nociceptive neurons seem to be more dense in the SII, 7b region than in SI (*see* chapter in this book by Dong). This raises the question regarding the sources of nociceptive inputs to SII. An anatomic study by Stevens *et al.* [25], using a 100 μm overlapping technique described by Gingold *et al.* [24], showed that SII is capable of receiving STT inputs, since the SII-projecting cells in VPI, VPL, anterior PO and CL had overlapping STT terminals within 100 μm of their somata. These putative spinothalamocortical pathways to SII are similar but not identical to those to SI. For the projections to SI [24], VPL is the major spinothalamocortical pathway (64% of total overlapped cells), followed by VPI (16%), CL (10%) and PO (3%). Stevens *et al.* showed that the spinothalamocortical inputs to SII are mainly from VPI (36.4%), and anterior PO (20.4%), followed by VPL (18.3%) and CL (11.4%) [25]. Other multisynaptic pathways that may convey nociceptive inputs to SII, for example a serial connection through SI [35], have been suggested. How nociceptive information accesses other cortical areas remains for the most part to be studied (*see* chapter by Craig).

Thalamic physiology

Single unit electrophysiologic experiments done in the thalamus have, for the most part, been limited to existence proof type studies. Neurons responsive to noxious thermal and mechanical stimuli were documented in the lateral and medial thalamus, classified as nociceptive specific (NS) or non-specific (wide dynamic range type, WDR), and their locations relative to nuclear boundaries identified. A large amount of the debate has concentrated on the location of these nociceptive neurons relative to nuclear boundaries, and their incidence within various nuclei. This debate has been confusing mainly because of anatomic differences in the spinothalamic inputs between species: rat, cat, monkey. The more recent studies indicate that the locations and incidences of thalamic nociceptive neurons correspond to the anatomic differences in STT inputs between species. In this section our physiologic findings and the recent studies by others are briefly reviewed.

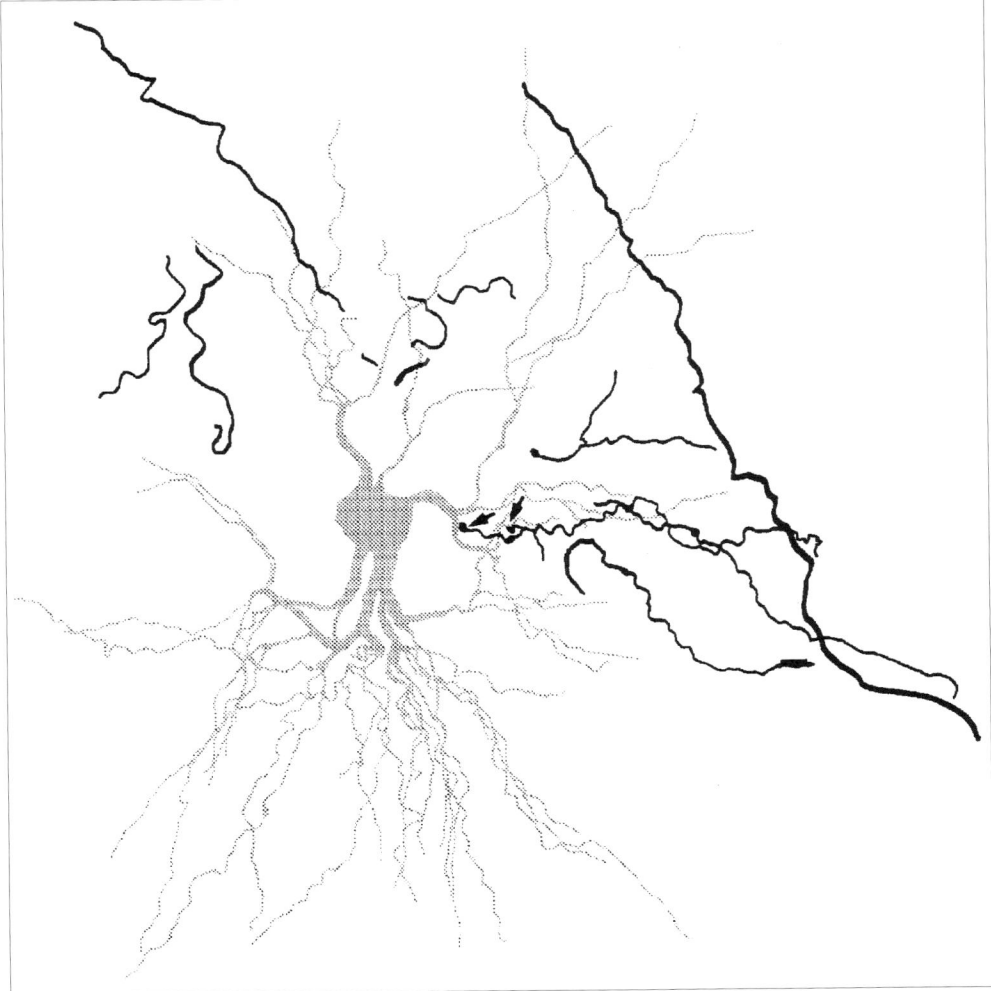

Figure 2. Drawing of an SI-projecting VPL neuron and spinothalamic terminals contacting the cell. Arrows point to contacts between the dendrites and the boutons. Scale bar = 20 μm. The cell was labeled retrogradely, and then injected intracellularly. The spinothalamic terminations were labeled anterogradely. From [34].

Somatic inputs

In the monkey lateral thalamus, VPL, VPI and PO are the primary nuclei to receive STT inputs. Correspondingly, these nuclei should contain nociceptive neurons. Indeed our single unit electrophysiologic studies in chloralose-nembutal anesthetized squirrel monkeys indicate functionally segregated representations of nociceptive inputs in the lateral thalamus [23]. Nociceptive neurons located in VPL and VPM (together termed VP) seem to be distinct from those located in VPI and PO. The incidence of different types of cells in these nuclei was approximately based on an objective sampling approach, *i.e.* every unit that could be isolated was tested systematically for nociceptive responses by mechanical stimuli. Nociceptive neurons in VP were mainly of WDR type. Nineteen of 203 neurons tested were nociceptive (10% of VP cells), all but two were of WDR type (90% of the nociceptive cells in VP). The incidence of nociceptive cells in VPI was higher than in VP. Twenty-three of 46 neurons tested responded to noxious stimuli (50% of VPI cells). Moreover, NS type neurons were found mainly in VPI, where 10 of all 14 NS cells recorded were located (10 of 23 nociceptive cells were NS type, 43%, in VPI). The incidence of nociceptive cells (8 of 21, 38%) and of NS cells (2 of 8) were both intermediate in PO as compared to VP and VPI. In this study, the electrodes were directed to the forelimb portion of VP; as a result, only a few electrode tracts were in VPM, passing through its lateral portion. Bushnell *et al.* reported the distribution of nociceptive and thermoceptive cells in the VPM of the awake macaque monkey [36].

In our study most cells determined to be nociceptive by mechanical stimulation were also tested for responses to thermal stimuli. Twenty-three of 40 cells (58%) with nociceptive responses to mechanical stimulation responded to noxious heating of their receptive fields, and 9 of 23 cells (39%) responded to noxious cooling. Seven WDR type and 2 NS type cells responded to both noxious heating and noxious cooling. One neuron in VPI responded to thermal but not to mechanical noxious stimuli. The thermal nociceptive neurons were evenly distributed between VP, VPI and PO. In VP, 6 of 17 cells (35% of mechanical WDR cells) were responsive to noxious heat, and 3 (18%) were responsive to both heating and cooling. In VPI, of 18 cells tested for thermal inputs, four WDR and two NS type units were heat responsive (altogether 33%), and three WDR and two NS (28%) were responsive to both heating and cooling. In PO, five cells were tested, three WDR cells (60%) were heat responsive, and one WDR cell (20%) responded to both heating and cooling.

The receptive field locations and sizes were determined for all units studied. Within VPL, the WDR type cells seemed randomly scattered between LT type cells. The receptive fields and locations of these WDR cells were similar and in continuity with the neighboring LT cells. As the recording electrodes traversed more ventrally into VPI the receptive field sizes and the incidence of nociceptive responses increased. Figure 3 shows one recording track where the electrodes travel through VPL and enter VPI; the responses of every unit that could be isolated is indicated. A few electrode tracks

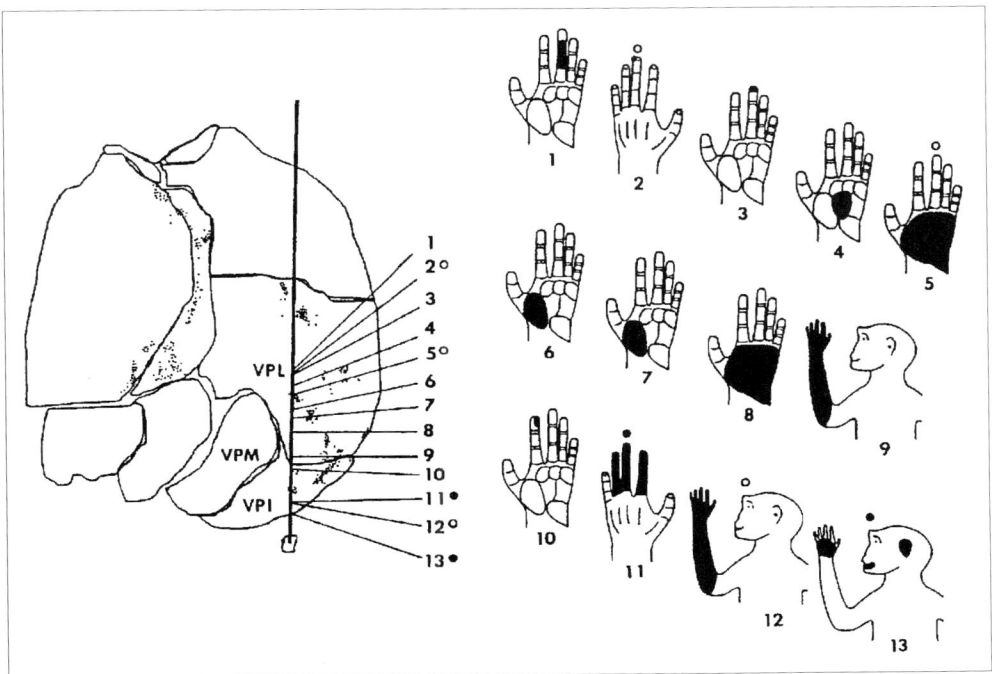

Figure 3. An electrode track passing through VPL and VPI. Thirteen units were isolated. Their receptive fields and response types are indicated. Three units were WDR type (open circles), two were nociceptive specific (solid circles), and the remainder did not respond to noxious stimuli. Spinothalamic terminal regions are shown with blak dots. Taken from [23].

traversed through the anterior portion of PO. The sequence of changes in receptive field locations indicated the presence of multiple body maps in PO.

The recording sites and receptive fields of 48 neurons were studied in VPI. Figure 4 shows the locations, response properties and receptive fields of these cells. Mediolaterally, the receptive fields are located on the face medially, on the hand and arm more laterally, and on the leg and foot even more laterally, mimicking the somatotopy of VP. However, the receptive fields often jump from one body part to another as the electrode moves from VP to VPI. Also more ventrally in VPI there seem to be a tendency for the receptive fields to include larger body regions. This somatotopy and the incidence of nociceptive responses in the squirrel monkey VPI closely agree with the results obtained by Vahle-Hinz et al. in the cat VPI [37]. In contrast to this similarity between the two species, there seems to be no nociceptive responsive neurons in the cat VP [7, 38], while 10% of the squirrel monkey VP cells were nociceptive.

The spinal cord of these squirrel monkeys were injected with the anterograde tracer WGA-HRP, a week prior to the recordings. The tissue was processed after the recording sessions and the relationship between recording sites and labeled spinothalamic

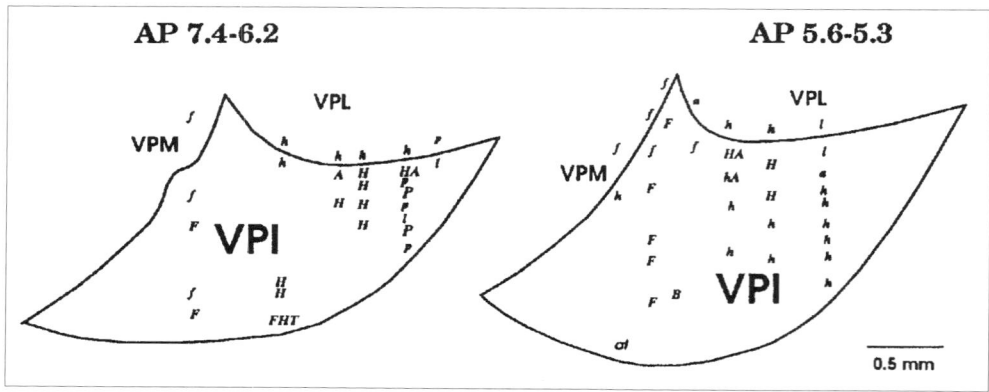

Figure 4. Organization of somatic representation within VPI. Body areas where the somatic receptive fields of the isolated units are indicated. All receptive fields were contralateral to the recordings. Receptive fields on the face are indicated as f, F; on the hand as h, H; on the arm as a, A; on the trunk as t, T; on the leg as l; and on the foot as p, P; on the half of the body as B. Upper case corresponds to cells with nociceptive inputs from the indicated body parts, while lower case corresponds to cells with low threshold type responses. Taken from [23].

terminations determined by counting the number of recording sites that were within (overlapping), or outside (non-overlapping), 100 µm of the spinothalamic terminals. Since the tracer was injected in the cervical enlargement, this relationship was determined only for cells with receptive fields that included proximal forelimb dermatomes. Only 20-26% of the LT cells in VPL and VPI were classified as overlapping. Nociceptive cells in VPL had a similar distribution. However, nociceptive cells in VPI were in closer proximity to STT terminals; 8 of 11 were classified as overlapping.

Overall, these results indicate that the organization of VPI is distinct from VP in the incidence of nociceptive cells, in its somatotopy, and the relationship of its cells to spinothalamic terminals. Given the strong connectivity of VPI to SII, these results also imply that SII should have NS and WDR type cells, while SI should have mostly WDR type nociceptive cells (*see* the chapter by Dong regarding nociceptive response differences between cortical cells). In this study we did not encounter an area resembling the properties described for VMpo by Craig *et al.* [26], and we remain uncertain of the location of such a region in the squirrel monkey.

Nociceptive inputs to the lateral thalamus has been studied in the past by a number of groups. However, to our knowledge this is the first systematic study of nociceptive inputs to the monkey VPI. Nociceptive neurons were observed in the squirrel monkey and macaque VP [39-43]. In both species most of these neurons were characterized as WDR type, although a small number of NS type cells were also found. Given our results in the squirrel monkey VPI, Chung *et al.* [39] reviewed the recording sites in their macaque study and concluded that none of the sites where NS type cells were found were in VPI. He also concluded that they seldom, if ever, have recorded from neurons in the macaque VPI. Thus, the incidence of NS type cells reported in the macaque (14% in Chung et al. [39]) must be compared to the incidence of NS type cells in VP of the squirrel monkey (2 of 19, 10% in our study), and they closely match. However, the properties of VPI cells in the macaque remain to be studied. The earlier studies of nociceptive cells in the squirrel monkey were conducted in awake animals [41-43]. It should be noted that the incidence of nociceptive cells in those studies was very similar to our results, done in anaesthetized animals. Thus, the anaesthesia used does not seem to effect the probability of encountering nociceptive cells. Morrow and Casey also found a few NS type cells [43], but, lacking accurate histologic verification, they were unable to accurately determine whether these were located in VPI, VPL, or on the border between VP and VPI. Thus, the overall incidence and properties of nociceptive cells seem to closely agree between the species and the conditions used for cells located primarily in VPL. There may be differences in location and response properties of nociceptive cells in VPM as compared to VPL; for details see the chapter by Bushnell in this book.

Visceral inputs

In a second group of squirrel monkeys the same lateral thalamic region was examined for responses to distention of various visceral organs [44]. To our surprise, yet in agreement with recent similar studies in the rat [45], we discovered that the lateral somatosensory region of the monkey thalamus receives a massive visceral input. The response properties of 106 lateral thalamic neurons were tested, 90 (85%) of these cells responded to distention of the urinary bladder, the distal colon, and/or the lower esophagus. The large majority of these visceroceptive cells also had convergent somatic and multivisceral responses (71% of the 85%). A small population (6%) was visceral specific, *i.e.* a somatic receptive fields were not found for these neurons. Most of the visceroceptive neurons were located in VPL (62 neurons), due to the search strategy. Visceroceptive cells were also found in: VPM, VPI, Zi, PO, R, Pulo, and VL. No segregation between neurons with inputs from the esophagus and the pelvic organs was observed. Also no segregation was observed between neurons characterized as visceral specific, somatovisceral, or pure somatic.

Neuronal responses to visceral stimulation were excitatory, inhibitory, mixed and non-responsive. The incidence of the response direction in relation to the three viscera tested was statistically highly significantly different from the expected random combination. The most common response was inhibition from the esophagus distention (91% were esophagus responsive, and 44 of 80 cells were inhibited by esophagus stimulation). Bladder and colon distention were less effective stimuli (51-56% responded). Excitatory responses were seen from all three viscera (13-25%) with no significant differences between the organs. The incidence of responses were significantly dependent on the organ distended. Based on visceral distention response thresholds and ability to respond to innocuous and noxious visceral pressures, the visceroceptive cells were classified as visceral WDR type, NS type, and LT type. Most were either visceral NS type (65%) or visceral WDR type (34%). The relative incidence of these two types of visceral responses was statistically highly significantly dependent on the organ distended. Most units were able to code visceral distention duration and intensity.

The inter-relation between various inputs for cells with multivisceral responses are shown in one recording track in Figure 5. The somatic and visceral convergence were classified as proper or improper according to the known spinal afferent input organization. This was necessary because a large number of the neurons had an unexpectedly high degree of convergence from viscera that do not follow the expected spinal cord convergence. In the track shown in Figure 5, units 5, 6, 12, 17, and 20 (5 of 11, 45%) had improper viscerovisceral convergences. With bladder stimulation, units 11, 12, 16, 17, and 18 had improper somatovisceral interactions (26%), while, for esophagus stimulation, units 10, 12, 13, 14 and 17 had improper somatovisceral interactions (55%). With a variety of other types of analysis, all indicated that generally the somatic receptive fields have no predictive value as to the visceral inputs that a given neuron receives. Similarly, inputs from one visceral organ could not predict the inputs and the direction of effect that another visceral organ stimulation might induce. Therefore, there seems to be an overall lack of visceral topography on thalamic neurons that have a highly organized somatotopy. We do not mean to imply that this organization is totally random. Clearly a number of parameters of the visceral inputs to the lateral thalamus are highly ordered as evidenced by the statistical dependence of these parameters on the organs stimulated. Moreover, this region seems to be specific for processing noxious but not innocuous visceral stimuli.

The high incidence of visceral responsive cells, when only three organs were tested, strongly implies that all neurons in the region respond to visceral stimuli, given the variety of visceral organs that were not tested. Therefore, the lateral thalamic somatosensory regions cannot be regarded as regions involved in processing solely somatosensory information, but rather multiplexing somatosensory and visceral information. Thus, it is more appropriate to label these areas as somato-visceral.

The distinct organization of the somatic and visceral inputs on these cells provides a mechanism by which the neuronal responses in the region can distinguish between visceral and somatic inputs. We have proposed that this distinction comes about by activating either a local homogeneous group of cells giving rise to somatic percepts, or activating a large distributed population of cells by excitation and inhibition which becomes associated with visceral, most likely nociceptive, percepts [46]. Moreover changes in these coding mechanisms may underlie the phenomenon of referred pain (for details see Apkarian *et al.* [47]). Chandler *et al.* studied visceral representation in the lateral thalamus of the macaque [48]. Unfortunately their study had a strong sampling bias: mainly thalamic cells with somatic nociceptive inputs were studied, resulting in conclusions seemingly contradictory to our results. We have explored visceral representation in two macaque monkeys, and observed little differences between macaques and squirrel monkeys in the organization of somatovisceral responsive cells in and around VP. Berkley *et al.* studied reproductive organ representation in the lateral

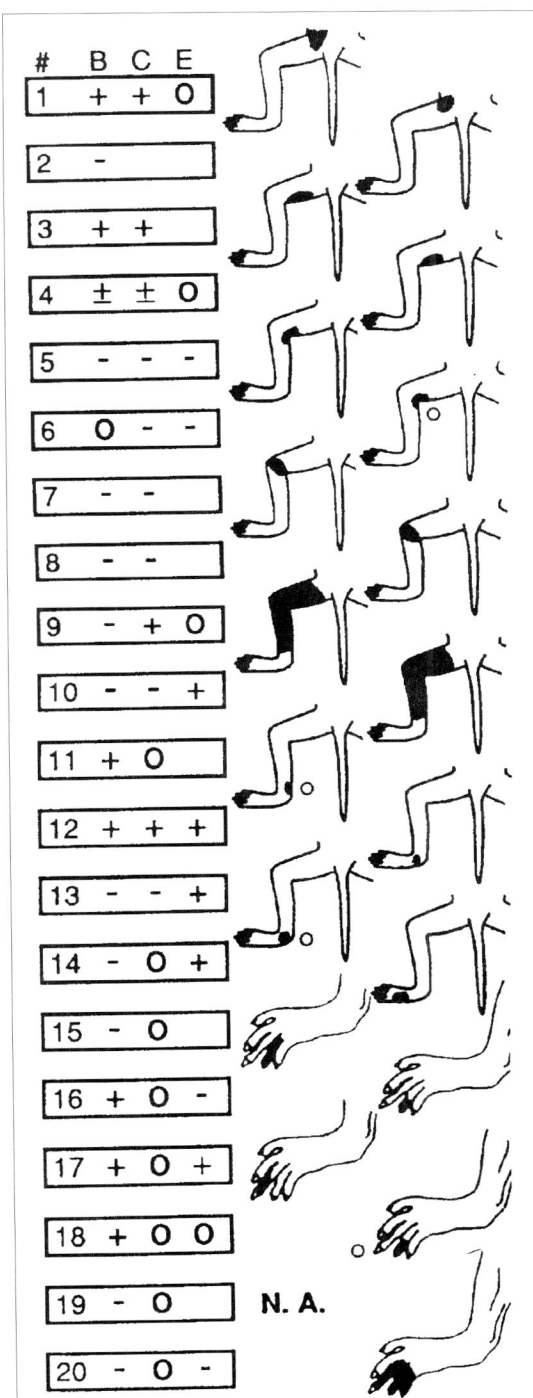

Figure 5. Viscero-somatic convergence in VPL. Somatic and visceral responses are shown for 20 neurons isolated in one track, the electrode traveling dorsoventrally through VPL. Somatic receptive fields are shown. Open circles next to the receptive fields indicate somatic nociceptive WDR type responses. Responses to bladder (B), colon (C), or esophagus (E) distentions are indicated by 0 = no response, + = excitation, - = inhibition, +/- = mixed responses. The combinations of interactions observed seem unpredictable. Taken from [44 ou 50 ?].

thalamus of the rat, and found an organization very similar to that seen in the squirrel monkey [45].

Akin to the species differences in somatic nociceptive inputs to the lateral thalamus, there seem to be important differences in visceral inputs between the monkey and the cat. In experiments performed in Dr. Kniffki's laboratory, visceral responsive cells have not been observed in the core of VP in the cat [49-51]. Most visceral responsive cells were found in areas surrounding the cat VP, in VPLvp, VPMvp, PO, ZI, and LP [51]. In this study visceral responsive cells were also found in a number of medial and intralaminar thalamic regions, such as MD, VMP, CL, CM, and PAC. Eight of 30 neurons studied responded to multiple viscera and 21 of 36 neurons tested responded to stimulation of visceral organs of the upper body (visceral organs tested were: esophagus, urinary bladder, colon, and baro- and chemoreceptors). The cells in MD were the only ones showing a certain somato-visceral organization, since most had inputs from baro- and chemoreceptors. Importantly, all cells but one with visceral inputs had nociceptive specific convergent input from small well-defined portions of the surface of the body. Interestingly, there was no significant difference between the extent of viscero-visceral convergence or the somatic receptive field sizes and somatic response properties between visceral responsive neurons found in the lateral as compared to the medial thalamic areas. There are no modern studies of visceral representation in the medial thalamus of the monkey, and species differences between cat and monkey are very significant in the lateral thalamus. Therefore, the studies in the cat medial thalamus do not clarify the organization of visceral inputs to the same region in the monkey.

We have also explored visceral representation in the primary somatosensory cortex (SI), an area receiving its main afferent inputs from VP, and have found that over 30% of the cells in the region have convergent visceral inputs over their known somatic responses [52]. Similar to the lateral thalamic cells, all these SI visceroceptive cells responded to visceral pressures in the noxious range. However, most responses were elicited only for the noxious pressures implying that most SI visceroceptive cells were of visceral nociceptive specific type. The incidence and the consistency of the visceral responses were highly dependent on depth of anaesthesia. These results confirm the notion that the VP-SI network is involved in processing both somatic and visceral information.

The thalamic studies in the squirrel monkey had hinted that some of the visceral inputs may play a modulatory role on somatic responses. Consequently, we investigated the interactions of the somatic and visceral inputs in halothane anaesthetized squirrel monkeys. In a third of the investigated VPL neurons, conditioning of responses to innocuous and noxious somatic stimuli with visceral stimuli (urinary bladder, colon, or esophagus distension) modulated the somatic responses. Altough the dominant interaction was an inhibition of the somatic responses, mixed excitatory/inhibitory and pure excitatory effects were also observed. In a subgroup of the neurons, visceral inputs were only revealed by conditioning, because visceral stimulation alone had no effect on the ongoing activity of these neurons. The results show strong modulatory effects of visceral stimulation on somatic responses. Because the visceral modulation is dominantly inhibitory on somatic responses, these effects enhance the processing of visceral information by the VPL neurons [51].

These results question whether there are any regions in the thalamus or cortex that process purely somatic information. Conversely, we surmise that thalamic and cortical regions thought to be involved in pure visceroception most likely also receive convergent somatic inputs. The type and relationship of the somatic convergence onto the visceral representations remain to be explored.

Temporal coding of somatic dimensions by thalamic WDR type cells

The exponential growth in computing power of the personal computer (PC) has enabled the physiologist to ask questions that, a few years ago, we could not imagine undertaking. Suddenly the price of computing is reduced to the development of the algorithms, since computing time is now equivalent to the price of electricity. Here we describe a series of computations where the algorithms themselves are simple, but the calculations are of the n^2 type. The calculations are achieved by dedicating our laboratory PC-s to run different parallel versions of the same programs overnight. With such an approach, we can perform exhaustive studies of a large list of statistical properties of spike trains within a few weeks. Differences in the temporal sequences of WDR type cells found in VPL and VPI are studied with these methods.

The definition of WDR type cells rests on their ability to increase their response rate to increasing intensity stimulation. We arbitrarily define them by requiring a statistically significant change in the mean firing rate (t-test with $p<0.05$), and at least 30% increase in the firing rate between brush, touch or pressure stimulus responses and the response to noxious thermal or mechanical stimulation. Implicit in the definition of WDR type cells, is their ability to discriminate among somatosensory dimensions, *i.e.* discriminate among different receptor types and thus participate in the perceptual distinctions associated with these distinct receptors. However, it has been repeatedly shown that the firing rate increase is not sufficient to distinguish among somatosensory dimensions, since vigorous brushing or touching of the receptive field of a WDR type neuron can increase the mean firing rate above and beyond that observed by noxious stimuli. We examine the ability of such cells in distinguishing between somatosensory dimensions using a temporal code that may be independent of the mean firing rate. The notion of temporal coding dates at least to the 1960-s, but it has not been seriously explored until very recently primarily because adequate tests for such coding mechanisms tend to be computationally very costly.

The WDR type neurons studied here are those isolated in the squirrel monkey study by Apkarian and Shi [23]. The response patterns of nine WDR type neurons located in VPI are compared to 11 WDR type neurons found in VPL, for somatic mechanical stimuli of increasing intensity. Standard parameters that were compared for the spike intervals between the two WDR populations under 4 conditions (spontaneous activity, and responses to brush, pressure and pinch) were mean rate, variance, interspike interval histograms (ISIH), and autocorrelation. By definition, the mean rate increased with the increasing intensity stimulation and, concomitantly, the variance decreased. The ISI histograms usually were multipeaked distributions, becoming more Poisson-like for the responses to pinch. The ratio of the variance to the mean (Fano coefficient, or coefficient of dispersion) was measured for all the data. For a Poisson process, this ratio should be 1.0. Statistical comparison showed highly significant difference between VPL and VPI WDR cells and a significant difference for different stimulus modalities, suggesting that the two types of WDR neurons can be differentiated by their extent of similarity, or dissimilarity, to a Poisson process. In both groups the spontaneous activity was closest to Poisson. Other measures of information content in the serial order of the spike trains included algorithmic complexity [34, 53, 54], second moment entropy in one dimensional embedding [53], pressing effect and pressing entropy [34]. All these metrics calculate the extent of information contained in the serial order of spike trains. These measures are compared to those obtained for corresponding null distributions, namely the shuffled spike interval train which should have a random ordering but possess the same mean, variance and ISIH. All these measures indicated, to different amounts, dependence on the location of the WDR cell (VPL *vs* VPI) and dependence on stimulus type (for details *see* Shi *et al.* [55]).

A simple but computationally costly method was the count of repeated patterns. For every spike train, every neighbor pair interval was taken as a template, compared to all neighbor intervals in the train, and the matches counted. The same was done for higher orders of intervals, up to 9 intervals. For the current data set, where the spike trains are collected over about 10 s, the majority of repeated intervals were of length less than 5 intervals. Null surrogate data was generated by again shuffling the intervals in each train and counting the repeated patterns in the null data. By repeating the shuffling 10 times for each interval, a mean and standard deviation of repeated counts could be calculated for the null data, providing a distance measure with which the original unshuffled repeat pattern counts could be tested. Figure 6 shows the repeat pattern counts for 2 intervals in the original spike trains *versus* the shuffled spike trains. Points along the diagonal indicate equality of repeated measures between the original and shuffled spike trains. Points above the diagonal indicate a larger number of repetitions in the original spike trains, as compared to the shuffled, while points below the diagonal indicate the patterns that should have been observed in the random distribution but are actually suppressed in the original spike trains. The figure shows that most spike trains of VPI WDR cells are found above the diagonal and those from VPL WDR cells below the diagonal. Figure 7 shows the pattern repetition distance metric (t-value) for the spike trains studied, when 4 interval repetitions are examined. The graph indicates that this distance decreases for VPI WDR type cells and increases for VPL WDR type cells, with increasing intensity stimulation (for details *see* Shi *et al.* [55]). Thus, not only are the temporal patterns different between WDR cells located in VPL *versus* VPI, but the kind of change in this temporal pattern is also different for their respective responses to innocuous and noxious mechanical stimuli. Currently these studies are proceeding in two directions. On the one hand we have begun identification and cataloguing of the significantly repeated patterns, and using these patterns to search their incidence throughout the data set and in other spike trains collected from the squirrel monkey lateral thalamus. The other work attempts to build computational models in search of mechanisms that can transform temporal patterns in spike trains of individual neurons into spatial activation patterns of populations of neurons, at the next level of processing.

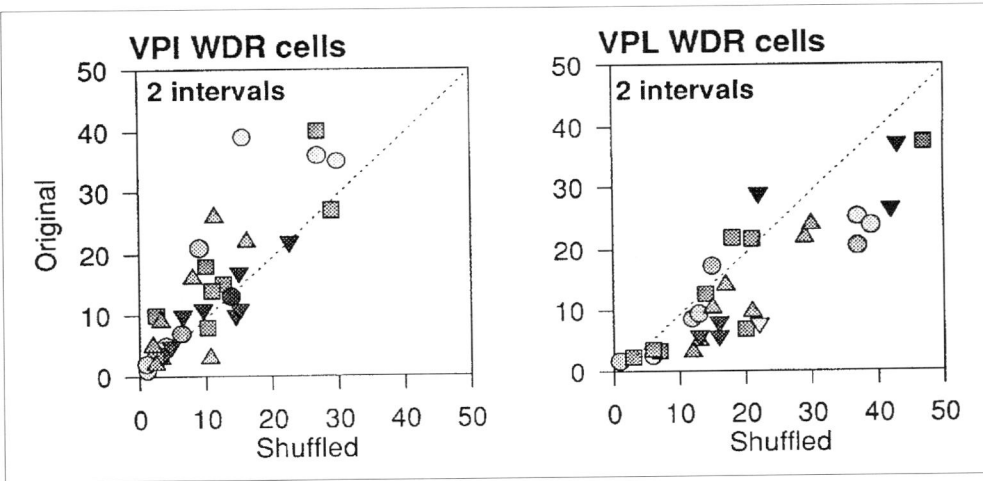

Figure 6. Two interval repeat patterns calculated in the original spike trains and in the trains following shuffling of the spike intervals. Points located above the 45° line indicate an excess of repeat patterns from that expected from the shuffled data, while those below the line indicate a decrease (suppression) of repeat patterns in the original train as compared to the shuffled train. Circles correspond to spike trains of spontaneous activity, squares to trains during brushing, upward triangles during pressure, downward triangle during pinching the receptive field of the unit. Note that for WDR cells in VPI, most points are above the diagonal, while for WDR cells in VPL, most points are below the diagonal.

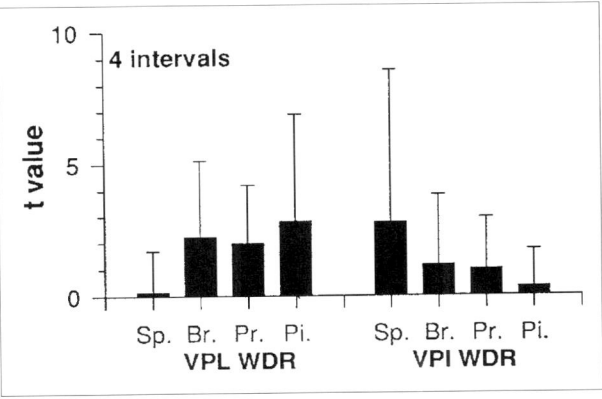

Figure 7. Differences in incidence of four interval repeat patterns between VPI and VPL WDR type cells, and between spontaneous activity (Sp.), and responses to brushing (Br.), pressure (Pr.) and pinch (Pi.). The mean and standard deviations of the t-values are calculated from the difference between the number of 4 interval repeats found in the original spike train subtracted from the mean repeats found in the 20 shuffled trains, and divided by the standard deviation of the repeats in the shuffled trains.

Spatial population dynamics for lateral thalamic neuronal nets

The first approach used to decode the relationships for populations of neurons in the lateral thalamus is a single electrode crosscorrelational study between an isolated unit and the rest of the neuronal activity recorded on the same electrode. The basic assumption is that activity below the well isolated unit, and above the instrumental noise, represents the summed activity of many nearby neurons. This so-called background noise activity and its relationship to the isolated neuron's activity would reveal properties shared between a small population of cells (estimated in the order of 10-15 neighbors), under different stimulus conditions.

Figures 8-10 illustrate the approach. The VPL neuron isolated was classified as somatic LT (LTs) type because its response to squeezing the somatic receptive field was much lower than to brushing, and visceral WDR (WDRv) type, because its activity increased with urinary bladder distention up to 60 mm Hg. During spontaneous activity (Figure 8), the neuron's autocorrelation, panel (LTs+WDRv)X(LTs+WDRv), shows that its mean rate is very low and it fires with preferred intervals. The autocorrelation of the background noise, panel NoiseXNoise, is flat, consistent with the assumption that it is noise. The crosscorrelation between the neuron and the noise, panel (LTs+WDRv)XNoise, shows a very early peak (< 10 ms), and many later peaks. The early peak is interpreted as evidence for co-activation of the neuron and the noise, and

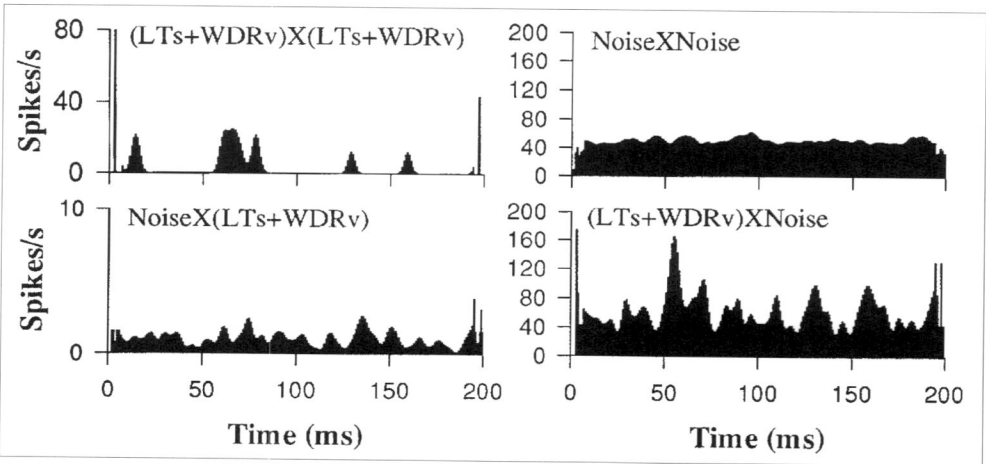

Figure 8. The interaction between a single neuron and the activity of its neighbors as monitored by the background activity on the same electrode. Auto- and cross-correlations of a neuron classified as somatic low threshold (LTs), and visceral wide dynamic range type (WDRv) based on its responses to bladder distention. The auto-correlations are indicated as (LTs+WDRv)X(LTs+WDRv) and NoiseXNoise, for the neuron and the background noise, respectively. The cross-correlations are shown in positive time only, and indicated as NoiseX(LTs+WDRv) for the effects of noise on the neuron, and as (LTs+WDRv)XNoise for the effects of the neuron on the noise.

the later peaks are contributing to thalamocortical-corticothalamic recurrent activity. During pinching of the somatic receptive field (Figure 9), the autocorrelation of the neuron is more uniform, and the mean rate of the noise has dramatically increased above that seen during spontaneous activity. The crosscorrelation shows a large prolonged early peak but the later peaks are reduced in size from the spontaneous activity case. Thus, during pinching, the neuron's activity pattern is changed, the background noise activity is increased, and the common activation between the background and the neuron is increased. Figure 10 shows the responses at the same recording site during bladder distension. The neurons autocorrelation is again changed, and shows preferred activity at very short intervals. The autocorrelation of the noise also shows preferred activity for short intervals, and a large decrease in the mean activity, as compared to spontaneous activity or to pinch. The crosscorrelations in both directions indicate a lack of early correlations, implying a decoupling between the isolated neuron and the background activity. These results agree with the hypothesis that the same neural networks are involved in coding for somatic and visceral inputs. However, the processing of somatic information is done by co-activating a local population of cells, while visceral inputs defractionate this population's coupling and, instead, activates a distributed group of cells widely separated from each other.

Another approach to studying population dynamics is to actually investigate the responses of many neurons located close to each other. We have started simultaneous recordings from four tungsten electrodes, with the tips located around 100 μm from each other. By using the Datawave data collection system, neuronal activity is collected on all four channels simultaneously. Whenever activity on any channel crosses its window discriminator, activity over a 1.5 ms period (0.5 ms prior to and 1.0 ms post trigger) are collected over all four channels at a 20,000 Hz sampling rate *per* channel.

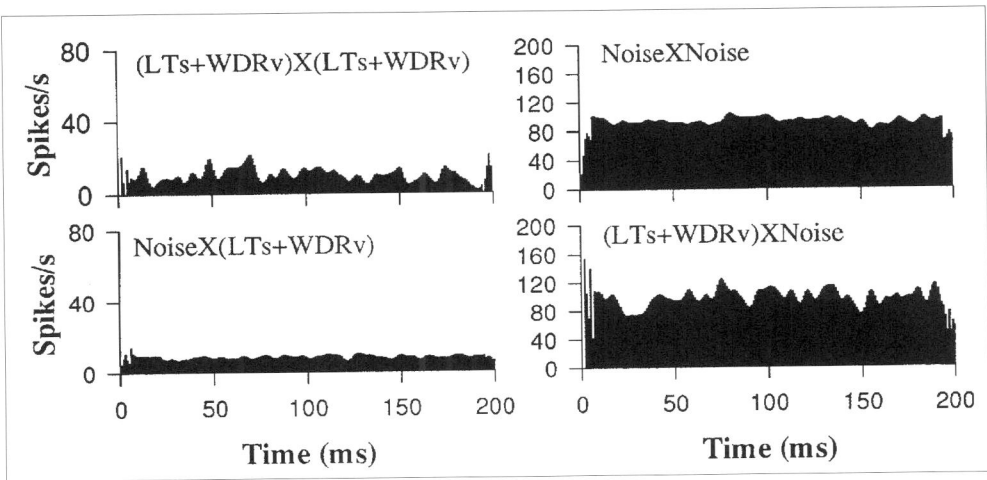

Figure 9. The interaction of the same neuron as in Figure 8 with the background activity during noxious squeezing of the somatic receptive field.

An off-line clustering method, where the size of the events captured over all channels are compared, results in identifying individual neurons (*see* [56]). With this technique, 5-10 individual neurons can be isolated *per* recording site. Once the neurons are identified, the mean amplitude of the action potential of each neuron is known at each tip. Given the electrode geometry, it is possible to uniquely calculate the exact position of each neuron from the four tips. Figure 11 shows the locations of eight neurons isolated at a single recording site in the squirrel monkey VPL. At this recording site the dominant activity was from a WDR type cell (unit 2). Somatic innocuous and noxious stimuli were applied within the somatic receptive field of this WDRs type cell. The responses of this neuron were monitored on-line and ascertained to the adequacy of the stimulus location on the skin. Off-line clustering then showed that 5 of the 8 neighbor neurons responded to the same innocuous and noxious thermal and mechanical stimuli, suggesting that nociceptive neuron in the lateral thalamus exist in bunches (Brüggemann *et al.* 1995 Neurosci Abst). The main advantage of this approach is the elimination of sampling bias that is inherent to single unit recordings. It seems that the mean distances between the identified cells approximate the mean separation of cells in the squirrel monkey VPL. Thus, very likely, we are recording from most if not all neurons in a 150 µm^3 box. Figure 12 indicates this network's effective connectivity, calculated from the strength of the crosscorrelations within 20 ms, and the mean firing rate of each neuron during spontaneous activity. Figure 13 shows the same network during squeezing the receptive field of neuron 2. There are both connectivity and firing rate changes, although the two are not obviously related to each other. The connectivity maps also indicate that nearby connections tend to be excitatory and connections at longer distances are more likely to be inhibitory. Interestingly, although the overall connection strengths increased during pinch as compared to spontaneous activity, the relative contribution of inhibitory connections increases as well.

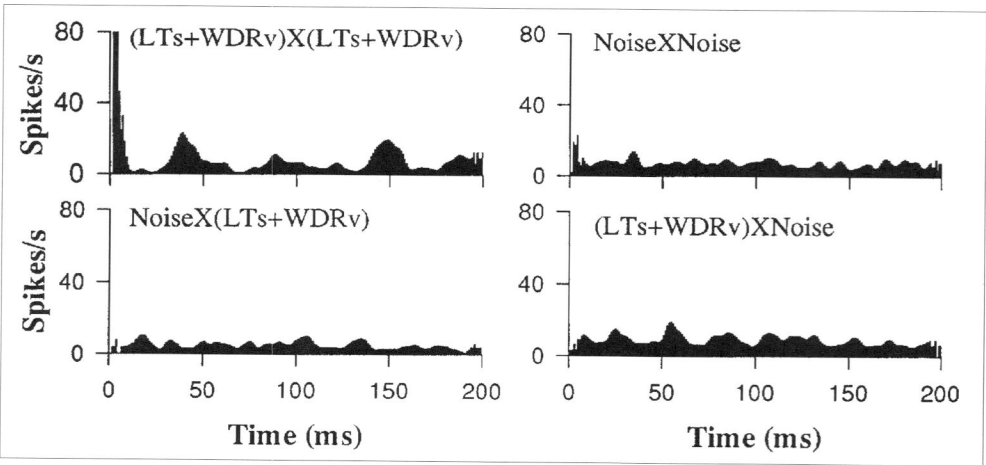

Figure 10. The interaction of the same neuron as in Figure 8 with the background activity during bladder inflation.

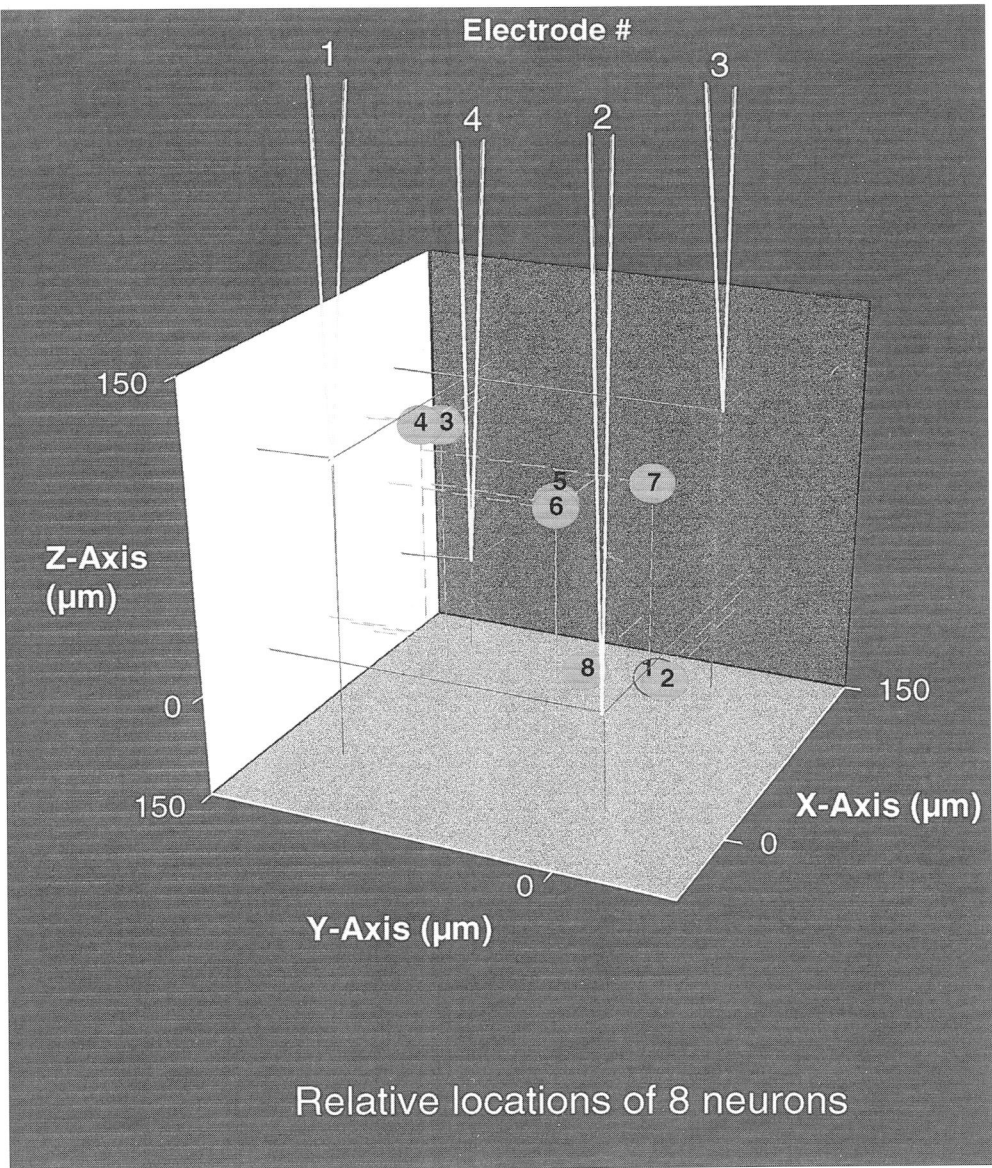

Figure 11. The locations of 8 neurons are shown relative to four Tungsten electrode tips, recorded in the VPL of the squirrel monkey. The receptive field and response properties were properly determined only for unit 2, which was somatic WDR type. However, many others also responded to the same stimuli. (See appendix for colour figures.)

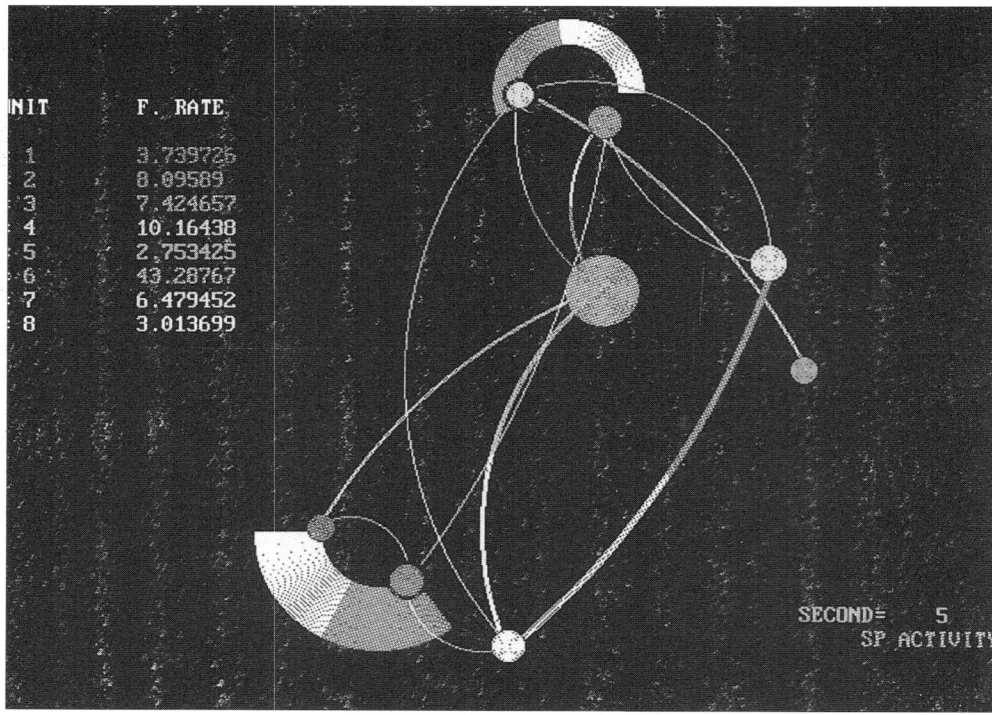

Figure 12. The connectivity and mean firing rate of the 8 neurons in Figure 11 are shown during spontaneous activity. The positions of the neurons are shown on the Z-X plane. The size of each neuron indicates its mean firing rate. The firing rates in spikes are displayed in the inset. The connectivity of the network is based on calculating the cross-correlations between the neurons. The thickness of the connection indicates connection strength. Connections ending in red are excitatory, in green are inhibitory. Direction of connectivity is from white to either red or green. (See appendix for colour figures.)

It should be emphasized that these are very preliminary results, and their interpretation relies on analyzing multiple such networks and comparing them under different stimulus conditions. However, given the present level of knowledge regarding the thalamic local and long distance connectivity, understanding the dynamics of information coding both in the spatial and temporal domains of the local neuron networks should enable the building of fairly constrained computational models of somatic and visceral information coding in the lateral thalamus. We, therefore, foresee that, in the next few years, much more realistic models of dynamical information coding systems should emerge, specifically for lateral thalamic networks.

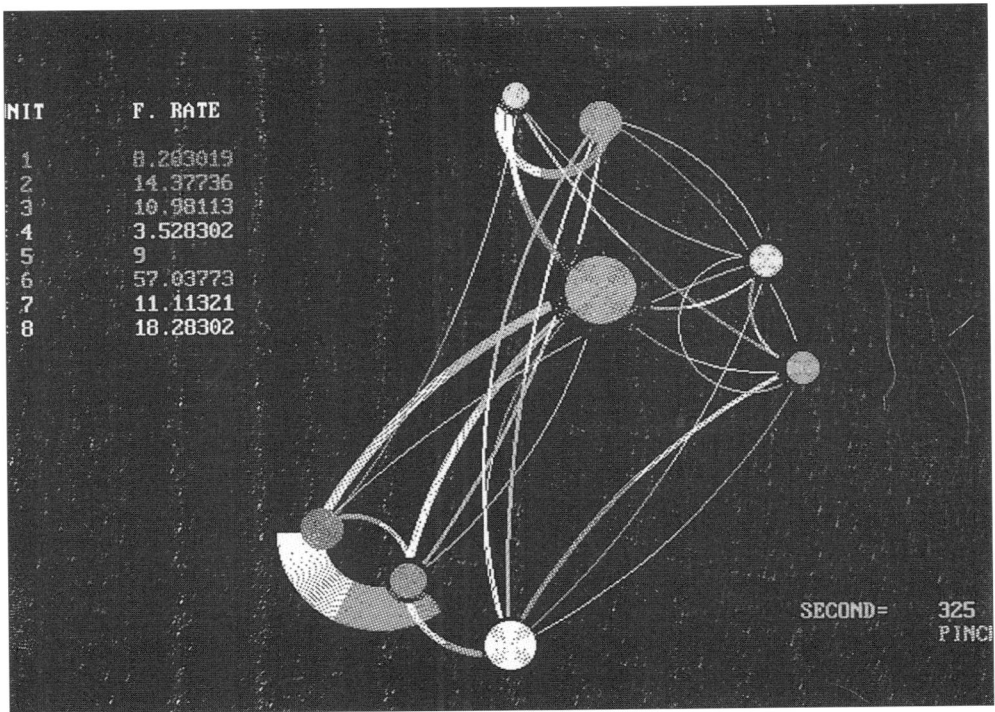

Figure 13. The connectivity and mean firing rate of the 8 neurons in Figure 11 are shown during pinching within the receptive field of unit 2. (See appendix for colour figures.)

Acknowledgments

The author thanks all the colleagues and students that have contributed to the work mentioned above. Special thanks go to RT Stevens, T Shi, J Brüggemann and L Airapetian for the help they provided for completing this manuscript. The author is grateful for the friendship and the scientifically exciting discussions with CJ Hodge, D Chialvo and KD Kniffki, which have significantly contributed to many parts of this work. Also, the constant support of the Department of Neurosurgery is greatly appreciated, without which most of this would not have been possible.

References

1. Newman HM, Stevens RT, Apkarian AV. Direct spinal projections to limbic and striatal areas: anterograde transport studies from the upper cervical spinal cord and the cervical enlargement in squirrel monkey and rat. 1995 (submitted).

2. Burstein R, Giesler GJ Jr. Retrograde labeling of neurons in spinal cord that project directly to nucleus accumbens or the septal nuclei in the rat. *Brain Res* 1989 ; 497 : 149-54.
3. Cliffer KD, Burstein R, Giesler GJ Jr. Distributions of spinothalamic, spinohypothalamic and spinotelencephalic fibers revealed by anterograde transport of PHA-L in rats. *J Neurosci* 1991 ; 11 : 852-68.
4. Giesler GJ. Direct spinal pathways to the limbic system for nociceptive information. *TINS* 1994 ; 17 : 244-50.
5. Apkarian AV, Hodge CJ. The primate spinothalamic pathways: II. The cells of origin of the dorsolateral and ventral spinothalamic pathways. *J Comp Neurol* 1989 ; 288 : 474-92.
6. Stevens RT, Hodge CJ Jr, Apkarian AV. Medial, Intralaminar, and lateral terminations of lumbar spinothalamic tract neurons: a fluorescent double-label study. *Somat Mot Res* 1989 ; 6 : 285-308.
7. Martin RJ, Apkarian AV, Hodge CJ Jr. Ventrolateral and dorsolateral ascending spinal cord pathway influence on thalamic nociception in cat. *J Neurophysiol* 1990 ; 64 : 1400-12.
8. Stevens RT, Apkarian AV, Hodge CJ Jr. The location of spinothalamic axons within spinal cord white matter in cat and squirrel monkey. *Somat Mot Res* 1991 ; 8 : 97-102.
9. Walker AE. The spinothalamic tract in man. *Arch Neurol Psychiat* 1940 ; 43 : 284-98.
10. Stookey B. Further light on the transmission of pain and temperature within the spinal cord: human cordotomy to abolish pain sense without destroying temperature sense. *J Nerv Ment Dis* 1929 ; 69 : 552-7.
11. Foerster O, Gagel O. Die Vorderseitenstrangdurchschneidung beim Menschen. Eine klinisch-patho-physiologisch-anatomische Studie. *Z Ges Neurol Psychiat* 1932 ; 138 : 1-92.
12. Kuru M. *Sensory paths in the spinal cord and brainstem in man.* Japan : Sogensya, 1949.
13. Friehs GM, Schröttner O, Pendl G. Evidence for segregated pain and temperature conduction within the spinothalamic tract. *J Neurosurg* 1995 ; 83 : 8-12.
14. Christensen BN, Perl ER. Spinal neurons specifically exited by noxious or thermal stimuli: marginal zone of the dorsal horn. *J Neurophysiol* 1970 ; 33 : 293-307.
15. Craig AD, Dostrovsky JO. Thermoreceptive lamina I trigeminothalamic neurons project to the nucleus submedius in the cat. *Exp Brain Res* 1991 ; 85 : 470-4.
16. McMahon SB, Wall PD. A system of rat spinal cord lamina I cells projecting through the contralateral dorsolateral funiculus. *J Comp Neurol* 1983 ; 214 : 217-23.
17. Apkarian AV, Stevens RT, Hodge CJ. Funicular location of ascending axons of lamina I cells in the cat. *Brain Res* 1985 ; 334 : 160-4.
18. Craig AD. Spinal location of ascending lamina I axons anterogradely labeled with *Phaseolus vulgaris* leucoagglutinin (PHA-L) in the cat. *J Comp Neurol* 1991 ; 313 : 377-93.
19. Jones MW, Hodge CJ Jr, Apkarian, AV, Stevens RT. A dorsolateral spinothalamic system in cat. *Brain Res* 1985 ; 335 : 188-93.
20. Apkarian AV, Hodge CJ. The primate spinothalamic pathways: I. A quantitative study of the cells of origin of the spinothalamic pathway. *J Comp Neurol* 1989 ; 288 : 447-73.
21. Dado RJ, Katter JT, Giesler GJ Jr. Spinothalamic and spinohypothalamic tract neurons in the cervical enlargement of rats. III. Locations of antidromically identified axons in the cervical cord white matter. *J Neurophysiol* 1994 ; 71 : 1003-21.
22. Norrsell U. Behavioural thermosensitivity after unilateral, partial lesions of the lateral funiculus in the cervical spinal cord of the cat. *Brain Res* 1989 ; 78 : 369-73.
23. Apkarian AV, Shi T. Nociceptive responsive neurons and their relations to spinothalamic terminals in the squirrel monkey lateral thalamus. *J Neurosci* 1994 ; 14 : 6779-95.
24. Gingold SI, Greenspan JD, Apkarian AV. Anatomic evidence of nociceptive inputs to primary somatosensory cortex: relationship between spinothalamic terminals and thalamocortical cells in squirrel monkeys. *J Comp Neurol* 1991 ; 308 : 467-90.

25. Stevens RT, London SM, Apkarian AV. Spinothalamocortical projections to the secondary somatosensory cortex (SII) in squirrel monkey. *Brain Res* 1993 ; 631 : 241-6.
26. Craig AD, Bushnell MC, Zhang ET, Blomqvist A. A thalamic nucleus specific for pain and temperature sensation. *Nature* 1994 ; 372 : 770-3.
27. Ralston HJ III, Peschanski M, Ralston DD. Fine structure of spinothalamic track axons and terminals in rat, cat and monkey demonstrated by the orthograde transport of lectin conjugated to horseradish peroxidase. In : Fields HL, Dubner R, Cervero F, eds. *Advances in pain research and therapy,* vol 9th. New York : Raven Press, 1985 : 269-75.
28. Ralston RD III, Ralston DD. Medial, lemniscal and spinal projections to the macaque thalamus: an electron microscopic study of differing GABAergic circuitry serving thalamic somatosensory mechanisms. *J Neurosci* 1994 ; 14 : 2485-502.
29. Ralston HJ III. Synaptic organization of spinothalamic tract projections to the thalamus with special reference to pain. In : Kruger L, Liebeskind JC, eds. *Advances in pain research and therapy*. New York : Raven Press, 1984 : 183-95.
30. Ma W, Peschanski M, Ralston III HJ. The differential synaptic organization of the spinal and lemniscal projections to the ventrobasal complex of the rat thalamus. Evidence of the convergence of the two systems upon single thalamic neurons. *Neuroscience* 1987 ; 22 : 925-34.
31. Jones EG. *The thalamus*. New York : Plenum Press, 1985.
32. Kaas JH, Pons TP. The somatosensory system of primates *Comp Prim Biol* 1988 ; 4 : 421-68.
33. Shi T, Stevens RT, Tessier J, Apkarian AV. Spinothalamocortical inputs nonpreferentially innervate the superficial deep cortical layers of SI. *Neurosci Lett* 1993 ; 160 : 209-13.
34. Shi T, Apkarian AV. Morphology of thalamocortical neurons projecting to the primary somatosensory cortex and their relationship to spinothalamic terminals in the squirrel monkey. *J Comp Neurol* 1995 ; 361 : 1-24.
35. Pons TP, Garraghty PE, Mishkin M. Serial and parallel processing of tactual information in somatosensory cortex of rhesus monkeys. *J Neurophysiol* 1992 ; 68 : 518-27.
36. Bushnell MC, Duncan GH, Termblay N. Thalamic VPM nucleus in the behaving monkey. I. Multimodal and discriminative properties of thermosensitive neurons. *J Neurophysiol* 1993 ; 69 : 739-52.
37. Vahle-Hinz C, Freund I, Kniffki K-D. Nociceptive neurons in the ventral periphery of the cat thalamic ventroposteromedial nucleus. In : Schmidt RF, Schaible H-G, Vahle-Hinz C, eds. *Fine afferent nerve fibers and pain*. Weinheim : VCH Verlagsgesellschaft, 1987 : 439-50.
38. Kniffki K-D, Craig AD. The distribution of nociceptive neurons in the cat's lateral thalamus: the dorsal and ventral periphery of VPL. In : Rowe M, Willis WD Jr, eds. *Development, organization and processing in somatosensory pathways*. New York : Alan R Liss Inc, 1985 : 375-82.
39. Chung JM, Lee KH, Surmeier DJ, Sorkin LS, Kim J, Willis WD. Response characteristics of neurons in the ventral posterior lateral nucleus of the monkey thalamus. *J Neurophysiol* 1986 ; 56 : 370-90.
40. Kenshalo DR, Giesler GJ, Leonard RB, Willis WD. Responses of neurons in primate ventral lateral nucleus to noxious stimuli. *J Neurophysiol* 1980 ; 43 : 1594-614.
41. Casey KL. Unit analysis of nociceptive mechanisms in the thalamus of the awake squirrel monkey. *J Physiol Lond* 1966 ; 29 : 727-50.
42. Casey KL, Morrow TJ. Nociceptive neurons in the ventral posterior thalamus of the awake squirrel monkey: observations on identification, modulation, and drug effects. In : Besson J-M, Guilbaud G, Peschanski M, eds. *Thalamus and pain*. Amsterdam : Elsevier Science Publishers BV (Biomedical Division), 1987 : 211-26.
43. Morrow TJ, Casey KL. State-related modulation of thalamic somatosensory responses in the awake monkey. *J Neurophysiol* 1992 ; 67 : 305-17.

44. Brüggemann J, Shi T, Apkarian AV. Squirrel monkey lateral thalamus: II. Viscero-somatic convergent representation of urinary bladder, colon and esophagus. *J Neurosci* 1994 ; 14 : 6796-814.
45. Berkley KJ, Guilbaud G, Benoist J-M, Gautron M. Responses of neurons in and near the thalamic ventrobasal complex of the rat to stimulation of uterus, cervix, vagina, colon and skin. *J Neurophysiol* 1993 ; 69(2) : 557-68.
46. Brüggemann J, Shi T, Apkarian AV. Viscero-somatic interactions in the thalamic ventral posterolateral nucleus (VPL) of the squirrel monkey. *Neurosci Lett* 1995 (submitted).
47. Apkarian AV, Brüggemann J, Shi T, Airapetian L. A thalamic model for true and referred viscera pain. In : Gebhart GF, ed. *Progress in pain research and management*, Vol 5. Seattle : IASP Press, 1995 : 217-59.
48. Chandler MJ, Hobbs SF, Qing-Gong Fu, Kenshalo DR, Blair RW, Foreman DR. Responses of neurons in ventroposterolateral nucleus of primate thalamus to urinary bladder distension. *Brain Res* 1992 ; 571 : 26-34.
49. Brüggemann J, Vahle-Hinz C, Kniffki K-D. Representation of the urinary bladder in the lateral thalamus of the cat. *J Neurophysiol* 1993 ; 17 : 482-91.
50. Brüggemann, J, Vahle-Hinz, C, Kniffki, K-D. Projections from the pelvic nerve to the periphery of the cat's thalamic ventral posterolateral nucleus and adjacent regions of the posterior complex. *J Neurophysiol* 1994 ; 72 : 2237-45.
51. Brüggemann J, Vahle-Hinz C, Apkarian AV, Kniffki K-D. Somato-visceral convergence in thalamic regions of the cat. *J Neurophysiol* 1995 (submitted).
52. Brüggemann J, Shi T, Apkarian AV. Viscerosomatic neurons in the primary somatosensory cortex (SI) of the squirrel monkey. *J. Neurosci* 1995 (submitted).
53. Rapp PE, Goldberg G, Albano AM, Janicki MB, Murphy D, Niemeyer E, Jiménez-Montaño MA. Using coarse-grained measures to characterize electromyographic signals. *Int J Birfurc Chaos* 1993 ; 3 : 525-41.
54. Rapp PE, Zimmerman ID, Vining EP, Albano AM, Jiménez-Montaño MA. The algorithmic complexity of neural spike trains increases during focal seizures. *J Neurosci* 1994 ; 14 : 4731-9.
55. Shi T, Airapetian LR, Brüggemann J, Apkarian AV. Evidence for spike interval patterns differentiating among somatosensory dimensions. *Pain* 1995 (submitted).
56. Wilson MA, McNaughton BL. Dynamics of the hippocampal ensemble code for space. *Science* 1993 ; 261 : 1055-8.

8

The region postero-inferior to the human thalamic principal sensory nucleus (Vc) may contribute to the affective dimension of pain through thalamo-corticolimbic connections

F.A. LENZ

Department of Neurosurgery, Johns Hopkins Hospital, Baltimore, USA.

The region at the postero-inferior aspect of the primate principal sensory nucleus is an important structure in pain signalling pathways. In the past, this suggestion rested on the observation that the spinothalamic tract (STT) terminated in this region [1, 2] and that the sensation of pain could be evoked by stimulation of this area [3-5]. Recent studies have demonstrated that cells responding to painful stimuli are located both postero-inferior to (postero-inferior region) [6] and within the core of Vc (core region) [6, 7]. The location of cells responding to painful stimuli was significantly correlated with sites where stimulation evoked pain, demonstrating that these cells signal pain [6, 8]. These observations demonstrate that cells at the postero-inferior aspect of Vc signal pain. However, the functional significance of pain related activity in the region postero-inferior to the core of Vc has remained unclear.

The present review speculates that the region postero-inferior to the core of Vc (postero-inferior region) is involved in the affective dimension of pain and memory for pain through thalamo-corticolimbic connections. This suggestion rests on several lines of evidence. Recent reports document that pain with a strong affective dimension can be evoked by stimulation postero-inferior to the core of Vc in patients with prior experience of such pain [9-11]. Similar pain without a strong affective component is evoked by stimulation in patients without experience of pain with a strong affective dimension [11]. These results suggest that the coupling of pain and a strong affective component is conditioned by prior experience. Anatomic studies suggest that the region postero-inferior to Vc is connected to secondary somatosensory cortex and insular cortex [12, 13] which may be involved in somatosensory memory through corticolimbic connections [14]. Therefore the region posterior to Vc may be involved in the affective dimension of pain, particularly those aspects based on learning through prior experience [15].

Cells in the region of Vc responsive to painful mechanical and thermal stimuli

There is now good evidence that cells in the region of human Vc respond to painful stimuli. Cells responding to noxious heat have been located close to the postero-inferior aspect of the core region or in the postero-inferior region while cells responding to innocuous cooling were located only within the postero-inferior aspect of the core. A response to painful heat significantly greater than that to innocuous mechanical and thermal stimuli was observed for 6% of cells studied in the core of Vc [6]. Half of the cells responding to noxious heat stimuli also exhibited significant phasic responses to cold stimuli. Responses to noxious heat were significantly greater than control for 5% of cells studied in the postero-inferior area. None of the cells in the postero-inferior area responded to innocuous stimuli.

The production of pain by threshold microstimulation was significantly correlated with the location of neurons which responded to noxious heat stimuli [6]. Cells responsive to noxious heat were recorded at a significantly greater proportion of sites where microstimulation evoked pain (66%) than sites where sensations other than pain were evoked (1.5%). Innocuous thermal sensations were not evoked by microstimulation at any of the sites where cells responsive to noxious heat were recorded. These results demonstrate that cells responsive to noxious thermal stimuli probably signal pain and are located in the postero-inferior aspect of the core and in the postero-inferior area.

A recent study demonstrated that one third of cells in the core of human Vc responded maximally to painful mechanical but not thermal stimuli [7]. None of the cells in the postero-inferior region exhibited the same response pattern. Stimulation at the site where these cells were recorded evoked the sensation of pain for only 14% of these cells. Since their stimulus response functions extend into the painful range, these cells might encode painful mechanical stimuli. A shift in the stimulus response function of these cells might mediate mechanical hyperalgesia. Therefore, these cells may signal pain and hyperalgesia in response to mechanical stimuli. The location of cells responsive to noxious thermal or mechanical stimulation is consistent with the conclusion that they receive input from the STT.

The thalamic termination of the STT has been studied in patients at autopsy following lesions of the STT [1, 2, 16]. These studies show that the human STT terminates in the magnocellular medial geniculate [1, 16] which projects to the inferior parietal lobule [17] plus superior temporal gyrus and insula at the posterior sylvian fissure [18]. The STT also terminates in limitans and Vc portae nuclei [2] which may project to parietal operculum [18]. There is a dense STT termination in the caudal portion of Vc [1] or dorsal Vc parvocellularis [2] which projects to anterior insula [18]. Finally, the STT makes its most dense termination contralaterally in Vc complex [1, 2, 19-21] which projects to postcentral parietal cortex [18].

A pattern of STT termination similar to that in humans has been reported in old world monkeys. Recent studies of acetyl choline esterase and neurokinin immunohistochemistry have demonstrated that "apart from differences in size of the nuclei, human and (old world) monkey thalamus are remarkably similar" [22, 23]. In monkeys, STT terminates in VP, corresponding to human Vc, [19, 24-27] with less dense terminations in nuclei located postero-inferior to VP including VPI [26], corresponding to Vcpc [23], and the posterior nuclear group including posterior nucleus [24, 25, 27-29], pulvinar oralis [26], limitans [26, 27], magnocellular medial geniculate [24] suprageniculate nuclei [24, 26, 27, 29] and VMpo, posterior inferior and medial to the medial division of VP [30]. Therefore anatomic studies support involvement of the region postero-inferior to the core of Vc in pain signalling pathways.

Sensations evoked by microstimulation in the region of Vc

Microstimulation studies suggest there is partitioning of thermal/pain sensations at different locations in the region of Vc. Thermal/pain sensations were evoked by stimulation over a relatively large area extending up to 4mm posterior of the core and up to 4mm below the ACPC line. Within the core of Vc, sites where stimulation evoked thermal/pain sensations were located near the border with the postero-inferior area. Thermal/pain sensations were evoked at a significantly greater percentage of all sites located in the postero-inferior area (30%) than at sites in the core area (5%). Sites where pain sensations were evoked made up a small minority of thermal/pain sensations evoked by stimulation in both the core and postero-inferior region. Threshold current for evoking sensation did not vary with location of the stimulation site (core/postero-inferior) or with quality of sensation (paresthesia or thermal/pain). Therefore, the difference between the proportion of sites in the core and postero-inferior areas where thermal/pain and paresthesia sensations were evoked is not explained by differences in thresholds. Previous reports suggest that pain but not nonpainful thermal sensations can be evoked by stimulation posterior to Vc [3-5].

Modalities of thermal/pain sensations are anatomically segregated within the region of Vc. For example, stimulation sites where thermal/pain sensations are evoked were located at the medial aspect of the cutaneous core of Vc, between the representation of cutaneous structures on the face and hand. The sensation of warmth was evoked by stimulation at sites which were located significantly posterior to sites where pain or cool sensations were evoked. The location of the evoked sensation or projected field (PF) also varies with thalamic location of the stimulation site. Thus, the sensation of paresthesia was more likely to be evoked in a large PF, by stimulation in the postero-inferior area (11% of sites) than in the core (3%). Differences in the size of the PF were related to descriptor quality within the thermal/pain category. The sensation of cool was usually evoked in small PFs located on the lips. The sensation of warmth or pain was in PFs that were larger than those where cool sensations were evoked on the same part of the body [8]. Locations of PFs in terms of depth relative to the skin also varied relative to location of the stimulation site. Evoked sensations were more likely to be referred to deep than superficial structures at stimulation sites in the postero-inferior (56%) than in the core area (28%).

In summary, a population of cells in the postero-inferior aspect of the core and in the postero-inferior area respond to noxious heat. Thermal/pain sensations are evoked at a significantly greater proportion of sites in the postero-inferior region than in the core region. Sites where pain is evoked by stimulation are significantly correlated with sites where cells respond to noxious stimuli. These results demonstrate that cells in the postero-inferior part of the core area and the postero-inferior area signal pain.

Pains with a strong affective dimension evoked by microstimulation in the region of Vc

Visceral pain can also be evoked by stimulation in the region of Vc [9]. The sensation of angina was evoked by stimulation at the postero-inferior aspect of Vc in a woman undergoing implantation of a deep brain stimulating electrode for treatment of pain secondary to arachnoiditis. She had a past history of unstable angina which was stable following coronary balloon angioplasty. At and posterior to the location of cells with cutaneous receptive fields on the left chest wall, in Vcpc, stimulation coincided precisely with the sensation of angina (stimulation-associated angina). Pain was described using a pain questionnaire with forty-five descriptors [9]. The descriptors chosen for the stimulation-associated angina were almost identical to those chosen for the patient's usual angina, including the affective dimension described as "frightful" and "fatiguing". Stimulation-evoked pains described with emotion descriptors in the questionnaire were said to have a strong affective dimension.

Stimulation-associated angina began and stopped instantaneously with stimulation, typical of sensations evoked by thalamic microstimulation [8], but quite unlike her usual angina which usually lasted for minutes and began and ended gradually [31, 32]. The sensation of angina was associated with a tingling sensation in the left leg. Tingling in the arm but not the leg is often associated with angina of cardiac origin [31, 32].

However, microstimulation at sites located posterior and inferior to Vc frequently evoke sensations simultaneously in more than one part of the body [8]. Clinical, hemodynamic, electrophysiologic and biochemical measures of cardiac function showed no evidence of myocardial strain or injury related to stimulation-associated angina. For example, no tachycardia or ST segment changes, such as those often observed with angina of cardiac origin [31, 33, 34], were observed in this patient. The absence of angina over a period of two months around the time of the procedure argues strongly against the possibility of unstable angina [35]. In summary, the characteristics of stimulation-associated angina and lack of cardiac findings strongly suggest that the sensation was related to the thalamic stimulation.

Similar observations have been made during stimulation posterior to Vc in a woman with a history of previous episodes of both labor pain and dyspareunia, pain during intercourse [10]. In this patient, stimulation at the postero-inferior aspect of Vc and adjacent to Vcpor reproduced her a pain which was "like the pain she experiences during sexual intercourse". At another site in Vcpor, stimulation produced pain which the patient described as "like having a baby, like the contractions". During stimulation at both sites, the patient became very "agitated" and "emotional". The patient started to cry during stimulation at the first site. In this patient and the patient with angina, the stimulation evoked pain was related to stimulation, was associated with a strong affective dimension and reproduced visceral pain which the patient had previously experienced.

In another case, atypical chest pain, a medically unexplained pain associated with panic attacks, was evoked by stimulation in the area posterior to Vc, in Vcpor [11]. A man with a diagnosis of panic disorder underwent a stereotactic thalamotomy for treatment of disabling essential tremor. He suffered weekly panic attacks characterized by chest pain, heart pounding, flushing, tinnitus, shortness of breath and the urge to escape from the situation. During the thalamotomy, stimulation posterior to Vc evoked a sensation which was determined by the questionnaire to be almost identical to his atypical chest pain, including the affective dimension. The patient's heart rate was stable throughout the procedure including the intervals of stimulation which produced his atypical chest pain. The postoperative cardiovascular exam, enzymes and EKGs, including an EKG done postoperatively during atypical chest pain, were within normal limits. During a postoperative thallium stress test, the patient experienced neither chest pain, nor EKG, nor thallium scan abnormalities. Thus a thorough cardiac evaluation failed to reveal evidence of a cardiac disease to explain his atypical chest pain or stimulation-evoked chest pain.

In each of the cases described above the patient had a severe episodic preoperative pain with a strong affective dimension. In each case, the preoperative pain was reproduced by stimulation posterior to Vc, suggesting that a memory for the preoperative pain was evoked by stimulation. In each case, the preoperative pain had a strong affective dimension which was reproduced by stimulation. In three of the four cases, the pain had a significant visceral component. Any mechanism attempting to explain stimulation-evoked pain with a strong affective component must account for visceral pain sensations, memory for pain and the affective dimension of the evoked pain.

Thalamic mechanisms of visceral pain

Anatomic and physiologic studies are consistent with involvement of the region posterior and inferior to Vc in signalling visceral sensations. STT tract cells in the upper thoracic spinal cord projecting to VP, the monkey nucleus equivalent to Vc respond to coronary artery occlusion [36] and intracardiac injection of bradykinin ([37] cf [38]). Additionally, cells at the posterior aspect of the nucleus equivalent to Vc in the cat respond to intracardiac injections of bradykinin [39] and stimulation of cardiac sympathetic nerves [40]. Neurons in the thalamic principal sensory nucleus also encode visceral inputs from gastrointestinal and genitourinary systems in rats and monkeys [41, 42]. Therefore experimental studies suggest that cells in the thalamic principal sensory nucleus encode noxious visceral stimuli. Finally, this region projects to insular cortex [12, 13, 18] where stimulation evokes both visceral sensations in humans [43] and alterations in visceral function in monkeys [44, 45]. In combination with these experimental results, the human reports described above [9, 10] argue forcefully that the region of human Vc signals painful visceral sensation.

Speculation concerning the reproduction of pain with a strong affective dimension by stimulation posterior to Vc

Angina, dyspareunia, labor pain and atypical chest pain all have a strong affective dimension. In each case described above, the sensation, including the affective dimension was reproduced by stimulation in the region postero-inferior to Vc [9-11]. In contrast to the results in the patient with atypical chest pain, stimulation during explorations in 100 patients without a history of chest pain with a strong affective dimension never evoked chest pain with an affective dimension [11]. Sharp chest pain, like that in the patient with atypical chest pain but without the affective dimension [11] was evoked at 3 sites demonstrating that sharp chest pain and the affective dimension can be dissociated. Stimulation evoked pain with a strong affective dimension is not particularly associated with the thalamic representation of the chest, since pain is only evoked by stimulation at 5% of sites in that area [9], comparable to other parts of the body [8]. In the thalamic representation of the part of the body where patients have not experienced recurrent or chronic pain (n = 6 sites), stimulation-evoked pain never included a strong affective dimension [8]. Neither was a strong affective dimension found for pain evoked by stimulation at 29 sites in the representation of the part of body where patient experienced chronic pain without a strong affective dimension [46]. Thus, in the Hopkins experience [8, 9, 11, 46], stimulation evoked chest pain with a strong affective dimension was only evoked by stimulation postero-inferior to Vc in patients who had prior experience of pain with a strong affective dimension. Chest pain without a strong affective component can be evoked in patients without prior experience of chest pain having a strong affective dimension [9]. Therefore stimulation evoked pain and a strong affective dimension may be coupled following conditioning by a prior experience of pain with a strong affective dimension.

The fact that stimulation reproduces a previously experienced pain suggests that stimulation in the region postero-inferior to Vc evokes a memory for pain including the affective dimension. Memory for pain might be mediated by the projection from the region postero-inferior to Vc to SII, insular cortex and related areas. These cortical areas have been implicated both in nociceptive processing and in the mechanism of somatosensory memory through corticolimbic connections [14]. Thus thalamic stimulation may reproduce pain with a strong affective dimension by activation of corticolimbic connections involved in somatosensory memory and conditioned by prior experience of the pain.

The cortical projections of thalamic regions where stimulation reproduces pain with a strong affective dimension have been studied in man. Vcpc projects to anterior insular cortex [1, 18] whereas Vcpor projects to the inferior parietal lobule, including the parietal operculum and secondary somatosensory cortex - SII [18]. Studies in monkeys provide a more detailed picture of cortical projections of monkey thalamic nuclei corresponding to human thalamic nuclei [23] where stimulation evokes pain with an affective dimension (posterior Vc, Vcpc and Vcpor). VP is well known to project to SI and SII cortex [13, 47, 48], while VPI, corresponding to Vcpc [23] projects to SII and insular dysgranular cortex [12, 49]. The posterior nuclear group projects to temporo-parietal cortical zones including: medial posterior nucleus to retroinsular cortex, lateral posterior nucleus to granular and retroinsular plus posterior auditory cortex and parietal operculum, suprageniculate and limitans nuclei to granular insular and retro-insular cortex, medial and oral division of pulvinar, corresponding to human Vc portae [23], to 7b [12, 13]. Thus the thalamic area where stimulation evokes sensations having a strong affective component projects to SII and parietal operculum and insula posterior to SII. These cortical areas have been implicated in nociceptive processing and in somatosensory memory [14].

Involvement of SII and insular cortex in pain processing is demonstrated by projections from thalamic areas involved in such processing and by responses in cells in SII [49-54] and granular insular cortex [50] to noxious stimuli. Cells responding to noxious stimuli tend to be clustered suggesting a sub-modality specific area within and posterior to SII [50, 52]. Positron emission tomography demonstrates a significant insular activation during painful as compared with control tactile stimuli [55, 56]. Lesions of insula impair emotional responses to painful stimuli [57]. Stimulation of insula normally evokes visceral sensations but not pain [43]. However, stimulation of these areas might evoke pain in patients who have experienced chronic or recurrent pain, as in other cortical and thalamic areas [8, 58]. Therefore much evidence supports involvement of SII and insular cortex in pain processing.

Mishkin has defined criteria for identifying cortical areas involved in sensory memory through corticolimbic connections [14]. These criteria describe the properties of the inferior temporal cortex which is known to be involved in visual memory. By these criteria, areas involved in sensory memory through corticolimbic connections should exhibit modality specificity and higher order function. Higher order function is identified by lesion related deficits of higher order perceptual function rather than primary sensory function. The cortical area should exhibit bilateral primary sensory input and cells in the area should have bilateral sensory input. Interhemispheric transfer of learning related to the sensory modality should be demonstrated behaviorally. Finally the cortical area should have output to the limbic system. A cortical area meeting these criteria may be involved in sensory memory through corticolimbic connections, by analogy to the role of inferior temporal cortex to visual memory [14].

Many of the criteria for identification of cortical areas involved in corticolimibic connections [14] have been fulfilled for SII and insular cortex where cells respond to noxious stimuli. Cells responding to noxious stimuli tend to be clustered suggesting that there is a submodality selective area within and posterior to SII [50, 52]. In monkeys, SII cortex projects to insular dysgranular cortex projecting to enterorhinal cortex and insular dysgranular and granular cortex projecting to perirhinal cortex and amygdala [59]. Cells in SII-7b cortex responding to noxious stimuli commonly have bilateral representation [52, 54, 60]. Bilateral primary sensory input to this cortical area is suggested by evoked potentials recorded in this area in response to both ipsilateral and contralateral stimulation [54], and by the presence of neurons with similar properties in thalamic regions projecting to this cortical area [61, 62]. Anatomic studies demonstrate commissural connections raising the possibility that there is interhemispheric transfer of nociceptive information [63, 64]. Interhemispheric transfer of tactile information has been demonstrated by physiologic and behavioral studies [65]. These studies have demonstrated that transfer of training in tactile discrimination tasks from the trained to the untrained hand was dramatically slower in animals with callosal section. However, similar studies have not been carried out for nociceptive discrimination tasks. Nevertheless, SII and insular cortex satisfy many of the criteria for cortical structures involved in corticolimbic connections [14].

The results of human thalamic studies demonstrate that stimulation evokes pain with a strong affective dimension in patients who have previously experienced such pain. Similar pains without a strong affective dimension were evoked by stimulation in patients without prior experience of pain with a strong affective dimension. This suggests that the coupling of pain and a strong affective dimension are conditioned by prior experience of the pain. The basic studies reviewed above suggest that stimulation postero-inferior to Vc may have activated cortical areas involved in somatosensory memory through corticolimbic connections. On this basis, we speculate that thalamic stimulation at and posterior to the principal sensory nucleus indirectly activates limbic structures conditioned by prior experience of pain. This conditioning process might be the substrate for the affective dimension of chronic pain syndromes which follow recurrent or severe episodes of pain. Reproduction of previously experienced pain by stimulation of somatosensory pathways suggests that peripheral stimuli activating those same pathways could reproduce the pain, including the affective dimension.

Acknowledgements

Supported by grants to FAL from the Eli Lilly Corporation and the NIH (NS28598, K08 NS01384, P01 NS32386).

References

1. Mehler WR. The anatomy of the so-called "pain tract" in man: an analysis of the course and distribution of the ascending fibers of the fasciculus anterolateralis. In : French JD, Porter RW, eds. *Basic research in paraplegia*. Springfield : Thomas, 1962 : 26-55.
2. Mehler WR. The posterior thalamic region in man. *Confin Neurol* 1966 ; 27 : 18-29.
3. Dostrovsky JO, Wells FEB, Tasker RR. Pain evoked by stimulation in human thalamus. In : Sjigenaga Y, ed. *International symposium on processing nociceptive information*. Amsterdam : Elsevier, 1991.
4. Halliday AM, Logue V. Painful sensations evoked by electrical stimulation in the thalamus. In : Somjen GG, ed. *Neurophysiology studied in man*. Amsterdam : Excerpta Medica, 1972 : 221-30.
5. Hassler R, Reichert T. Klinische und anatomische Befunde bei stereotaktischen Schmerzoperationen im Thalamus. *Arch Psychiat Nerverkr* 1959 ; 200 : 93-122.
6. Lenz FA, Seike M, Lin YC, Baker FH, Rowland LH, Gracely RH, Richardson RT. Neurons in the area of human thalamic nucleus ventralis caudalis respond to painful heat stimuli. *Brain Res* 1993 ; 623 : 235-40.
7. Lenz FA, Gracely RH, Rowland LH, Dougherty PM. A population of cells in the human principal sensory nucleus respond to painful mechanical stimuli. *Neurosci Lett* 1994 ; 180 : 46-50.
8. Lenz FA, Seike M, Lin YC, Baker FH, Richardson RT, Gracely RH. Thermal and pain sensations evoked by microstimulation in the area of the human ventrocaudal nucleus (Vc). *J Neurophysiol* 1993 ; 70 : 200-12.
9. Lenz FA, Gracely RH, Hope EJ, Baker FH, Rowland LH, Dougherty PM, Richardson RT. The sensation of angina can be evoked by stimulation of the human thalamus. *Pain* 1994 ; 59 : 119-25.
10. Davis KD, Tasker RR, Kiss ZHT, Hutchison WD, Dostrovsky JO. Visceral pain evoked by thalamic microstimulation in humans. *Neuroreport* 1995 ; 6 : 369-74.
11. Lenz FA, Gracely RH, Romanoski AJ, Hope EJ, Rowland LH, Dougherty PM. Pain with a strong affective dimension reproduced by stimulation of the human somatosensory thalamus. *Soc Neurosci Abstr* 1995 (in press).
12. Burton H, Jones EG. The posterior thalamic region and its cortical projection in new world and old world monkeys. *J Comp Neurol* 1976 ; 168 : 249-302.
13. Burton H. Second somatosensory cortex and related areas. In : Jones EG, Peters A, eds. *Cerebral cortex Vol 5. Sensory-motor areas and aspects of cortical connectivity*. New York and London : Plenum Press, 1986 : 31-98.

14. Mishkin M. Analogous neural models for tactual and visual learning. *Neuropsych* 1979 ; 17 : 139-51.
15. Price D, Harkins S. The affective-motivational dimension of pain. *APS J* 1992 ; 4 : 229-39.
16. Mehler WR. Some neurological species differences - *a posteriori*. *Ann N Y Acad Sci* 1969 ; 167 : 424-68.
17. Locke S, Angevine JB, Marin OSM. Projection of magnocellular medial geniculate nucleus in man. *Anat Rec* 1961 ; 139 : 249-50.
18. Van Buren JM, Borke RC. *Variations and connections of the human thalamus*. Berlin : Springer Verlag, 1972.
19. Mehler WR, Feferman ME, Nauta WHJ. Ascending axon degeneration following anterolateral cordotomy. An experimental study in the monkey. *Brain* 1960 ; 83 : 718-50.
20. Bowsher D. Termination of the central pain pathway in man: the conscious appreciation of pain. *Brain* 1957 ; 80 : 606-20.
21. Walker AE. Central representation of pain. *Res Publ Assoc Res Nerv Ment Dis* 1943 ; 23 : 63-85.
22. Hirai T, Jones EG. Distribution of tachykinin-and enkephalin-immunoreactive fibers in the human thalamus. *Brain Res Rev* 1989 ; 14 : 35-52.
23. Hirai T, Jones EG. A new parcellation of the human thalamus on the basis of histochemical staining. *Brain Res Rev* 1989 ; 14 : 1-34.
24. Berkley KJ. Spatial relationships between the terminations of somatic sensory and motor pathways in the rostral brainstem of cats and monkeys. I. Ascending somatic sensory inputs to lateral diencephalon. *J Comp Neurol* 1980 ; 193 : 283-317.
25. Boivie J. An anatomic reinvestigation of the termination of the spinothalamic tract in the monkey. *J Comp Neurol* 1979 ; 168 : 343-70.
26. Apkarian AV, Hodge CJ. Primate spinothalamic pathways: III. Thalamic terminations of the dorsolateral and ventral spinothalamic pathways. *J Comp Neurol* 1989 ; 288 : 493-511.
27. Mantyh PW. The spinothalamic tract in primate: a re-examination using wheatgerm agglutinin conjugated with horseradish peroxidase. *Neuroscience* 1983 ; 9 : 847-62.
28. Burton H, Craig AD Jr. Spinothalamic projections in cat, raccoon and monkey: a study based on anterograde transport of horseradish peroxidase. In : Macchi G, Rustioni A, Spreafico R, eds. *Somatosensory integration in the thalamus*. Amsterdam : Elsevier, 1983 : 17-41.
29. Ralston HJ, Ralston DD. The primate dorsal spinothalamic tract: evidence for a specific termination in the posterior nuclei [Po/SG] of the thalamus. *Pain* 1992 ; 48 : 107-18.
30. Craig AD, Bushnell MC, Zhang ET, Blomqvist A. A specific thalamic nucleus for pain and temperature sensation in macaques and humans. *Nature* 1994 ; 372 : 770-3.
31. Roughgarden JW. Circulatory changes associated with spontaneous angina pectoris. *Am J Med* 1966 ; 41 : 947-61.
32. Matthews MB. Clinical diagnosis. In : Julian DG, ed. *Angina pectoris*. Edinburgh, London, Melbourne and New York : Churchill Livingstone, 1985 : 62-83.
33. Friesinger GC, Robertson RMS. Haemodynamics in stable angina pectoris. In : Julian DG, ed. *Angina pectoris*. Edinburgh, London, Melbourne and New York : Churchill Livingstone, 1985 : 25-37.
34. Hauser AM, Vellappillil G, Ramos RG, Gordon S, Timmis GC, Dudlets P. Sequence of mechanical, electrocardiographic and clinical effects of repeated coronary artery occlusion in human beings: echocardiographic observations during coronary angioplasty. *JACC* 1985 ; 5 : 7.
35. Rutherford JD, Braunwald E. Chronic ischemic heart disease. In : Braunwald E, ed. *Cardiac disease*. Philadelphia : W.B.Saunders, 1992 : 1292-363.
36. Blair RW, Ammons WS, Foreman RD. Responses of thoracic spinothalamic and spinoreticular cells to coronary artery occlusion. *J Neurophysiol* 1984 ; 51 : 636-48.

37. Blair RW, Weber N, Foreman RD. Responses of thoracic spinothalamic neurons to intracardiac injection of bradykinin in the monkey. *Circ Res* 1982 ; 51 : 83-94.
38. Meller ST, Gebhart GF. A critical review of the afferent pathways and the potential chemical mediators involved in cardiac pain. *Neuroscience* 1992 ; 48 : 501-24.
39. Horie H, Yokota T. Responses of nociceptive VPL neurons to intracardiac injection of bradykinin in the cat. *Brain Res* 1990 ; 516 : 161-4.
40. Taguchi H, Masuda T, Yokota T. Cardiac sympathetic afferent input onto neurons in nucleus ventralis posterolateralis in cat thalamus. *Brain Res* 1987 ; 436 : 240-52.
41. Berkley KJ, Guilbaud G, Benoist J-M, Gautron M. Responses of neurons in and near the thalamic ventrobasal complex of the rat to stimulation of the uterus, cervix, vagina, colon and skin. *J Neurophysiol* 1993 ; 69 : 557-68.
42. Bruggemann J, Shi T, Stea RA, Stevens RT, Apkarian AV. Representation of bladder, colon and esophagus in the lateral thalamus of the squirrel monkey. *Soc Neurosci Abstr* 1992 ; 18 : 495.
43. Penfield W, Rasmussen T. *The cerebral cortex of man*. New York : Macmillan, 1955.
44. Anand BK, Dua S. Circulatory and respiratory changes induced by electrical stimulation of the limbic system. *J Neurophysiol* 1956 ; 19 : 393-400.
45. Hoffman BL, Rasmussen T. Stimulation studies of insular cortex in *Macaca mulata*. *J Neurophysiol* 1953 ; 16 : 343-51.
46. Lin YC, Gracely RH, Lenz FA, Baker FH, Rowland LH, Dougherty PM. Sensations evoked by microstimulation in the area of the ventrocaudal nucleus of thalamus (Vc) in patients with chronic pain. *Soc Neurosci Abstr* 1993 ; 19 : 1572.
47. Jones EG. *The thalamus*. New York : Plenum, 1985.
48. Kenshalo DR Jr, Willis WD Jr. The role of the cerebral cortex in pain sensation. In : Peters A, Jones EG, eds. *Cerebral cortex, vol 9. Normal and altered states of function*. New York and London : Plenum Press, 1991 : 153-212.
49. Friedman D, Murray E. Thalamic connectivity of the second somatosensory area and neighboring somatosensory fields of the lateral sulcus of the macaque. *J Comp Neurol* 1986 ; 252 : 348-73.
50. Robinson CJ, Burton H. Somatic submodality distribution within the second somatosensory (SII), 7b, retroinsular, postauditory and granular insular cortical areas of *M. fascicularis*. *J Comp Neurol* 1980 ; 192 : 93-108.
51. Chudler E, Dong W, Kawakami Y. Cortical nociceptive responses and behavioral correlates in the monkey. *Brain Res* 1986 ; 397 : 47-60.
52. Dong W, Salonen L, Kawakami Y, Shiwaku T, Kaukoranta E, Martin R. Nociceptive responses of trigeminal neurons in SII-7b cortex of awake monkeys. *Brain Res* 1989 ; 484 : 314-24.
53. Chudler E, Dong W, Kawakami Y. Tooth pulp-evoked potentials in the monkey: cortical surface and intracortical distribution. *Pain* 1985 ; 22 : 221-33.
54. Chatrian G, Canfield R, Knauss T, Lettich E. Cerebral responses to electrical tooth pulp stimulation in man. *Neurology* 1975 ; 25 : 745-57.
55. Coghill RC, Talbot JD, Evans AC, Meyer E, Gjedde A, Bushnell MC, Duncan GH. Distributed processing of pain and vibration by the human brain. *J Neurosci* 1994 ; 14 : 4095-108.
56. Casey KL, Minoshima S, Koeppe RA, Weeder RJ, Morrow TJ. Temporo-spatial dynamics of human forebrain activity during noxious heat stimulation. *Soc Neurosci Abstr* 1994 ; 20 : 1573.
57. Berthier M, Starkstein S, Leiguarda R. Asymbolia for pain: a sensory-limbic disconnection syndrome. *Ann Neurol* 1988 ; 24 : 41-9.
58. Lewin W, Phillips CG. Observations on partial removal of the post-central gyrus of pain. *J Neurol Neurosurg Psychiatry* 1952 ; 15 : 143-7.
59. Friedman D, Murray E, O'Neill J, Mishkin M. Cortical connections of the somatosensory fields of the lateral sulcus of marcaques: evidence for a corticolimbic pathways of touch. *J Comp Neurol* 1986 ; 252 : 323-47.

60. Dong W, Chudler E, Sugiyama K, Roberts V, Hayashi T. Somatosensory, multisensory and task-related neurons in cortical area 7b (PF) of unanesthetized monkeys. *J Neurophysiol* 1994 ; 72 : 1-23.
61. Perl ER, Whitlockk DG. Somatic stimuli exciting spinothalamic projections to thalamic neurons in cat and monkey. *Exp Neurol* 1961 ; 3 : 256-96.
62. Casey KL. Unit analysis of nociceptive mechanisms in the thalamus of the awake squirrel monkey. *J Neurophysiol* 1966 ; 29 : 727-50.
63. Jones E, Powell T. Connections of the somatic sensory cortex of the rhesus monkey II. Contralateral cortical connections. *Brain* 1969 ; 92 : 717-30.
64. Pandya D, Vignolo L. Interhemispheric projections of the parietal lobe in the rhesus M monkey. *Brain Res* 1969 ; 15 : 49-65.
65. Myers R, Ebner F. Localization of functions in corpus callosum: tactual information transmission in *Macaca mulatta. Brain Res* 1976 : 103 : 455-62.

9

The role of excitatory amino acid receptors in thalamic nociception

S.A. EATON, T.E. SALT

Department of Visual Science, Institute of Ophthalmology, London, U.K.

The ventrobasal thalamus (VBT) is the principal thalamic nucleus involved in the transfer and processing of somatosensory information ascending to the somatosensory cortex [1]. In addition to the vast majority of neurons which respond to low threshold somatosensory stimulation (*e.g.* [2]), the VBT also contains a population of nociceptive neurons and it has been proposed that these neurons play an important role in the sensory-discriminative aspect of nociception [3]. Neurons located in the thalamus immediately dorsal to the VBT, in the posterior nuclear complex (PO) and in the laterodorsal thalamic nucleus (LD), also respond to noxious sensory stimulation [4, 5]. The VBT and PO not only project to the somatosensory cortex, but also receive a massive projection from the somatosensory cortex. The role of the cortico-thalamic projection in general is not clear, although recent evidence and speculation indicate that this projection may serve to lock on to specific stimulus features and function as a neuronal spotlight [6, 7]. Until recently, the thalamus has generally been considered to be a simple relay station for information ascending from the periphery to the cerebral cortex.

It has since become clear that, in fact, a considerable degree of integration occurs within the thalamus, including the VBT (*e.g.* [8]). It has also been suggested that the PO serves not as a thalamic relay for information transfer from the periphery to the neocortex, but, instead, as an integral component of a cortico-thalamo-cortical loop [9] which may act to regulate the level of communication between columns in the barrel cortex [10].

Ionotropic excitatory amino acid receptors are thought to mediate synaptic transmission throughout the vertebrate central nervous system [11], and these receptors can be subclassified broadly into N-methyl-D-aspartate (NMDA) and non-NMDA (AMPA/kainate) receptor types. It has become apparent that excitatory amino acids can also act at receptors coupled to second messenger systems, the so-called metabotropic receptors. Currently, metabotropic glutamate receptors can be divided into 3 subgroups on the basis of sequence homology and second messenger coupling, as well as agonist and antagonist preference [12]. Metabotropic receptor group I consists of $mGluR_1$ and $mGluR_5$; these receptors are coupled to inositol phosphate metabolism, can be activated by (1S,3R)-1-aminocyclopentane-1,3-dicarboxylic acid ((lS,3R)-ACPD) and antagonized by a range of novel phenylglycine derivatives, including (S)-4-Carboxy-3-hydroxyphenylglycine ((S)-4C3HPG). Although there is some electrophysiological evidence for the involvement of ACPD-activated metabotropic receptors in the corticofugal input to the visual thalamus [13], any direct pharmacological demonstration has not been possible until recently due to the lack of selective antagonists.

We have previously shown, using intracellular and extracellular recording techniques *in vivo*, that both NMDA and non-NMDA (AMPA/kainate) ionotropic receptors mediate the synaptic responses of neurones in the VBT to natural, low-threshold somatosensory stimulation [14, 15]. Group I metabotropic receptors do not, however, appear to contribute to these sensory synaptic responses [16]. The types of receptors involved in synaptic transmission of nociceptive information to neurons in the VBT, PO and LD have not been determined. We have therefore used iontophoretic application of glutamate receptor antagonists to determine which receptor sub-types mediate synaptic input to the thalamus, evoked by noxious sensory stimulation.

The results presented here suggest that NMDA receptors and group I metabotropic receptors mediate the synaptic response to noxious stimulation. This combination of receptors also mediates cortical input to the VBT. Additional experiments showed that the synaptic response to noxious stimulation was virtually abolished by cooling the somatosensory cortex. Taken together, these findings suggest an important role for the neocortex in the generation of synaptic responses in the thalamus to peripheral stimulation and contribute to the growing body of evidence which suggests that the thalamus is not a simple sensory relay, but rather the site of complex integrative control over sensory information flow.

Experimental procedures

Animal preparation

Experiments were performed on adult, male Wistar rats (weight 310-530g), as described in detail previously [17].

Anaesthesia was induced with diethyl ether or halothane and maintained with urethane (1.2g/kg) administered intraperitoneally. Electrocardiogram and electroencephalogram were recorded and displayed continuously as monitors of adequate anaesthesia. Tracheal cannulation aided respiration and correct body temperature was maintained using a thermostatically controlled heating blanket. All wound margins were infiltrated with lignocaine (1% with 1:200000 adrenaline). The head of the animal was held in a stereotaxic frame, a discrete craniotomy was made (ca. 9mm^2, centred above the proposed recording site) and the dura cleared to allow electrode entry. Recordings were made 2.5 - 3mm lateral, 2 - 2.5mm posterior to bregma according to the atlas of Paxinos and Watson [18]. In cortical cooling experiments, a discrete craniotomy was made above the somatosensory cortex and the cortex was cooled by deposition of ice on the cortical surface.

Recording, iontophoresis and sensory stimulation

Extracellular single neurone recordings and iontophoretic application of drugs were made in the thalamus using multibarrel electrode assemblies. Conventional 5- or 7-barrelled glass electrodes were used, or electrode assemblies, consisting of a tungsten-in-glass recording electrode glued alongside a 7-barrelled iontophoretic electrode. Each barrel of the electrode contained either a different drug solution or NaCl solution for neuronal recording or automatic current balancing.

Iontophoretic barrels contained one of Na N-methyl-D-aspartate (NMDA, 50mM, pH 8), Na N-methyl-D,L-aspartate (NMA, 100mM, pH 8), Na (RS)-α-amino-3-hydroxy-5-methyl-4-isoxazolepropionate (AMPA, 10mM in 150mM NaCl, pH 8), Na kainate (50mM, pH 8), Na quisqualate (25mM in 75mM NaCl, pH 8), (1S,3R)-1-aminocyclopentane-1,3-dicarboxylic acid ((1S,3R)-ACPD, 50mM, pH 8.5), Na 3-((±)-2-carboxypiperazin-4-yl) propyl-1-phosphonate (CPP, 20mM in 75mM NaCl, pH 8), 6-cyano-7-nitroquinoxaline-2,3-dione (CNQX, 1mM in 50mM NaCl, pH 8), (S)-4-carboxy-3-hydroxyphenylglycine ((S)-4C3HPG, 50mM, pH 8). CPP, CNQX and (S)-4C3HPG were generous gifts from Sandoz (Berne), Ferrosan (Soeborg) and Professor JC Watkins (Bristol), respectively.

NMDA, AMPA, (1S,3R)-ACPD, kainate and quisqualate were obtained from Tocris (Bristol). All remaining drugs were obtained from Sigma. One barrel routinely contained pontamine sky blue (PSB) dye (2.5% w/v in 0.5M Na acetate / 0.5M NaCl) which could be used for the histological verification of selected recording sites. Automatic current balancing could be performed through a barrel containing 1M NaCl or the PSB solution. However, no qualitative differences were seen between experiments with or without current balancing.

Conventional extracellular recording and amplification techniques were used to record action potentials. These potentials were gated by a waveform discriminator and timed by a computer system in order to generate peristimulus time histograms (PSTHs).

Responses were quantified by counting the number of action potentials occurring during the response period. Excitatory amino acid receptor agonists were iontophoretically applied in computer-generated, time-locked cycles. Responses to agonists were recorded before, during and after concurrent, continuous iontophoretic application of an antagonist. Whenever necessary, multiple antagonist ejections were made in order to determine the appropriate ejection currents and durations which would cause the most selective antagonism of the desired agonist. When the effects of the antagonist against the agonists had been ascertained, reproducible responses to noxious sensory stimulation were challenged by the antagonist, ejected at the same current magnitude and for the same duration. Sensory stimulation consisted of immersion of the whole tail in water at 52 °C for 15 - 60 seconds duration [4].

Results

As reported previously [3-5], nociceptive neurons were located in the ventrobasal thalamus (VBT), the laterodorsal thalamic nucleus (LD) and in the region between these two nuclei, designated the posterior nuclear group (PO) according to the atlas of Paxinos and Watson [18].

The effects of CPP on responses to excitatory amino acids and noxious sensory stimulation

On 24 neurons, CPP was tested against the responses to N-methyl-D,L-aspartate (NMA) and one or more non-NMDA receptor agonists. CPP abolished or greatly reduced the responses to NMA, with little or no effect against responses mediated by agonists acting at other receptor types (Table I and Figure 1).

At these NMA-selective ejection currents, CPP markedly reduced the action potential responses to noxious sensory stimulation of the same neurons (Table I; Figure 1).

The effects of CNQX on responses to excitatory amino acids and noxious sensory stimulation

The AMPA/kainate receptor antagonist, CNQX, was tested against responses to noxious stimulation and a variety of iontophoretically applied excitatory amino acid receptor agonists on 17 neurons.

On all of the neurons tested, CNQX greatly reduced the responses to AMPA and/or kainate compared with responses to NMA, yet had little or no effect against the synaptic response to noxious sensory stimulation (Figure 2; Table I).

EXCITATORY AMINO ACID RECEPTORS IN THALAMIC NOCICEPTION

Table I. The effects of CPP, (S)-4C3HPG and CNQX on responses to excitatory amino acids and noxious sensory stimulation.

	Kainate	Quisqualate	AMPA	NMA or NMDA	Heat 52 C
CPP	97.7 ± 21.0 (8) n = 8	91.5 ± 24.5 (13) n = 18		19.0 ± 20.0 (24) n = 29	24.1 ± 18.2 (24) n = 29
(S)-4C3HPG		159.5 ± 33.2 (2) n = 2	103.7 ± 28.3 (10) n = 10	118.5 ± 47.7 (12) n = 12	38.5 ± 26.3 (12) n = 12
CNQX	26.6 ± 14.9 (16) n = 18	119.7 ± 69.0 (3) n = 3	57.2 ± 38.0 (12) n = 14	87.5 ± 24.4 (17) n = 19	97.7 ± 13.6 (17) n = 19

Values are mean percentage responses relative to control values, ± standard deviation of *n* trials. Values in parentheses represent the number of neurons.

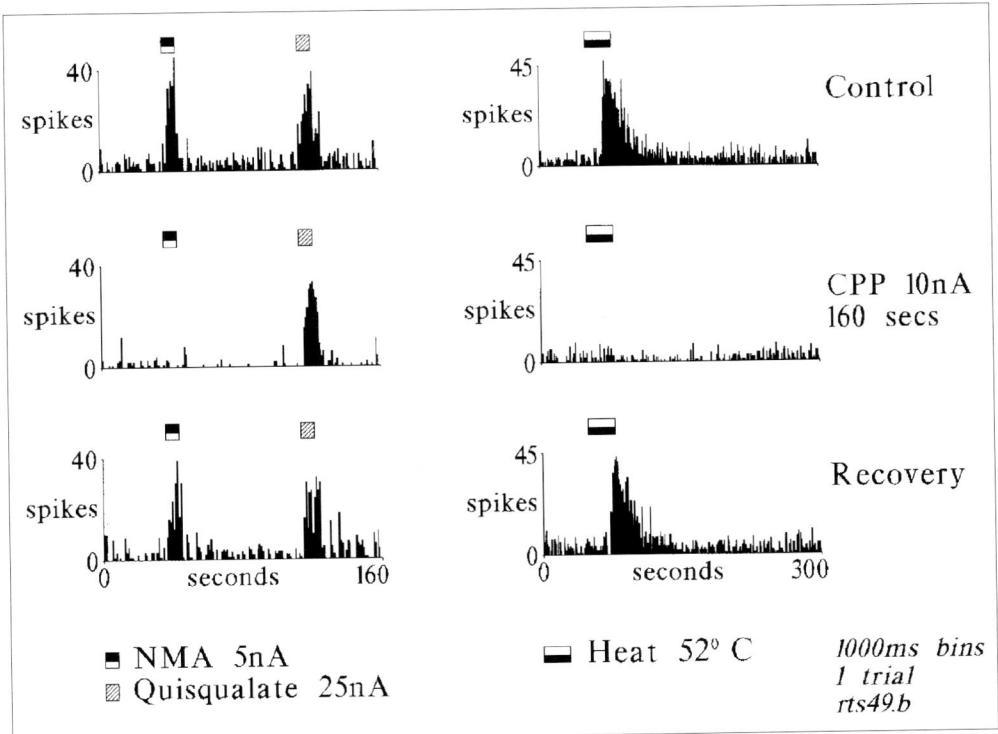

Figure 1. Antagonism of responses to NMA and noxious thermal stimulation by CPP. Records are PSTHs of action potential spikes counted into one-second epochs. The bars above the records correspond to the timing and duration of agonist applications or thermal stimulation (*see* key). Upper panels: control responses to iontophoresis of NMA and Quisqualate, and to noxious thermal stimulation. Middle panels: responses to the same stimuli but during the concurrent iontophoresis of CPP at 10nA for 160 seconds. Note that the antagonist blocked responses to both NMA and noxious thermal stimulation. Bottom panels: recovery from the effects of CPP after the termination of the ejection.

The effects of (S)-4C3HPG on responses to excitatory amino acids and noxious sensory stimulation

The group I metabotropic receptor antagonist, (S)-4C3HPG, attenuated the responses to (1S,3R)-ACPD on all of the 12 neurons tested in this study and concurrently enhanced or had little effect against the responses to NMDA, AMPA or quisqualate (Figure 3; Table I). (S)-4C3HPG reduced the synaptic responses to noxious stimulation on all but one of the 12 neurons tested.

The effects of cortical cooling on responses to noxious sensory stimulation

Cooling the somatosensory cortex attenuated the sensory response to noxious stimulation on all of the five neurones tested. Figure 4 shows typical synaptic responses before, during and after cortical cooling.

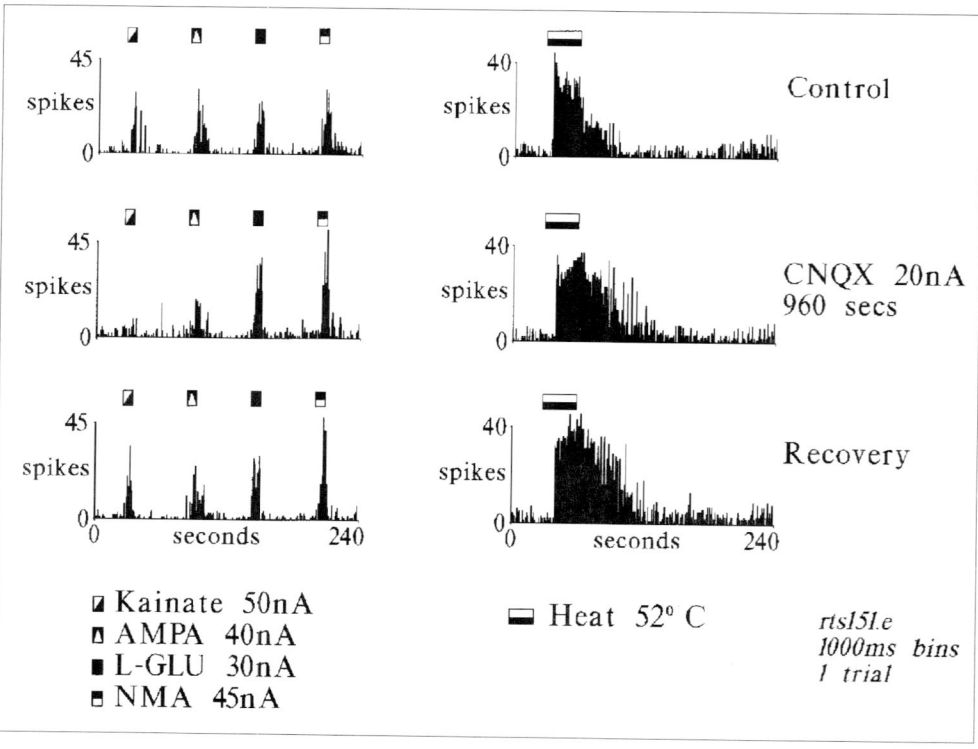

Figure 2. CNQX reduced the responses to kainate and AMPA, but not the synaptic response to noxious stimulation. For figure details *see* Figure 1. Upper panels: control responses to kainate, AMPA, L-glutamate, NMA and thermal stimulation. Middle panels: effects of concurrent ejection of CNQX; responses to kainate and AMPA are attenuated, but the response to NMA and the synaptic response are not reduced. Bottom panels: recovery after the end of the CNQX ejection.

Discussion

In these experiments, care has been taken to test the selectivity of the antagonists for their appropriate receptor(s), to ensure that any reduction in the synaptic response by the antagonist is associated with an action of the antagonist at the appropriate receptor type. The group I metabotropic receptor antagonist, (S)-4C3HPG, selectively antagonized ACPD responses and the synaptic response to noxious sensory stimulation. Similarly, CPP reduced the synaptic response at ejection currents which selectively antagonized responses to the NMDA receptor agonist, NMA. In contrast, CNQX had little or no effect against the sensory response, despite reducing responses mediated at AMPA/kainate receptors on the same neurons. These findings suggest that the synaptic response to noxious sensory stimulation is mediated by NMDA receptors and group I metabotropic receptors, whilst CNQX-sensitive AMPA/kainate receptors make little or no contribution to the sensory response.

The finding that NMDA receptors and group I metabotropic receptors are so substantially involved in this synaptic response is unusual and distinctive. In particular, the utilization of this combination of glutamate receptor subtypes is very different to the

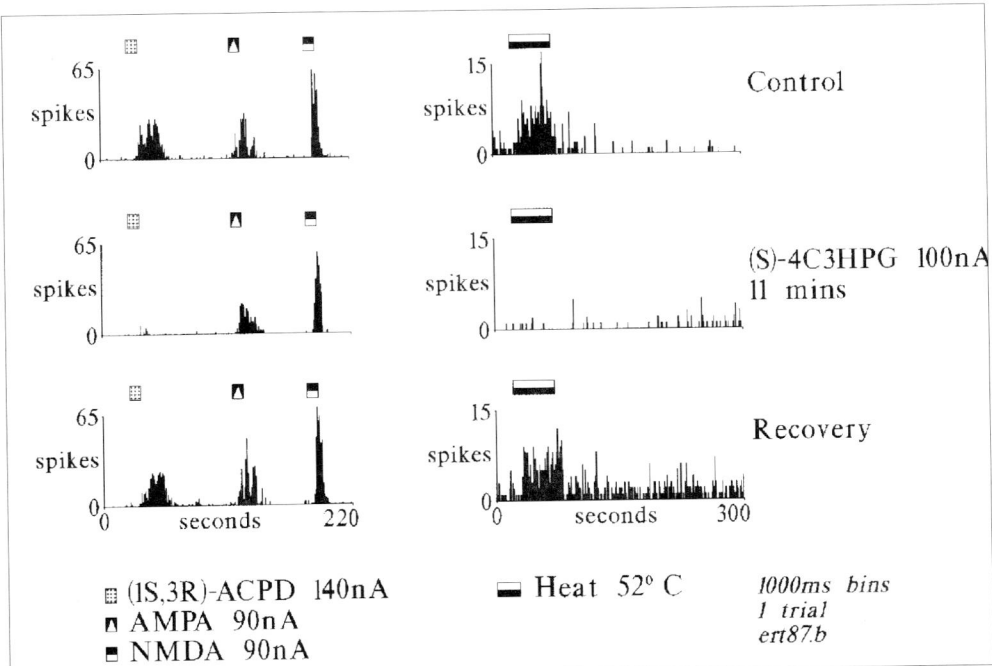

Figure 3. Antagonism of responses to (1S,3R)-ACPD and noxious thermal stimulation by the metabotropic receptor antagonist (S)-4C3HPG. For figure details see Figure 1. Upper panels: control responses to (1S,3R)-ACPD, AMPA, NMDA and noxious heat. Middle panels: the same series of stimuli during the ejection of (S)-4C3HPG. Bottom panels: recovery from the effects of the antagonist.

combination of glutamate receptor subtypes which mediate non-noxious somatosensory afferent input to VBT neurons. In the VBT, synaptic responses evoked by low threshold, air jet stimulation of the peripheral receptive field are mediated by AMPA/kainate receptors and by NMDA receptors, but not by group I metabotropic receptors [14-16]. It appears, therefore, that different somatosensory modalities utilise different combinations of glutamate receptor subtypes. These findings might be important in the development of novel centrally-acting analgesic agents.

In this study, nociceptive neurons were recorded in the VBT and in the thalamus dorsal to the VBT, although the majority of nociceptive neurons were recorded in thalamic regions dorsal to the VBT, mainly in the PO. It has also been suggested on anatomical grounds that the PO serves not as a thalamic relay for information transfer from the periphery to the neocortex, but instead, as part of a cortico-thalamo-cortical loop [9]. Electrophysiological evidence also indicates that PO may have such a function [10]. The effects of cooling the somatosensory cortex on the synaptic response to noxious sensory stimulation, presented here, also indicate that these sensory responses are strongly dependent upon the somatosensory cortex. Reports from other laboratories

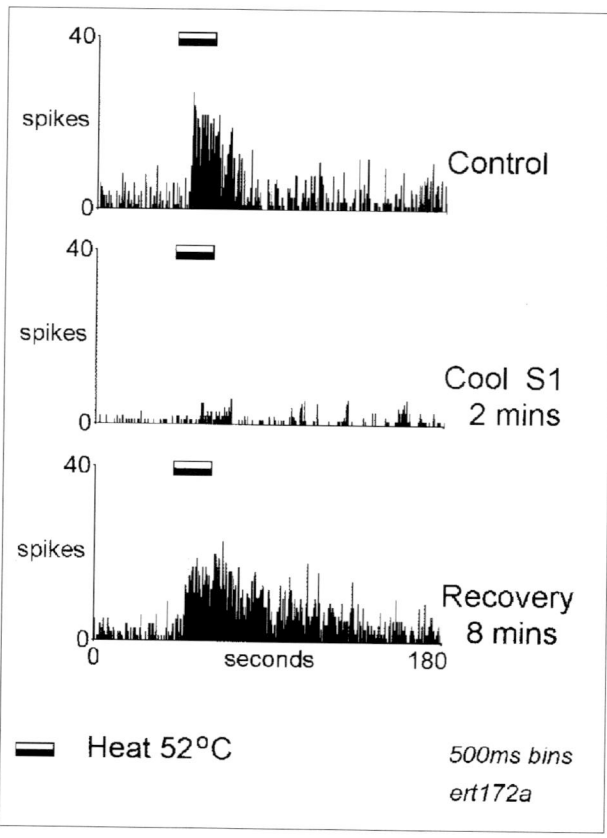

Figure 4. Reduced synaptic response to noxious thermal stimulation during cooling of the somatosensory cortex. For figure details see Figure 1. Upper panel: control response to noxious thermal stimulation. Middle panel: synaptic response of the same neuron during cooling of the somatosensory cortex. Note the marked reduction in the sensory synaptic response. Bottom panels: recovery of the synaptic response on re-warming of the somatosensory cortex.

have shown the response of thalamic neurons to sensory stimulation can be attenuated by cortical inactivation [10, 19].

In addition, in our previous experiments where the somatosensory cortex had been deliberately ablated, neurons which we would have expected to have nociceptive receptive fields appeared to have none (unpublished observations). In this respect it is interesting that cortical input to the VBT is mediated by the same combination of receptors that mediate synaptic responses to noxious sensory stimulation: in recent experiments we have combined intracellular recording with iontophoretic application of drugs onto the same neuron, *in vivo*. Electrical stimulation of the somatosensory cortex typically evokes an excitatory postsynaptic potential (EPSP) which is rapidly curtailed by a sequence of inhibitory postsynaptic potentials (IPSPs). Preliminary results show that the cortically-evoked EPSP could be reduced by an NMDA receptor antagonist and by a group I metabotropic receptor antagonist, but not by the AMPA/kainate receptor antagonist, CNQX (unpublished data). The similarity between the receptor types which mediate cortical input to the VBT and the synaptic response to noxious sensory stimulation is readily apparent.

Taken together with the strong dependency of the response to noxious sensory stimulation on the somatosensory cortex, it would seem that the thalamic response to noxious stimulation seen in this study may in fact be generated predominantly by the neocortex, perhaps resulting from a reverberative activity in the proposed cortico-thalamo-cortical loop.

It has been observed that the responses of VBT nociceptive neurons are subject to long term enhancement following a relatively short period of inflammation of the receptive field [20] and that possibly central, rather than peripheral, modifications may account for changes in thalamic neuronal activity [21]. Given that NMDA receptors have been specifically implicated in synaptic plasticity in several brain areas [22], it is interesting to speculate that the substantial contribution of NMDA receptors in synaptic transmission of nociceptive information to the thalamic neurons in this study might correlate with recently observed changes in their activity in a model of hyperalgesic inflammation [21].

Considering the substantial contribution to the noxious synaptic response made by group I metabotropic receptors, it is also conceivable that activation of intracellular second-messenger systems may play a role in such adaptive processes. Furthermore, if this thalamic sensory response is dependent upon the somatosensory cortex, then changes in synaptic plasticity within the somatosensory cortex itself (*e.g.* [23]) could lead to modified response properties within the thalamus.

Conclusions

In conclusion, synaptic transmission to nociceptive thalamic neurones appears to be mediated predominantly by NMDA receptors and group I metabotropic excitatory amino acid receptors. The involvement of CNQX-sensitive non-NMDA receptors, if any, is not extensive. These data show that the combination of excitatory amino acid receptor types utilized in synaptic transmission of noxious somatosensory information differ from those previously reported to mediate non-noxious somatosensory information to the VBT. The sensory response to noxious stimuli appears to be strongly dependent upon the somatosensory cortex and shares a similar synaptic pharmacology, suggesting that the thalamic response to noxious stimulation may be generated predominantly by the neocortex, perhaps resulting from a reverberative activity in a cortico-thalamo-cortical loop.

Acknowledgements

This work was supported by the Medical Research Council and Wellcome Trust.

References

1. Jones EG. *The thalamus*. New York : Plenum Press, 1985.
2. Waite PME. Somatotopic organization of vibrissal responses in the ventro-basal complex of the rat thalamus. *J Physiol* 1973 ; 228 : 527-40.
3. Peschanski M, Guilbaud G, Gautron M, Besson J-M. Encoding of noxious heat messages in neurons of the ventrobasal thalamic complex of the rat. *Brain Res* 1980 ; 197 : 401-13.
4. Hill RG, Pepper CM. Selective effects of morphine on the nociceptive responses of thalamic neurons in the rat. *Br J Pharmac* 1978 ; 64 : 137-43.
5. Guilbaud G, Peschanski M, Gautron M, Binder D. Neurons responding to noxious stimulation in VB complex and caudal adjacent regions in the thalamus of the rat. *Pain* 1980 ; 8 : 303-18.
6. Sillito AM, Jones HE, Gerstein GL, West DC. Feature-linked synchronization of thalamic relay cell firing induced by feedback from the visual cortex. *Nature* 1994 ; 369 : 479-82.
7. Koch C. The action of the corticofugal pathway on sensory thalamic nuclei: a hypothesis. *Neuroscience* 1987 ; 23 : 399-406.
8. Lee SM, Friedberg MH, Ebner FF. The role of GABA-mediated inhibition in the rat ventral posterior medial thalamus. I. Assessment of receptive field changes following thalamic reticular nucleus lesions. *J Neurophysiol* 1994 ; 71 : 1702-15.
9. Nothias F, Peschanski M, Besson J-M. Somatotopic reciprocal connections between the somatosensory cortex and the thalamic PO nucleus in the rat. *Brain Res* 1988 ; 447 : 169-74.
10. Diamond ME, Armstrong-James M, Budway MJ, Ebner FF. Somatic sensory responses in the rostral sector of the posterior group (POm) and VPM of the rat thalamus: dependence on the barrel field cortex. *J Comp Neurol* 1992 ; 319 : 66-84.
11. Mayer ML, Westbrook GL. The physiology of excitatory amino acids in the vertebrate central nervous system. *Prog Neurobiol* 1987 ; 28 : 197-276.
12. Watkins JC, Collingridge G. Phenylglycine derivatives as antagonists of metabotropic glutamate receptors. *Trends Pharmacol Sci* 1994 ; 15 : 333-42.

13. McCormick DA, Von Krosigk M. Corticothalamic activation modulates thalamic firing through glutamate "metabotropic" receptors. *Proc Natl Acad Sci USA* 1992 ; 89 : 2774-8.
14. Salt TE, Eaton SA. Function of non-NMDA receptors and NMDA receptors in synaptic responses to natural somatosensory stimulation in the ventrobasal thalamus. *Exp Brain Res* 1989 ; 77 : 646-52.
15. Salt TE, Eaton SA. Sensory excitatory postsynaptic potentials mediated by NMDA and non-NMDA receptors in the thalamus *in vivo*. *Eur J Neurosci* 1991 ; 3 : 296-300.
16. Salt TE, Eaton SA. The function of metabotropic excitatory amino acid receptors in synaptic transmission in the thalamus: studies with novel phenylglycine antagonists. *Neurochem Internat* 1994 ; 24 : 451-8.
17. Salt TE. Excitatory amino acid receptors and synaptic transmission in the rat ventrobasal thalamus. *J Physiol* 1987 ; 391 : 499-510.
18. Paxinos G, Watson C. *The rat brain in stereotaxic co-ordinates*. Sydney : Academic Press, 1982.
19. Condes-Lara M, Zapata IO. Suppression of noxious thermal evoked responses in thalamic central lateral nucleus by cortical spreading depression. *Pain* 1988 ; 35 : 199-204.
20. Guilbaud G, Kayser V, Benoist JM, Gautron M. Modifications in the responsiveness of rat ventrobasal thalamic neurones at different stages of carrageenin-produced inflammation. *Brain Res* 1986 ; 385 : 86-98.
21. Guilbaud G, Benoist JM, Eschalier A, Kayser V, Gautron M, Attal N. Evidence for central phenomena participating in the changes of responses of ventrobasal neurons in arthritic rats. *Brain Res* 1989 ; 484 : 383-8.
22. Collingridge GL, Singer W. Excitatory amino acid receptors and synaptic plasticity. *Tr Pharmacol Sci* 1990 ; 11 : 290-6.
23. Lee SM, Ebner FF. Induction of high frequency activity in the somatosensory thalamus of rats *in vivo* results in long-term potentiation of responses in the SI cortex. *Exp Brain Res* 1992 ; 90 : 253-61.

10

Brain neural images of persistent pain states in rats using 2-DG autoradiography

D.D. PRICE, J. MAO, D.J. MAYER

Department of Anesthesiology, Medical College of Virginia, Richmond, Virginia, U.S.A.

Until recently, understanding of the role of the forebrain in pain has remained elusive, partly for methodological reasons. For example, attempts to record from cortical neurons selectively or differentially responsive to nociceptive stimuli have resulted in few numbers of characterized neurons even within somatosensory cortical areas [1-3]. However, though few in number, cortical nociceptive neurons clearly exist and their responses to controlled graded nociceptive stimuli parallel several psychophysical attributes of pain, including exquisite discriminability of heat stimuli in the noxious range [2, 3]. Similarly, it has been difficult to elicit pain sensations by electrical stimulation of cortical sites within the somatosensory cortex of awake human patients. The paucity of such sites (11 of 426 stimulation sites) led neurosurgeons to the view that pain is a diencephalic phenomenon and that the cerebral cortex has no direct role in nociception [4, 5]. Paradoxically, other types of evidence indicate that pain is associated with multiple activation of cortical regions. Indeed, widespread cortical activation by painful stimuli has been observed electroencephalographically and by means of increases in blood flow over wide areas of the cerebral cortex, especially frontal cortical areas [6]. These responses are consistent with results of studies showing that lesions or damage to various cortical regions result in distinct deficits in some aspect of pain experience in man, for example the reduction in some aspect of pain-associated suffering in frontal lobotomy patients [7, 8]. Thus, there are several lines of indirect evidence that the human cerebral cortex is involved in different dimensions of pain, though the exact cortical representations of these various dimensions remain poorly understood. The problem, as pointed out by Willis [6], is that it is far more likely that the cerebral cortex has multiple representations of pain than it has none.

Recent advances in functional imaging in both human and other animal species provide a potentially powerful tool for helping to determine the functional role of thalamic and cortical structures in pain processing and thereby resolving these disparate views of the roles of forebrain areas in pain. In this chapter, we present a comparison of our results of mapping neural activity of brain regions in sciatic nerve injured rats with results of other groups of investigators who have mapped human and/or animal brain activity in response to various types of pain conditions. Based on this comparison, we contend that the cortical representation of pain is spatially distributed over regions likely to be involved in sensory, affective, and cognitive-evaluative aspects of pain, that this spatial distribution is at least generally consistent across different species and mapping techniques, and that the extent of this spatial distribution is greater than that which occurs in non-painful somatosensory processing.

Mapping 2-DG metabolic activity in sciatic nerve constricted rats

Peripheral nerve injury sometimes results in a chronic neuropathic pain syndrome characterized by hyperalgesia, spontaneous pain, radiation of pain, and nociceptive responses to normally innocuous stimulation (allodynia) [9]. Most of these symptoms have been recently observed in a rodent model of painful peripheral mononeuropathy induced by loose ligation of the rat's common sciatic nerve (chronic constrictive injury, CCI) [10]. For example, one prominent change seen in CCI rats is the appearance of ongoing behaviors such as typical hind paw guarding positions following sciatic nerve ligation, suggesting the presence of persistent spontaneous pain [10, 11]. However, based on these behaviors alone, it is difficult to determine whether CCI rats truly experience spontaneous pain or these ongoing behaviors simply occur as a defense against pains evoked by mechanical or thermal stimuli from the affected area. Some evidence indicating the presence of spontaneous pain in CCI rats derives from recent [^{14}C]-2-deoxyglucose (2-DG) autoradiographic studies that show that spinal cord neural activity (inferred from increased local glucose utilization rate) increases substantially in the absence of overt peripheral stimulation in CCI rats 10 days after sciatic nerve ligation [12, 13]. Consistent with spontaneous increases in spinal cord neural activity in CCI rats, electrophysiological studies have indicated increases in spontaneous neuronal discharges both in spinothalamic tract neurons [14] and in the ventrobasal thalamic complex [15] of CCI rats 2-3 weeks after peripheral nerve injury. In view of the critical roles of supraspinal structures in nociceptive processing, more conclusive evidence for the existence of spontaneous pain in CCI rats should be provided if increased neural activity occurs in brain regions that have been implicated in pain. Furthermore, a three-dimensional mapping of such activity could help characterize the relative contribution of various forebrain structures to persistent pain states.

Using the 2-DG metabolic mapping technique, we examined the spatial distribution of neural activity throughout the entire brain of CCI rats, examining brain structures implicated in supraspinal nociceptive processing. The advantage of using this technique is that it allows examination of relative intensities of activation of multiple central nervous system areas affected by a stimulus or behavioral condition, by measuring local glucose utilization rates during a relatively long period (30 - 40 min) [16-22]. Thus, the 2-DG technique is particularly suitable for mapping neural activity during prolonged noxious stimulation [20] or ongoing nociception such as in this CCI model [12, 13]. Comparable electrophysiological single unit examinations of the spatial distribution of neural activity within the entire nervous system would be impossible. Spatial patterns of increased spinal cord neural activity in CCI rats, also determined by the 2-DG technique, served as guidelines for examining spatial patterns of increases in neural activity in specific brain regions of CCI rats. For instance, spinal cord regions showing increased neural activity in these CCI rats include superficial laminae I-II, deep dorsal horn laminae V-VI, and the ventral horn lamina VII [12, 13], regions highly implicated in spinal cord nociceptive processing and representing the main origin of ascending spinothalamic, spinoreticular, and spinomesencephalic tracts. These pathways transmit somatosensory information to many brain structures involved in supraspinal nociceptive processing [6, 21].

The possibility that structures activated by impulses in these ascending pathways were investigated in CCI rats 10 days after sciatic nerve injury [22]. The discovery that striking increases in 2-DG metabolic activity occurred in widespread brain regions of CCI rats represented the first functional mapping of supraspinal neural activity resulting from a chronic pain condition. These increases in 2-DG metabolic activity, shown in Figure 1, occurred in CCI rats with demonstrable thermal hyperalgesia and spontaneous pain behaviors. The fact that peak increases in metabolic activity occurred in contralateral brain regions previously implicated in supraspinal nociceptive processing suggests a causal relationship between increases in brain neural activity (as measured by 2-DG metabolic activity) and neuropathic pain behaviors in CCI rats. These striking increases in neural activity, which occur in the absence of overt peripheral stimulation, provide further evidence that ongoing pain behaviors reflect persistent spontaneous pain in CCI rats and are not exclusively defensive behaviors directed toward avoiding pain.

Functional relationships to brain regions implicated in nociceptive processing

The extensive activation of brain regions of a CCI rat in comparison with a sham operated control is shown in Figure 1. The pattern of activation shown is representative of results based on statistical analysis of group data [22]. This pattern of activation most likely reflects central nervous system processing of neuropathic pain and not non-specific elevation of neural activity in CCI rats for several reasons. First, increases in brain neural activity of CCI rats reflect the anatomic and functional continuation of ascending spinal cord somatosensory pathways (e.g. spinoreticular, spinomesencephalic, and spinothalamic tracts), whose spinal cord origins (laminae I-IV, V-VI, VII) exhibit substantially elevated neural activity in these same CCI rats (*cf.*

results in [12] and [13]). Second, brain regions that are very unlikely to be involved in pain, such as those within the visual pathway (lateral geniculate body, occipital cortex) and the vestibular pathway (medullar vestibular nuclei) remained unchanged in CCI rats as compared to sham-operated rats. Third, a large body of evidence indicates that the increase in brain neural activity in CCI rats exhibits regional specificity with respect to known anatomical and electrophysiological involvement of these regions in supraspinal nociceptive processing.

The pattern of elevation in 2-DG activity shown in Figure 1 is likely to reflect mainly excitatory processes related to action potential generation and conduction for several reasons. First, studies of combined 2-DG measurement and physiological recording of primate somatosensory cortex strongly suggest that neural excitation is a major contribution to increases in 2-DG metabolic activity [23], and, in fact, inhibitory neural events are shown to decrease local glucose utilization in these studies. Second,

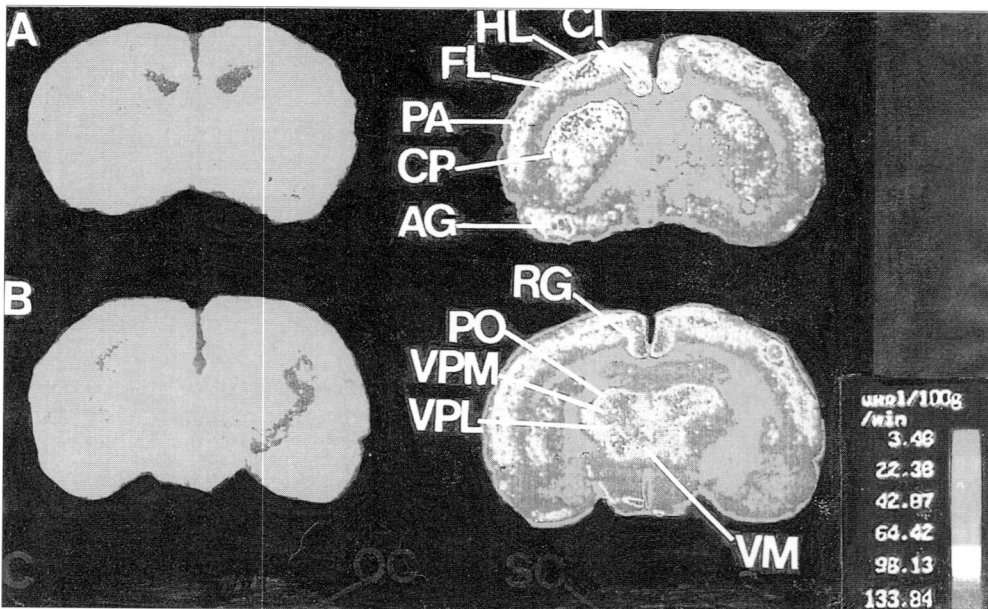

Figure 1. Topographic presentation of coronal sections showing local glucose utilization in the brain of a CCI rat (right column) and a sham-operated rat (left column). Sciatic nerve ligation produced substantial increases in metabolic activity within cortical hind limb (HL) and fore limb (FL) area, retrosplenial granular cortex (RG), cingulate cortex (CI), parietal area (PA), caudate-putamen complex (CP), amygdala (AG), ventral posterolateral thalamic nucleus (VPL), ventral posteromedial thalamic nucleus (VPM), ventral medial thalamic nucleus (VM), as compared to corresponding regions of sham-operated rats. This increase was more pronounced on the contralateral side (left side of an image) of CCI rats than on the ipsilateral side.

The anteroposterior coordinates (from Bregma) of each coronal section (from pair A to pair E) are -0.80 mm, -3.14 mm, -7.80 mm, -9.80 mm, and -11.96 mm, respectively, based on the Paxinos and Watson's Atlas (Paxinos and Watson, 1986). The middle-bottom color bar represents the calibration of the local glucose utilization rate (μmoles/100g/min) for these images. (See appendix for colour figures.)

consistent with these observations, recent electrophysiological studies have reported increased background neuronal discharges within the lumbar spinal cord [14] and the thalamic ventrobasal complex [15] of CCI rats, in which substantial increases in 2-DG metabolic activity are detected under comparable conditions [12, 13]. Third and finally, the 2-DG technique is based on the well-understood mechanism that the increase in local cerebral glucose utilization is proportional to the increase in neural activity, particularly to processes related to action potential generation and the sodium-potassium pump [17].

Thus, the patterns of increased metabolic activity can be at least generally interpreted as representing relative density of excitatory neural processes. The relationships between observed increases in neural activity and evidence for involvement in nociceptive processing or pain modulation will be discussed for individual brain regions in turn.

Thalamus and hypothalamus

The role of thalamic somatosensory relay nuclei and their adjacent regions in brain nociceptive processing has been well documented [6, 21, 24-27]. Accordingly, the ventral posterolateral thalamic nucleus, posterior thalamic nucleus, ventral lateral and medial thalamic nuclei, and central medial and lateral thalamic nuclei were shown to be highly activated in the 2-DG/brain study. Moreover, results from our 2-DG labeling are also consistent with the data derived from a recent electrophysiological study [15]. In that study, abnormal neuronal responses within the ventrobasal thalamic complex (regions corresponding to major thalamic relay nuclei in our 2-DG labeling) were observed in the same CCI model used in the present 2-DG experiment, including increased spontaneous neuronal activity, fading of the response with repetitive stimulation, and prolonged after discharges [15].

Consistent with the involvement of the hypothalamic arcuate nucleus in pain modulation, increases in 2-DG metabolic activity are also seen in this hypothalamic nucleus in CCI rats. Direct spinohypothalamic projections from both superficial spinal laminae I-II and the base of dorsal horn has been recently reported [28]. This direct spinohypothalamic pathway may at least partially account for the activation of hypothalamic nuclei in CCI rats. The hypothalamic arcuate nucleus is the major origin of β-endorphinergic neurons in the brain and β-endorphin is known to play important roles in pain modulation. Thus, the activation of the hypothalamic arcuate nucleus may have a descending inhibitory influence on nociceptive processing in CCI rats. On the other hand, since the hypothalamic arcuate nucleus has numerous connections with brainstem structures and the pituitary [29], and is therefore involved in regulation of many physiological reactions including stress and emotional reactions, its activation in CCI rats may reflect possible roles of this hypothalamic nucleus in the affective-motivational dimension of pain in CCI rats.

Cortex and subcortical areas

Regions activated at the cortical level such as parietal areas and the hind limb somatosensory area, areas corresponding to the rat's primary somatosensory area (SI) [30] are consistent with those thalamic somatosensory relay nuclei showing increased neural activity in CCI rats. Of particular interest is the fact that peak activity occurred within the hind limb area of the somatosensory cortex (Figure 1). Nociceptive neuronal responses within these cortical areas have been reported in previous animal and human studies [6, 21, 31, 32]. It should be emphasized that the activation of cortical areas in CCI rats presents a general laminar organization (Figure 1). Thus, increased neural activity occurs mainly within middle and deep layers of the cortex, a feature consistent with the heavy concentration of wide dynamic range and nociceptive-specific neurons found in these cortical layers in electrophysiological studies [32].

The caudate and putamen complex is part of the subcortical basal ganglia which is known as a central region involved in coordination of motor activity [30]. Several recent reports, however, have indicated its role in pain modulation. Given the abnormal motor activity resulting from abnormal guarding postures in CCI rats, the activation of the caudate and putamen complex may be related to pain modulation and/or pain-related abnormal motoric activity [33].

It is surprising that the greatest increase in 2-DG metabolic activity occurs within the retrosplenial granular cortex of CCI rats (Figure 1). The retrosplenial granular cortex is an association cortex which has numerous reciprocal connections with the thalamus, hypothalamus, limbic structures, and other cortical areas [34, 35]. To our knowledge, the role of this cortical area in nociceptive processing has not yet been investigated. This area is known to play important roles in learning and memory in many species [34, 35]. Of interest is that intracellular changes of spinal cord neurons similar to those during mammalian learning and memory processes have been reported in CCI rats. This striking increase in neural activity within the retrosplenial granular cortex, which is involved in learning and memory, lends further support to the hypothesis that neural mechanisms of post-injury neuropathic pain may be related to central nervous system neuronal plastic changes similar to those occurring in learning and memory.

The activation of the cingulate cortex and amygdala may be related to general arousal, anxiety, and stress [34, 35], although these areas have also been implicated in nociceptive processing and pain modulation [31, 36-39]. The activation of the cingulate cortex and amygdala may primarily reflect neural processing related to pain, particularly the affective-motivational dimension of chronic neuropathic pain. The activation of the amygdala is highly expected in view of the now well characterized spinopontoamygdaloid pathway [38, 39]. Indeed, the parabrachial nucleus, which has been shown to be an integral part of this pathway also has been shown to have significant elevations in 2-DG metabolic activity [22]. In fact, the feature of bilateral activation of the amygdala, cingulate cortex, and retrosplenial granular cortex in CCI rats is consistent with the clinical observation that the affective-motivational dimension of persistent pain in human patients, including neuropathic pain patients, can be partially relieved after bilateral lesions of frontal cortical areas that include these cortical structures [40, 41]. Thus, it will be of interest to determine whether the activation of the cingulate cortex, amygdala, and retrosplenial granular cortex contributes to the immediate unpleasantness stage or the secondary stage (related to long-term implications and suffering) of the affective dimension of pain [42].

Patterns of increased brain activity between acute and persistent pain and implications for mechanisms of neuropathic pain

Patterns of increased brain neural activity following CCI are similar in many respects to those induced by acute noxious heat or formalin stimulation [31, 43, 44]. First, lower brainstem regions activated in CCI rats overlap primarily with those activated by hind paw formalin injection, both including medullar and pontine reticular nuclei, nucleus raphe magnus, dorsal raphe nucleus, and central grey matter. These regions receive input from spinoreticular and spinomesencephalic pathways, the spinal cord origins of which are highly activated in similar 2-DG studies [12, 13, 44]. Second, the increase in 2-DG metabolic activity is bilateral in most sampled brainstem regions, but with greater increases within the contralateral side following either unilateral sciatic nerve injury or unilateral hind paw formalin stimulation, a feature consistent with bilateral increases in spinal cord 2-DG metabolic activity in both cases [12, 13, 43, 44]. The bilateral activation of brain structures following unilateral sciatic nerve ligation is consistent with behavioral observations that mechanical hyperalgesia occurs in hind paws of CCI rats both ipsilateral and contralateral to the side of nerve ligation [11]. Bilateral activation also occurs in the spinal cord of rats exposed to noxious heat stimulation [20], although much higher contralateral spinal cord neural activity is seen in CCI rats [13] than in rats stimulated with noxious heat. Third, cortical areas with increased neural activity in CCI rats are generally consistent with those activated by noxious heat stimulation in awake human subjects [31], including cortical somatosensory regions and the cingulate cortex. Thus, at least the same general brain regions involved in central nervous system nociceptive processing appear to be activated under both acute and chronic pain conditions.

An important aspect of spatial patterns of brain neural activity is that brain regions activated in CCI rats appear to be multiple, perhaps even more than during formalin or noxious heat stimulation [31, 43, 45]. For example, the activation of the brain is bilateral in many thalamic and cortical regions of CCI rats including the ventral posterolateral thalamic nucleus, posterior thalamic nucleus, cortical hind limb area, fore limb area, and parietal areas. The existence of large and bilateral receptive fields of nociceptive neurons within spinal cord lamina VII may have conceivably contributed to such bilateral activation in CCI rats. On the other hand, the bilateral activation of brain regions (e.g., the cortical fore limb area) in CCI rats may result from the divergence of neural responses at both spinal and supraspinal levels. For instance, propriospinal connections have been shown to extend from caudal spinal cord segments up to the cervical enlargement, a region receiving fore limb somatosensory input [6, 21].

Consistent with these anatomical connections, elevations of spontaneous neural activity are observed across the entire sampled spinal cord lumbar segments (L_1-L_5) with little decrease at both rostral (L_1) and caudal (L_5) extremes in CCI rats [12, 13]. Thus, it is likely that changes in neural activity within the spinal cord may extend well beyond the primary afferent terminations of the ligated sciatic nerve in CCI rats and may even include the forelimb area. The divergence of spinal cord activity may, thereby, account for much of the widespread activity in thalamic and cortical somatosensory regions.

In addition to the extensive activation of many brain regions related to processing of the sensory-discriminative dimension of pain, a number of structures within the limbic system (retrosplenial granular cortex, amygdala, cingulate cortex), the motor system (caudate-putamen complex), and the autonomic system (medullary reticular formation, hypothalamic areas) are also highly activated in CCI rats. Such a multiple-system activation is consistent with clinical characteristics of chronic neuropathic pain syndromes which involve disorders associated with sensory, motor, and autonomic systems [9]. Similar pathological changes are seen in CCI rats including thermal hyperalgesia, spontaneous pain behaviors (abnormal guarding positions), and asymmetry of hind paw skin temperature [10, 11]. These symptoms are likely to be mediated by activation of multiple brain regions and their anatomic interconnections.

It is important to point out that sciatic nerve injury in CCI rats activates not only those brain regions implicated in afferent processing of sensory-discriminative and affective-motivational dimensions of pain but also those associated with centrifugal modulation of pain. The latter structures may include the medullary reticular formation, nucleus raphe magnus, parabrachial nuclei, dorsal raphe nucleus, central grey matter, and hypothalamic arcuate nucleus. Such a dual-functional activation of both afferent and efferent nociceptive processing systems in CCI rats may reflect central nervous system mechanisms of adaptation to a persistent pain condition. Thus, this CCI-induced increase in neural activity across extensive brain regions implicated in both sensory-discriminative and affective-motivational dimensions of pain as well as centrifugal modulation of pain may represent patterns of supraspinal processing related to chronic pain conditions.

The use of the 2-DG functional activity mapping technique provides a three-dimensional view of the entire picture of brain nociceptive processes under a persistent pain condition. Such an approach is likely to lead to improved understanding of central nervous system processing related to acute and chronic pain. For instance, the as yet unexplained activation of certain brain regions such as the retrosplenial granular cortex and caudate-putamen complex suggests that studies of the role of these brain regions in the neural processing of pain might provide new insights into the neurobiology of neuropathic pain and pain in general. Thus, results derived from this functional (2-DG) activity mapping study may serve as guidelines for future electrophysiological and anatomic studies to determine the physiological nature of neurons activated in neuropathic pain as well as to delineate the neural circuitry involving supraspinal nociceptive processing under chronic pain conditions.

Implications for supraspinal nociceptive coding mechanisms

The combination of observations from single neuron recording, 2-DG mapping, and spinal anterolateral quadrant stimulation experiments in awake humans [20, 46] provides strong evidence that the number of spinal cord neurons activated by peripheral stimuli and their action potential frequencies are both crucial factors that combine to encode the distinction between innocuous and nociceptive somatosensory events as well as the intensity of nociceptive stimulation [46]. This combination of spatial and temporal factors provides a mechanism by which wide dynamic range neurons that respond to both innocuous and nociceptive stimuli can encode pain. Indeed, it is the distinctive receptive field organization of WDR neurons that directly led to the various tests of this hypothesis [21]. WDR neuron receptive fields have a relatively small area of skin within which increasing stimulus intensities ranging from those that are extremely gentle to those that are frankly nociceptive produce graded differential responses (hence the term "wide dynamic range"). Surrounding this small zone is usually a much larger zone wherein only intense and often nociceptive stimuli are effective in evoking impulse discharge. Given this common receptive field organization and a rostro-caudal somatotopic organization of WDR neurons within the dorsal horn along various spinal segments (e.g. L-2 to S-1), one would predict that a nociceptive stimulus would recruit a much larger number of WDR neurons than a non-nociceptive stimulus. This prediction is consistent with both spinal cord 2-DG mapping of metabolic activity in response to graded levels of nociceptive stimulation and with human anterolateral quadrant stimulation studies which clearly indicate that both the number of axons stimulated and stimulation frequency interact to produce both threshold pain sensations as well as graded levels of pain sensation intensity.

The spatial organization of receptive fields of WDR neurons at VPL_c and S-1 cortical areas is precisely similar to that of dorsal horn WDR neurons, including the central zone differentially responsive to innocuous and nociceptive stimulation and the surrounding zone responsive mainly to nociceptive stimuli. Even the total receptive field areas are similiar among spinal, VPL_c- thalamic, and S-1 cortical neurons [6, 21]. Taken in light of encoding mechanisms just proposed for dorsal horn neurons, a nociceptive stimulus would be expected to activate more VPL_c and more S-1 WDR nociceptive neurons than an innocuous stimulus and, thus, such neuronal recruitment may contribute to supraspinal intensity encoding of nociceptive information. The concept that neuronal recruitment is a salient factor in neural representation of pain at telencephalic levels is also supported by other recent lines of evidence. A recent PET study comparing cortical responses to vibration and heat induced pain in awake human volunteers, shows activation of more cortical regions in the case of pain [46]. A patient with total corpus callosum section showed reduction in pain sensitivity when low to moderate nociceptive skin temperature stimuli (45 °C - 47 °C) were presented ipsilateral to the responding cerebral hemisphere, but reported high intensity ipsilateral nociceptive stimuli (49 °C to 51 °C skin temperatures) as distinctly painful [47]. This pattern of responses suggests that at high enough nociceptive levels, recruitment of pathways other than the classical crossed spinothalamic-cortical pathway may make up for the pain sensory deficit which occurs when one cerebral hemisphere is no longer able to share nociceptive information with the other *via* the corpus callosum. A similar pattern of results has been reported in a patient with a lateral thalamic lesion [48].

Indeed, the extensive anatomical collateralization of ascending pathways known to be important for pain has long been regarded as a mechanism of providing diffuse activation of numerous brain regions during pain states and has long been suspected as a basis for the extreme difficulty in producing long term reductions in clinical pain by lesions. The extensive spatial distribution metabolic activity seen in Figure 1 is both consistent with this view and with some degree of specificity of central structures activated during a painful neuropathic condition. As discussed above, the specific telencephalic structures activated in the rat and the overall widespread distribution of increased neural activity as a consequence of chronic constriction of the sciatic nerve is generally consistent with that obtained in rats after intradermal formalin injection and with the structures activated during acute pain conditions in human volunteers.

References

1. Kenshalo DR Jr, Isensee O. Responses of SI cortical neurons to noxious stimuli. *J Neurophysiol* 1983 ; 50 : 1479-96.
2. Chudler EH, Anton F, Dubner R, Kenshalo DR. Responses of nociceptive S-1 neurons in monkeys and pain sensation in humans elicited by noxious thermal stimulation: effect of interstimulus interval. *J Neurophysiol* 1990 ; 63 (3) : 559-69.
3. Kenshalo DR Jr, Chudler EH, Anton F, Dubner R. SI nociceptive neurons participate in the encoding process by which monkeys perceive the intensity of noxious thermal stimulation. *Brain Res* 1988 ; 454 : 378-82.
4. Penfield W, Boldrey E. Somatic motor and sensory representation in the cerebral cortex of man. *Brain* 1937 ; 60 : 116-26.
5. Head H, Holmes G. Sensory disturbances from cerebral lesions. *Brain* 1911; 34 : 102-54.
6. Willis WD. *The pain system. The neural basis of nociceptive transmission in the mammalian nervous system.* Basel : Karger, 1985.
7. Hardy JD, Wolff HG, Goodell H. *Pain sensations and reactions.* Baltimore : Williams and Wilkins, 1952.
8. White JC, Sweet WH. *Pain and the neurosurgeon.* Springfield, Illinois : Thomas, 1969.
9. Bonica JJ. Causalgia and other reflex sympathetic dystrophies. In : Bonica JJ, Liebeskind JC, Albe-Fessard DG, eds. *Advances in pain research and therapy.* New York : Raven Press, 1979 : 141-66.
10. Bennett GJ, Xie YK. A peripheral mononeuropathy in rat that produces disorders of pain sensation like those seen in man. *Pain* 1988 ; 33 : 87-107.
11. Attal N, Jazat F, Kayser V, Guilbaud G. Further evidence for "pain-related" behaviors in a model of unilateral peripheral mononeuropathy. *Pain* 1990 ; 41: 235-51.
12. Price DD, Mao J, Coghill RC, d'Avella D, Cicciarello R, Fiori M, Mayer DJ, Hayes RL. Regional changes in spinal cord glucose metabolism in a rat model of painful neuropathy. *Brain Res* 1991 ; 564 : 314-8.
13. Mao J, Coghill RC, Price DD, Mayer DJ, Hayes RL. Spatial patterns of spinal cord metabolic activity in a rodent model of peripheral mononeuropathy. *Pain* 1992 ; 50 : 89-100.

14. Palecek J, Paleckova V, Dougherty PM, Willis WD, Carlton SM. Responses of spinothalamic tract cells to mechanical and thermal stimulation of skin in rats with experimental peripheral neuropathy. *Soc Neurosci Abstr* 1991 ; 17 : 437.
15. Guilbaud G, Benoist JM, Jazat F, Gautron M. Neuronal responsiveness in the ventrobasal thalamic complex of rats with an experimental peripheral mononeuropathy. *J Neurophysiol* 1990 ; 64 : 1537-54.
16. Kennedy C, Des Rosiers MH, Jehle JW, Reivich M, Sharpe F, Sokoloff L. Mapping of functional neural pathways by autoradiographic survey of local metabolic rate with (14C) deoxyglucose. *Science* 1975 ; 187 : 850-3.
17. Sokoloff L, Reivich M, Kennedy C, Des Rosiers MH, Patlak CS, Pettigrew KD, Sakurada O, Shinohara M. The [14C]deoxyglucose method for the measurement of local cerebral glucose utilization: theory, procedure, and normal values in the conscious and anesthetized albino rat. *J Neurochem* 1977 ; 28 : 897-916.
18. Singer P, Mehler S. 2-Deoxy[14C]glucose uptake in the rat hypoglossal nucleus after nerve transection. *Exp Neurol* 1980 ; 69 : 617-26.
19. DiRocco, RJ, Kageyama, GH, Wong-Riley, MTT. The relationship between CNS metabolism and cytoarchitecture: a review of ^{14}C-deoxyglucose studies with correlation to cytochrome oxidase histochemistry. *Comput Med Imaging Graphics* 1989 ; 13 : 81-92.
20. Coghill RC, Price DD, Hayes R, Mayer DJ. Spatial distribution of nociceptive processing in the rat spinal cord. *J Neurophysiol* 1991 ; 65 : 33-140.
21. Price DD. *Psychological and neural mechanisms of pain*. New York : Raven Press, 1988.
22. Mao, J, Mayer, DJ, Price, DD. Patterns of increased brain activity indicative of pain in a rat model of peripheral mononeuropathy. *J Neurosci* 1993 ; 13(6) : 2689-702.
23. Juliano SL, Whitsel BL. A combined 2-deoxyglucose and neurophysiological study of primate somatosensory cortex. *J Comp Neurol* 1987 ; 263 : 514-25.
24. Dostrovsky JO, Guilbaud G. Nociceptive responses in medial thalamus of the normal and arthritic rat. *Pain* 1990 ; 40 : 93-104.
25. Lenz FA, Dostrovsky JO, Tasker RR, Yamashiro K, Kwan HC, Murphy JT. Single-unit analysis of the human ventral thalamic nuclear group: somatosensory responses. *J Neurophysiol* 1988 ; 59 : 299-316.
26. Guilbaud G, Peschanski M, Briand A, Gautron M. The organization of spinal pathways to ventrobasal thalamus in an experimental model of pain (the arthritic rat). An electrophysiological study. *Pain* 1986 ; 26 : 301-12.
27. Chung JM, Lee KH, Surmeier DJ, Sorkin LS, Kim J, Willis WD. Response characteristics of neurons in the ventral posterior lateral nucleus of the monkey thalamus. *J Neurophysiol* 1986 ; 56 : 370-90.
28. Burstein R, Cliffer KD, Giesler GJ. Direct somatosensory projections from the spinal cord to the hypothalamus and telencephalon. *J Neurosci* 1987 ; 7 : 4159-64.
29. Sim LJ, Joseph SA. Arcuate nucleus projections to brainstem regions which modulate nociception. *J Chem Neuroanat* 1991 ; 4 : 97-109.
30. Mountcastle VB, Darian-Smith I. Neural mechanisms in somesthesia. In : Mountcastle VB, ed. *Medical physiology*. Saint Louis : Mosby, 1968 : 1372-423.
31. Talbot JD, Marrett S, Evans AC, Mayer E, Bushnell MC, Duncan GH. Multiple representations of pain in human cerebral cortex. *Science* 1991 ; 251 : 1355-8.
32. Lamour Y, Willer JC, Guilbaud G. Rat somatosensory (SmI) cortex: I. Characteristics of neuronal responses to noxious stimulation and comparison with responses to non-noxious stimulation. *Exp Brain Res* 1983 ; 49 : 35-45.
33. Chudler EH, Dong, WK. The role of the basal ganglia in nociception and pain. *Pain* 1995 ; 60(1) : 3-38.

34. Groen TV, Wyss JM. Connections of the retrosplenial dysgranular cortex in the rat. *J Comp Neurol* 1992 ; 315 : 200-16.
35. Thompson S, Robertson RT. Organization of subcortical pathways for sensory projections to the limbic cortex I. Subcortical projections to the medial limbic cortex in the rat. *J Comp Neurol* 1987 ; 265 : 175-88.
36. Jones AK, Brown WD, Friston KJ, Qi LY, Frackowiak RS. Cortical and subcortical localization of response to pain in man using positron emission tomography. *Proc R Soc Lond (Biol)* 1991 ; 244 : 39-44.
37. Hylden JL, Anton F, Nahin RL. Spinal lamina I projection neurons in the rat: collateral innervation of parabrachial area and thalamus. *Neuroscience* 1989 ; 28 : 27-37.
38. Bernard JF, Peschanski M, Besson JM. A possible spino (trigemino)-ponto-amygdaloid pathway for pain. *Neurosci Lett* 1989 ; 100 : 83-8.
39. Bernard JF, Besson JM. The spino(trigemino)pontoamygdaloid pathway: electrophysiological evidence for an involvement in pain processes. *J Neurophysiol* 1990 ; 63 : 473-90.
40. Foltz EL, White LE. Pain "relief" by frontal cingulumotomy. *J Neurosurg* 1962 ; 19 : 89-100.
41. Hurt RW, Ballantine HT. Stereotactic anterior cingulate lesions for persistent pain: a report on 68 cases. *Clin Neurosurg* 1973 ; 21 : 334-51.
42. Price DD, Harkins SW. The affective-motivational dimension of pain: a two stage model. *J APS* 1992 ; 1(4) : 229-39.
43. Porro CA, Cavazzuti M, Galetti A, Sassatell L. Functional activity mapping of the rat brainstem during formalin-induced noxious stimulation. *Neuroscience* 1991 ; 41 : 667-80.
44. Porro CA, Cavazzuti M, Galetti A, Sassatelli L, Barbieri GC. Functional activity mapping of the rat spinal cord during formalin-induced noxious stimulation. *Neuroscience* 1991 ; 41 : 655-65.
45. Casey KL, Satoshi M, Berger KL, Koeppe RA, Morrow TJ, Frey K. Positron emission tomographic analysis of cerebral structures activated specfically by repetitive noxious heat stimuli. *J Neurophysiol* 1994 ; 71 : 802-7.
46. Coghill RC, Talbot JD, Evans AC, Meyer E, Gjedde A, Bushnell MC, Duncan GH. Distributed processing of pain and vibration by the human brain. *J Neurosci* 1994 ; 14(7) : 4095-108.
47. Stein BE, Price DD, Gazzaniga M. Pain perception in a man with total corpus callosum transection. *Pain* 1989 ; 38 : 51-6.
48. Greenspan JD, Winfield JA, Poe LA, Hodge CJ. Selective pain deficits associated with an extensive posterolateral thalamic lesion. *IASP Abtracts* 1993 ; 462 : 1246.

11

Hindbrain structures involved in pain processing as revealed by the evoked expression of immediate early genes in freely behaving animals

D. MENÉTREY

INSERM U 161, Paris, France.

Recent evidence shows that the study of the expression of immediate early gene (IEG)-encoded proteins is particularly suited to understanding nervous activity that takes place during sensory processing. The great advantage of such a functionally oriented anatomical approach is that the "activity" of large numbers of cells can readily be identified under natural living conditions and, at the same time, the information can be compared to parallel clinical observations. All structures involved simultaneously in parallel processing can be identified and studied in a comparative quantitative manner; such an approach opens onto true functional maps of activity. IEGs have a key function in stimulation-transcription coupling. They are cellular genes whose mRNA is induced even in the absence of protein synthesis and which encode DNA-binding proteins acting as transcription factors. The better known of these genes are members of the fos, jun and krox families. Fos and Jun proteins have analog structures that dimerize through a leucine zipper motif to act transcriptionally as various dimers; Krox proteins belong to a superfamily of transcription factors which act through a zinc finger motif. IEGs couple extracellular signals and long-term genomic responses; their transcription products are nuclear proteins which link short-term extracellular signals to long-lasting phenotypic changes by modulating the transcription rate of secondary target genes.

IEG-encoded proteins should be considered as third messenger molecules in the signal-transcriptional coupling cascade (for review *see* [1] and [2]].

Pain field studies at supraspinal levels may largely benefit from such a new approach especially if studies use a large array of IEG-encoded proteins. However, as it is now well-established that none of the IEG-encoded proteins can be considered as specific activity markers for any type of stimulation, in order to be valid, results must be obtained from extremely well-designed models of stimulation and analyzed in a way that considers the entire set of elements that constitute them. Only the "specificity" of the stimulus can result in the "specificity" of activation; only an interpretation that considers all the ins and outs of a question can approach real significance. Thus, there is a need for "pure" models of stimulation that are devoid of interfering conditions (anaesthesia, stress, surgery and introduction of a stimulating device) which may themselves evoke or modify levels of IEG expression. Models of stimulation which apply to freely behaving animals are evidently of particular value. In the study of nociception these models must:
 - associate mild and controllable pain for the shortest periods of time to agree, as much as possible, with ethical rules;
 - avoid, as much as possible, any interfering situation such as those mentioned above;
 - refer to pure organ disease such that clinical evolution can be monitored through histological observations;
 - include behavioral observations, preferentially of a quantitative type.

The present article gives some clues to the involvement of hindbrain structures in pain processing as recently obtained in our laboratory; similar information regarding forebrain areas is not presently available. Results consider both somatic pain in freely behaving animals [3, 4] and visceral pain in either freely behaving animals [5] or under general anaesthesia [6]. A report of results obtained at the spinal cord level will be given for better comprehension. The conclusion will be given in regard to data obtained in scientific fields more specifically designed to study the influences of vegetative- or stress-related inputs.

Somatic pain of inflammatory origin

Information regarding somatic pain in freely behaving animals refers to models of unilateral inflammation of either the plantar foot or the tibio-tarsal joint thus using the models initially described by Stein *et al.* [7] and Butler *et al.* [8], respectively. Results come from male Sprague-Dawley rats. Inflammation is a complex process which results in multifactorial disease having both local (nociception genesis, tissue alteration, functional loss) and systemic (circulating blood-borne substances built-up) consequences. Since there is presently no way of knowing to what extent any of these consequences are responsible for the central effects we have observed, we will consider our results as a whole with no attempt to distinguish between the respective implications of these different manifestations.

Models of stimulation

The inflammatory process that resulted in somatic pain was induced by local injection of complete adjuvant. Following injection, animals were allowed to behave freely over the full period of disease development. The evolution of the disease was followed clinically using a large panel of criteria *i.e.* the difference of paw or tibio-tarsal joint size between the injected and the non-injected side (size score); the degree of mobility of the animal (mobility score); the rat's willingness or not to put its affected limb on the floor during either rest or motion (withdrawal score), the degrees of ankle stiffness and toe retraction on the affected side (joint stiffness and toe retraction scores, respectively). Subcutaneous inflammation of the plantar foot was studied from 4 hours to 8 weeks post-injection; monoarthritis resulting from ankle injection was studied from one day to 15 weeks post-injection (Figures 1 and 2). Considering both the very long time course and the absence of a return to normal clinical aspects, only monoarthritis can be considered as a chronic disease model.

Spinal labeling

Only animals with unilateral local impairment were considered and with the non-injected side used as a control side. Each disease had specific characteristics in terms of patterns of evoked protein expression (Figures 1 and 2). All IEG proteins were expressed in both cases. Most of the staining was observed at midlumbar level in both superficial layers of the dorsal horn and deep dorsal horn (laminae V-VII and X). Monoarthritis was distinguished by a high level of total protein expression. Staining was especially dense in the deep dorsal horn. More labeled cells were observed at 1-2 days and at 2 weeks postinjection corresponding to the initiation and progressive phases of the disease, respectively. Subcutaneous inflammation was characterized by a moderate level of total IEG expression. More labeled cells were observed in the first day following injection. It is the relative degree of expression of each IEG-encoded protein with regard to the others that characterized the progression of the disease. Early stages of the disease coincided with the expression of all Fos and Jun proteins, while late stages showed an increase in Jun D and Fos B involvement; Krox-24 was induced mostly during the early phases and/or paroxystic periods of the disease. Persistent stimulation was characterized by a predominant expression in deep *versus* superficial layers of the dorsal horn. How these changes in genomic regulation may correlate with the electrophysiological and neurochemical ones [9-12] are still unknown.

Hindbrain labeling

In freely behaving animals, somatic pain of inflammatory origin evoked IEGs expression, mostly c-Fos and Krox-24, in only a restricted subset of discrete hindbrain subregions. As shown in Table I, staining in these areas evolved differentially throughout the post-injection survival time of the animal.

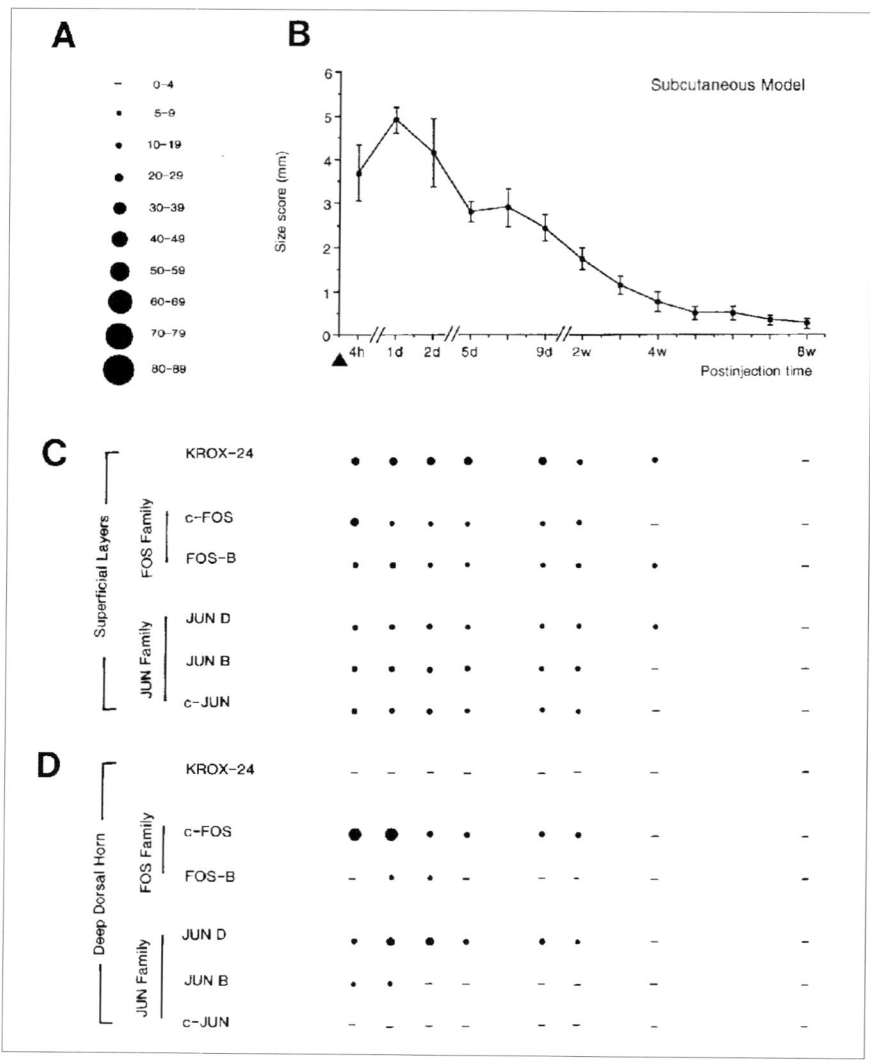

Figure 1. Time-course of subcutaneous inflammation as shown by the evolution of the size score (ordinate in B) from 4 hours to eight weeks postinjection (abscissa in B) and parallel schematic representations of the expression of IEG-encoded proteins in both the superficial layers (C) and deep dorsal horn (lamina V-VII and X; D). Mean-curve in B (size score expressed in millimeters as the difference of paw size between the injected and the non-injected side ± SE) comes from observations performed on animals which survived for the longest time (8 weeks). The abscissa is not a true linear scale; scale factor changes are indicated by a break in the horizontal line. Time of inoculation is shown by an arrow head on the abscissa in B. The inflammation was rapid in onset (2-4 hours, initiation phase), peaked at 24-48 hours (acute phase) and lasted for about 2-3 weeks with progressive decline (postacute phase). The numbers of protein positive cells (C and D) relate to 4 hours (h), 1, 2, 5, 9 days (d) and 2, 4 and 8 weeks (w) postinjection. The size of dots in C and D is proportional to the mean number of cells per L4/L5 section (A). Labeling in laminae III-IV (Krox-24) and lamina IX (Jun D and c-Jun) which were in the range of constitutive expression have not been counted (Reprinted from Figure 1 of [3] with kind permission from John Wiley and Sons, New York, USA).

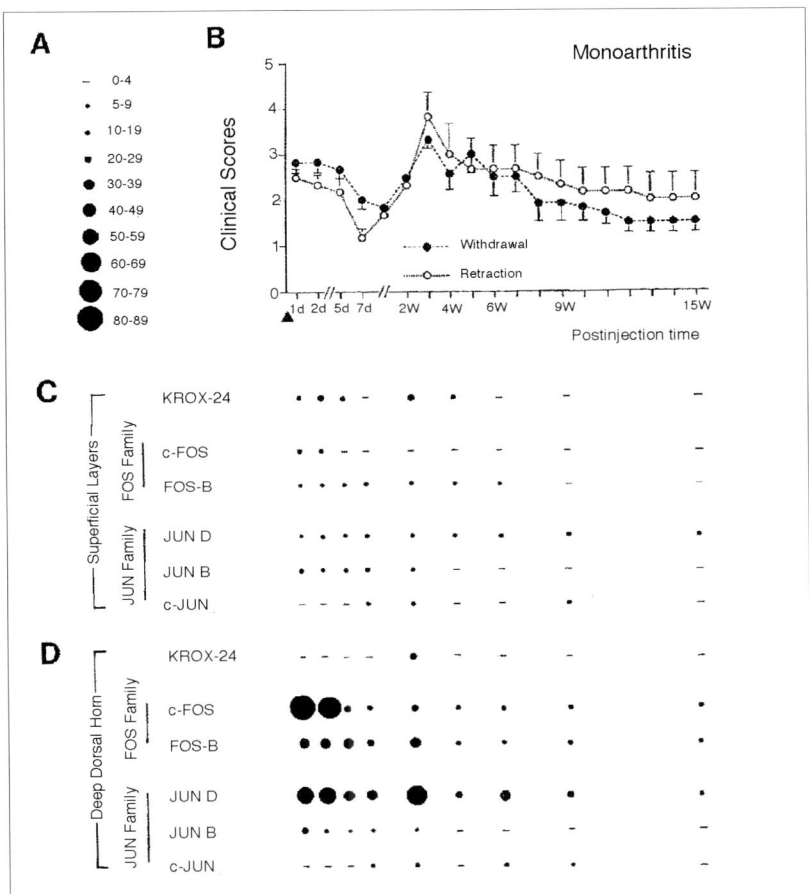

Figure 2. Time-course of monoathritic inflammation as shown by the evolution of the withdrawal and toe retraction scores (ordinate in B) from day one to fifteen weeks postinjection (abscissa in B) and parallel schematic representations of the expression of IEG-encoded proteins in both superficial layers (C) and deep dorsal horn (lamina V-VII and X; D). Mean-curves of toe retraction score (positive SE) and withdrawal score (negative SE) in B come from observations performed on animals which survived for the longest time (15 weeks). Clinical scores are from 0 (normal performance) to 6 (maximal impairment). The abscissa is not a true linear scale; scale factor changes are indicated by a break in the horizontal line. Time of inoculation is shown by an arrow head on abscissa in B. The initial phase of the disease included the very first days following injection and mainly corresponded to an acute reaction induced by the intra-articular injection itself. Transient similar clinical aspects were also obtained after injection of the vehicle mixture alone or in adjuvant injected animals that did not develop arthritis. Except for the severity of impairment this initial period did not differ intrinsically from the subsequent periods of monoarthritis. The end of the first week and the following days were characterized by a period of partial remission. Monoarthritis typically developed over the second and third weeks postinjection (progressive phase) and lasted for periods of weeks as a prolonged chronic phase. The fourth week marked the transition from progressive to chronic phases. This transitional phase sometimes coincided with a moderate drop in clinical scores. The biphasic evolution of monoarthritis allows clear distinction between post-acute (first week post-injection) and chronic (over two weeks post-injection) phases. The numbers of protein positive cells (C and D) relate to 1, 2, 5, 7 days (d) and 2, 4, 6, 9 and 15 weeks (w) postinjection. The size of dots in C and D is proportional to the mean number of cells (A) *per* section (Reprinted from Figure 3 of [3] with kind permission from John Wiley and Sons, New York, USA).

Survival Time	Constitutive n=5	Subcutaneous Inflammation 4 hours n=7		Monoarthritis 24 hours n=3		Monoarthritis 2 weeks n=3		Monoarthritis 6 to 15 weeks n=6	
		Contralateral	Ipsilateral	Contralateral	Ipsilateral	Contralateral	Ipsilateral	Contralateral	Ipsilateral
Caudal intermediate reticular n.	2,3 ± 1,1	11 ± 1,2***	7 ± 1,1**	13,3 ± 1,7****	11 ± 1,5****	4 ± 0,5	4 ± 0,5	2,5 ± 0,8	1,5 ± 0,4
Caudal Medulla									
Ventrolateral area	3,8 ± 2,1	19,5 ± 4,6**	17,4 ± 3,8**	29,3 ± 5,6***	24 ± 5***	7,3 ± 0,6	6 ± 0,5	7,3 ± 1,8	5,3 ± 1,3
Parabrachial Area	0,2 ± 0,5	30,1 ± 8,6**	18,2 ± 6,3*	26,3 ± 6,8*	12,6 ± 2,4	41,6 ± 10,9**	34 ± 9,1***	5,6 ± 2,4	4 ± 1,4
n. Cuneiformis	3,3 ± 2,3	34,2 ± 8,4**	25,4 ± 7,1**	32 ± 8*	20 ± 3,4	32,6 ± 6,3*	26,7 ± 4,3*	3,6 ± 1,8	2,3 ± 1,1
Central Gray	6,2 ± 2,5	20,4 ± 5,5*	17,8 ± 4,7*	33 ± 6**	23,3 ± 1,7**	25,6 ± 4,9*	22,6 ± 4,2*	4,6 ± 1,4	3,4 ± 1,4

Table I. Number of c-Fos positive cells in areas of the caudal medulla oblongata and pontomesencephalic structures (left column) that were activated by somatic inflammation. Results are expressed as mean value (m ± SE) of positive cells per section. Constitutive expression is indicated in the third column as the mean-value of positive cells encountered on both sides; evoked labeling is indicated in the following columns in regard to specific stimulating conditions (acute subcutaneous stimulation, 4 hours survival time) or monoarthritis (either 24 hours, 2 weeks or 6 to 15 weeks survival times). The numbers of positive cells on both contralateral (left) and ipsilateral (right) sides in regard to peripheral stimulation are given. Stars refer to degree of significance between constitutive and evoked labeling (1 to 4 stars for $p < 0.05$, 0.01, 0.001 and 0.0001, respectively) using Fisner's PLSD. (Reprinted from Table 3 of [4] with kind permission from Elsevier Science Ltd, Kidlington, UK.)

Two main sets of structures could be identified: one located caudally in the reticular formation of the medulla oblongata, the other situated more rostrally at the level of the pontomesencephalic junction. Structures involved in the caudal medulla oblongata (Figure 3) included the caudal intermediate reticular nucleus, the subnucleus reticularis dorsalis, the ventrolateral reticular formation and the lateral paragigantocellular nucleus. Staining in these areas was evident only at short survival times (4 and 24 hour survival times in the case of subcutaneous and monoarthritis models, respectively). Structures involved at the pontomesencephalic junction level (Figure 4) mostly included the superior and dorsal lateral subnuclei of the parabrachial area, the nucleus cuneiformis and the most caudal portions of the lateral central gray also including the laterodorsal tegmental nucleus; labeling in other lateral subnuclei of the parabrachial area always remained moderate. Staining in these nuclei was evident in all cases except for the very long survival periods (6 to 15 weeks) in monoarthritis. In all cases staining was bilateral with contralateral predominance with regard to the stimulated limb.

Visceral pain

IEGs-related studies regarding visceral pain processing at supraspinal levels in freely behaving animals are still unavailable from the literature. Studies of that type are presently in progress in our laboratory [5] using the model of cyclophosphamide cystitis recently developed by Lantéri-Minet et al. [13]. The only presently published information regarding the involvement of hindbrain structures in the case of visceral stimulation and using IEGs expression concerns colorectal distension under general anaesthesia [6].

Models

Repetitive colorectal distensions were applied through a flexible latex balloon. The balloon was introduced under deep anaesthesia (2% halothane) to be later kept in position and inflated with air for 20 sec *per* minute. Intraluminal distending pressure (80 mm Hg) was controlled through an in-line pressure transducer. Pressures above 40 mm Hg are considered nociceptive as they are accompanied by affective reactions in behaving rats [14]. Animals survived for 2 hours.

Cyclophosphamide was injected at the dose of 100mg/kg/ip. Cyclophosphamide is an antitumoral agent which is metabolized by the hepatic cytochrome P-450 to form inactive circulating metabolites, the renal cleavage of which by phosphamidases generates toxic byproducts mostly acrolein [15, 16]. It is the prolonged contact of acrolein with the bladder wall during urine accumulation and retention that generates disease. Cyclophosphamide cystitis is associated with abnormal behaviors such as lacrimation, piloerection, assumption of a peculiar "rounded-back" posture and episodes of tail hyperextension, abdominal retraction, licking of the lower abdomen and backward withdrawal movements. The animals develop these abnormal behaviors in

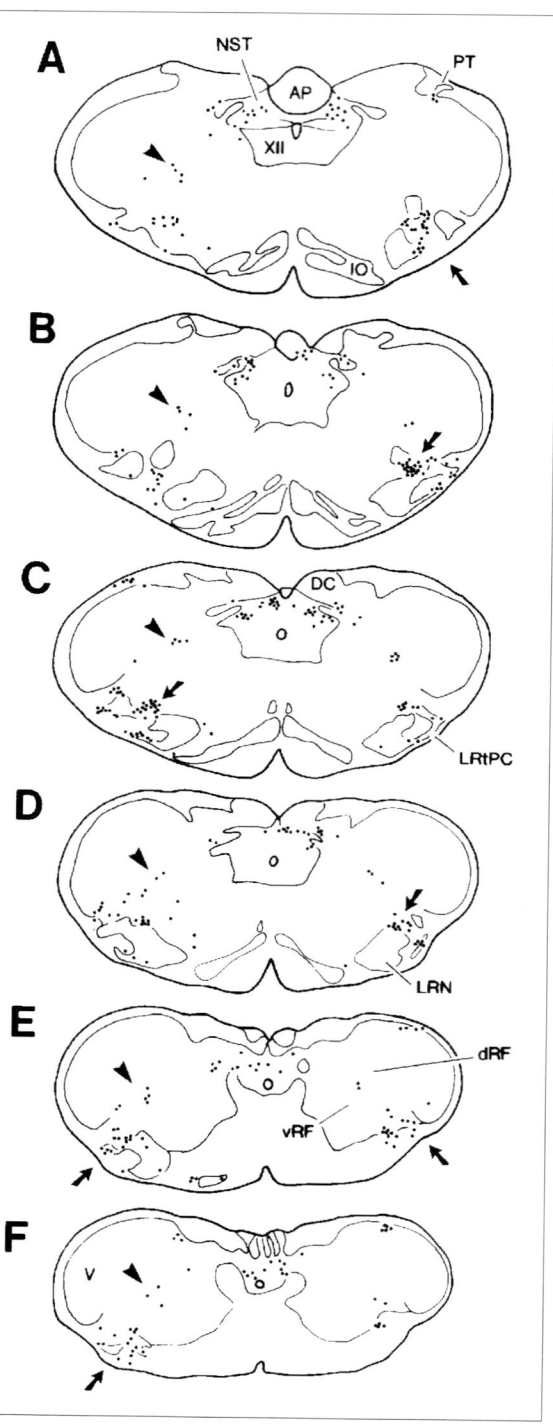

Figure 3. These drawings illustrate the distribution of c-Fos-immunoreactive cells in the medulla oblongata of a rat during unilateral subcutaneous inflammation (4 hours survival time; Freund's adjuvant injection in the plantar foot). Six levels from caudal (bottom) to rostral (top) are represented. Note that planes on the left side are slightly more rostral than those on the right. Level A passes just anterior (left) or through the anterior pole (right) of the lateral reticular nucleus (LRN). Level F is just caudal to (right) or passes through the caudal end (left) of LRN. Each diagram includes all labeled cells in one 40 μm section; each dot represents one labeled cell. In this case a unilateral injection resulted in bilateral staining in all nuclei. Arrows point to labeling in the ventrolateral medulla; arrow heads point to labeling in caudal intermediate reticular nucleus and subnucleus reticularis dorsalis. Labeling in the nucleus of the solitary tract and lateral reticular nucleus parvocellular was in the range of constitutive expression. Abbreviations: AP; area postrema; DC: dorsal column nuclei; dRF: dorsal reticular field; IO: inferior olive; PT: paratrigeminal nucleus; vRF: ventral reticular field; V: caudal trigeminal nucleus; XII: Hypoglossal nerve (Reprinted from Figure 1 of [4] with kind permission from Elsevier Science Ltd, Kidlington UK).

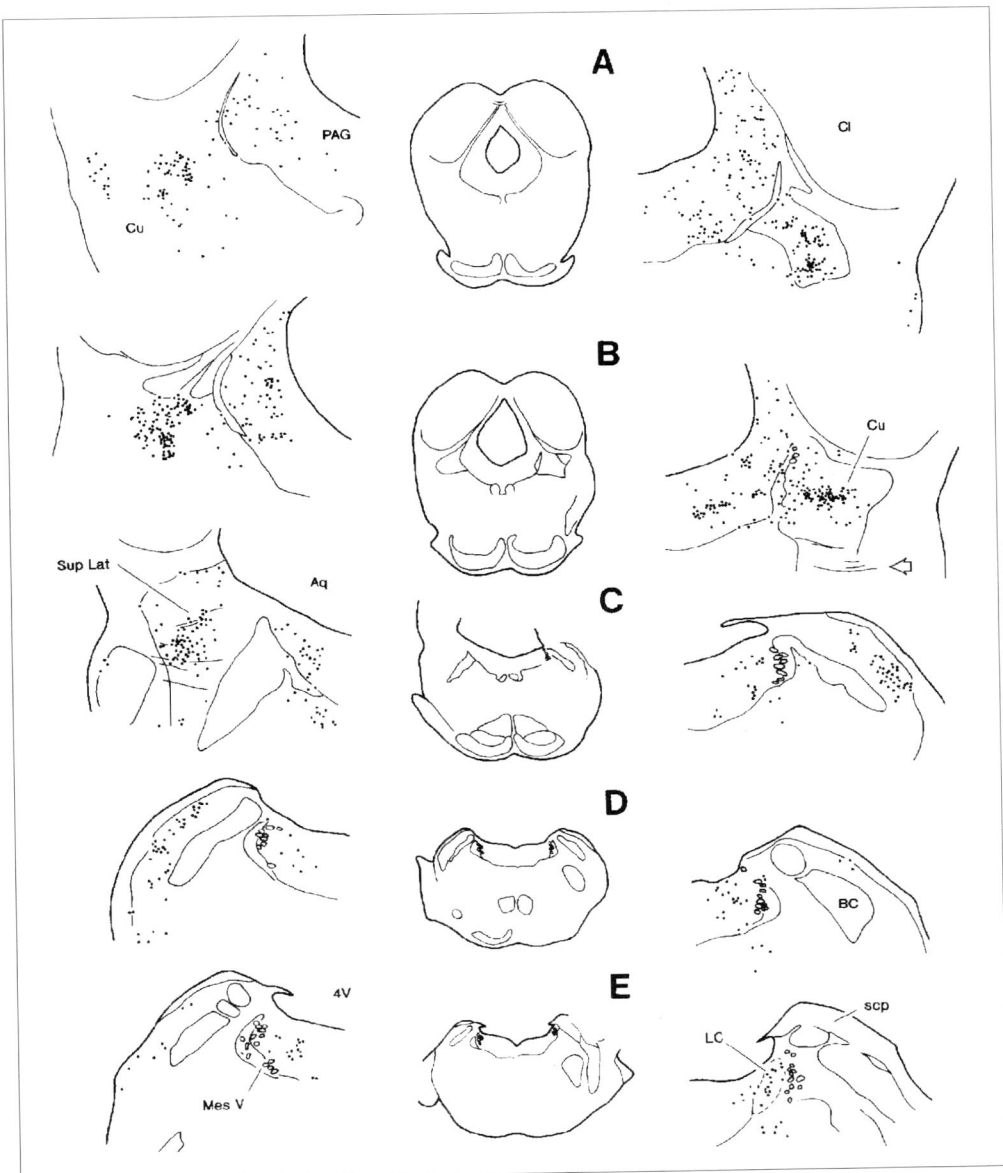

Figure 4. These diagrams illustrate the distribution of c-Fos-immunoreactive cells at the level of the pontomesencephalic junction (4 hour subcutaneous injection; same animal as in Figure 3). Five frontal levels from caudal (bottom) to rostral (top) are represented. Details as in Figure 3. Constitutive labeling in the inferior colliculi (CI) has not been displayed. Open arrows indicate fibers of the lateral lemniscus commissure. Frontal levels are indicated by low magnification drawings in the center column. Abbreviations: Aq: aqueduct; BC: brachium conjonctivum; Cu: cuneiformis nucleus; LC: locus coeruleus; Mes V: mesencephalic nucleus of the trigeminal complex; PAG: periaqueductal gray; scp: superior cerebellar peduncule; Sup Lat.: superior lateral nucleus of PBl; 4V: fourth ventricule. (Reprinted from Figure 3 of [4] with kind permission from Elsevier Science Ltd, Kidlington, UK.)

four hours as the bladder impairment progressively becomes more severe. The degree of bladder impairment can be assessed in a graded manner using chorionic oedema, fibrin deposit, epithelial thinning, desquamation, petechial haemorrhage and immunocompetent cell infiltration as criteria. The cyclophosphamide cystitis model has the following unique features compared to other visceral models. First, the stimulus is a "pure" visceral one confined to one viscus (bladder) and no somatic stimulation is induced either by introducing a stimulating device or from surgical wounds, and no anaesthesia is required; second, it is the exact replication of a human disease and its evolution can be efficently monitored through behavioral and histological observations.

Spinal labeling

Spinal labeling resulting from either repetitive colorectal distensions or cystitis clearly differed from that observed following somatic inflammation of the hindlimb. Only the following lumbosacral areas were stained: the parasympathetic column (SPN), the dorsal gray commissure (DGC as the caudal extent of lamina X) and superficial layers of the dorsal horn. As shown in Figures 5 and 6 in the case of evolutive cyclophosphamide cystitis and colorectal distension, respectively, these three discrete areas differentially reacted to visceral stimulation thus suggesting partly distinct but related functions. DGC which displays a high level of basal Krox-24 expression and in which both Krox-24 and c-Fos expressions are evoked in relation to the intensity of stimulation, would code for inputs from both physiological and all degrees of pathological conditions. SPN which, except for basal Krox-24 expression, responds like DGC and contains preganglionic motor cells, would code for inputs involved in eliciting visceral motor activity. Superficial layers would also reflect the physiopathological changes of the bladder including pain sensitivity but in a slightly different manner. Laminae I and II which respond like DGC and SPN regarding Krox-24 expression would both code for inputs from physiopathological changes, but only lamina I would be more primarily involved in pain processing as it is the only region in which c-Fos expression increases during the definitive inflammatory process. Labeling at the thoraco-lumbar junction was always moderate and only concerned colorectal distension.

Hindbrain labeling

Repetitive colorectal distensions under general anaesthesia (a mixture of 1/3 O_2, 2/3 N_2O, 0.5-0.75% halothane) evoked c-Fos and Krox-24 expression in only the caudal most part of the medulla oblongata and at transverse planes passing through, or just caudal to the caudal tip of the lateral reticular nucleus (Figure 7). Cells formed an oblique row (arrows) inserted between the ventral and dorsal reticular fields, and in a location that caudally prolonged that of the intermediate reticular nucleus. This nucleus has been refered to as the caudal intermediate reticular nucleus. No differential labeling was observed in either the nucleus of the solitary tract or the parabrachial area.

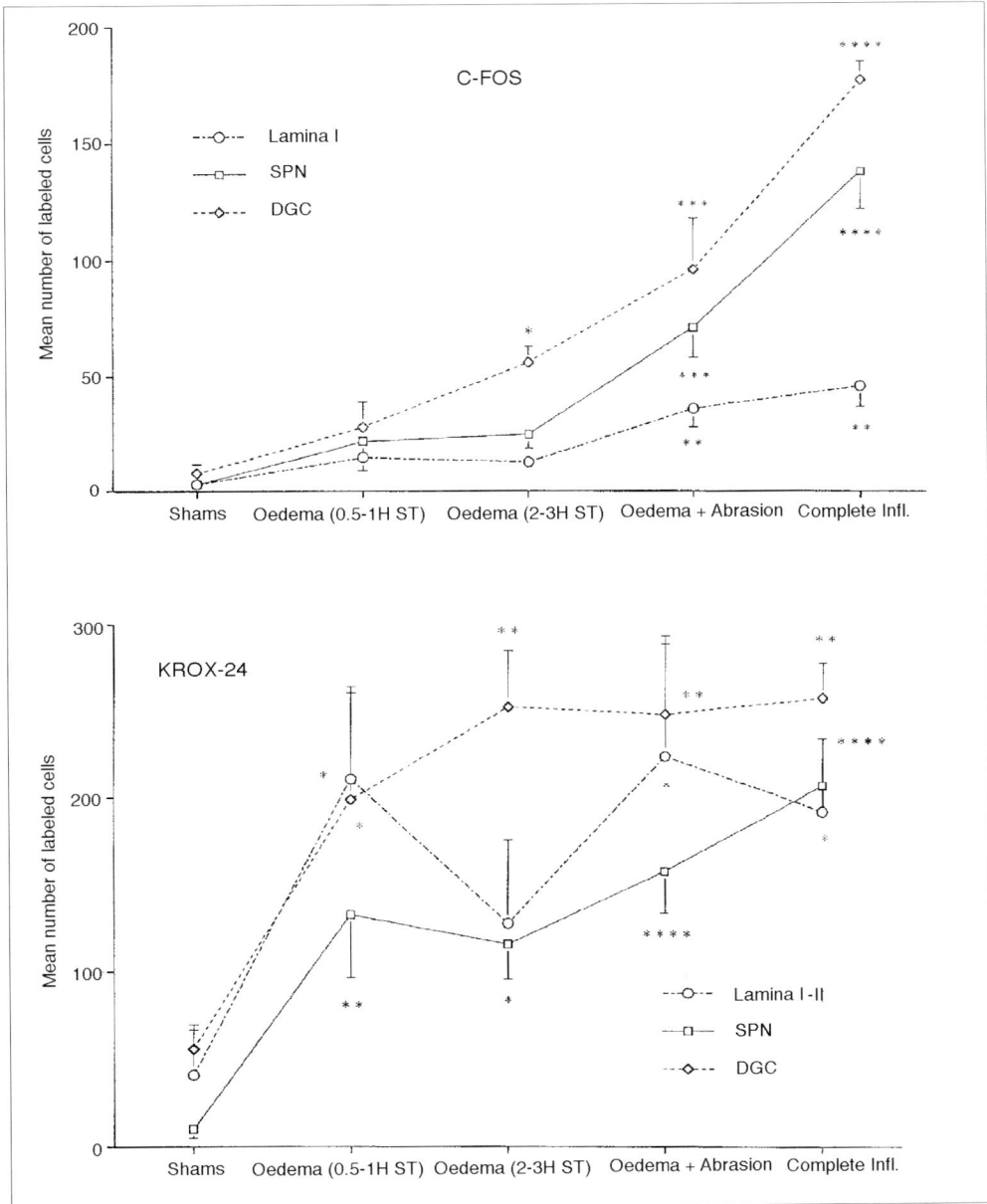

Figure 5. The number of lumbosacral c-Fos (A) or Krox-24 (B) positive cells (ordinate) in response to bladder stimulation (abscissa) for either controls or increasing degrees of bladder lesion (chorionic oedema, chorionic oedema and epithelial abrasion, complete inflammation). Results are expressed as mean number (m ± SE) of positive cells on both sides of the spinal cord (5 sections). Stars refer to the degree of significance between constitutive and evoked labeling (1 to 4 stars for $p < 0.05$, < 0.01, < 0.001 and < 0.0001, respectively) using Fisher's PLSD. (Reprinted from Figures 4 and 5 of [13] with kind permission from Springer-Verlag GmbH and Co Heidelberg, Germany.)

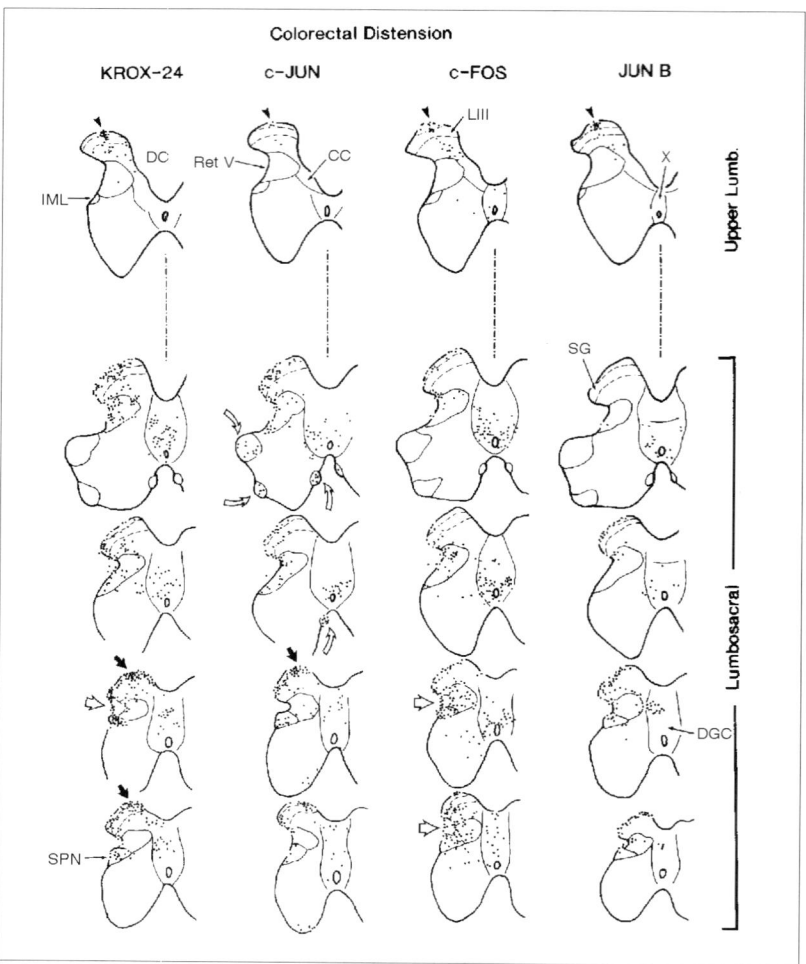

Figure 6. These illustrations show the distribution of Krox-24- (first column), c Jun- (second column), c-Fos- (third column) and Jun B- (fourth column) immunoreactive cells in the spinal cord of a rat with repetitive colorectal distension (80 mm Hg intraluminal pressure). Five segments are represented, including the upper lumbar level (first row) and four lumbosacral levels (four lower rows). Segments of the midlevel of the lumbar enlargement, which do not show consistent labeling, are marked by a dashed line. Each diagram includes all labeled cells in one 40 μm section; each dot represents one labeled cell. The boundaries of the reticular part of the neck of the dorsal horn (Ret.V), lamina X (X) and its caudal extension, the dorsal gray commissure (DGC), the intermediolateral (IML) and sacral parasympathetic nucleus (SPN), Clark's columns (CC) and lamina III (L III) have been outlined for orientation. Black arrows at caudal levels in both the Krox-24 and c-Jun columns point to the area of densest staining in the superficial layers of the dorsal horn, thus probably corresponding to the entry zone for afferent inputs; open arrows at caudal levels in both the Krox-24 and c-Fos columns point to the strands of fibers that run from the most lateral tip of the superficial layers of the dorsal horn to the sacral parasympathetic nucleus; arrow heads at upper lumbar level (first row) point to positive cells that insert between the superficial layers and the medial portion of the neck of the dorsal horn. Curved open arrows in the second column point to sacral motoneuronal groups (dorsolateral, retrodorsolateral nuclei and spinal nucleus of the bulbocavernosus) containing c-Jun constitutive expression. DC: dorsal columns (Reprinted from Figure 1 of [6] with kind permission from Elsevier Science Ltd, Kidlington, UK).

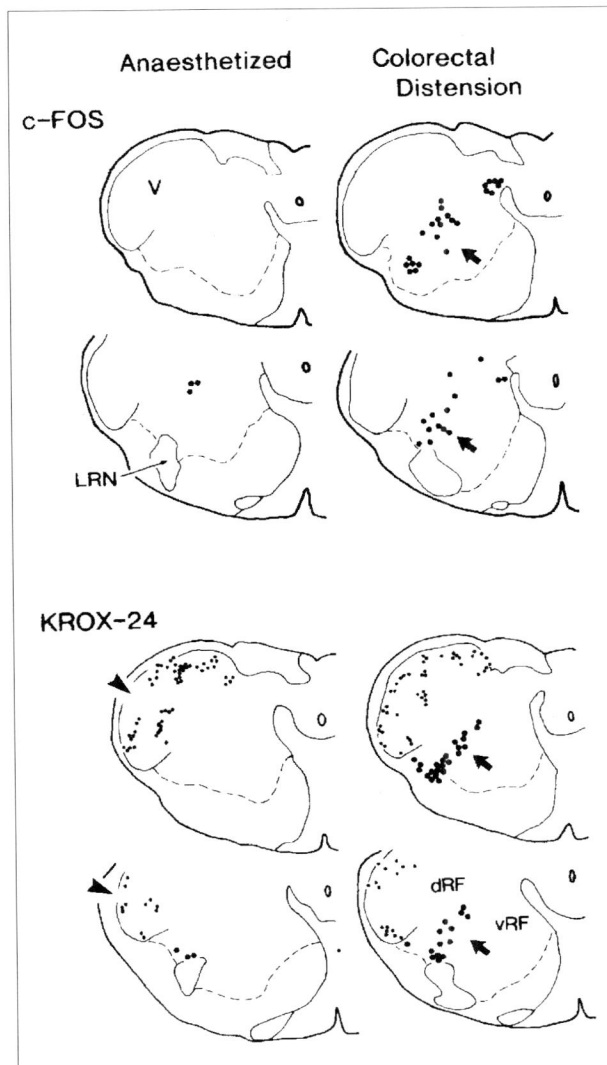

Figure 7. Illustrations of the distribution of c-Fos- (two upper rows) and Krox-24- (two lower rows) immunoreactive cells in the caudal part of the ventrolateral medulla. From left to right, are shown: anaesthesia- (first column) and colorectal distension (second column) stimulating conditions. Two frontal levels passing either through the posterior part of the lateral reticular nucleus (LRN) or just posterior to it are shown in each case. Visceronociceptive-evoked labeling (arrows) is concentrated in an area lying between the dorsal (dRF) and ventral (vRF) reticular fields; this region is devoided of anaesthesia-evoked staining (first column). (Reprinted from Figure 6 of [6] with kind permission from Elsevier Science Ltd, Kidlington, UK).

Fully developed cyclophosphamide cystitis (4 hours post-injection) maximally evoked IEGs in both the nucleus of the solitary tract and the caudal reticular formation but not in other parts of the hindbrain. In another group of hindbrain structures (nucleus O and central gray pars alpha, locus coeruleus, Barrington's nucleus, caudal parabrachial area mostly in its ventral and lateral subdivisions) the evoked expression of IEGs was maximum only at times corresponding to the earliest stages of cystitis development (1 to 2 hours) and thus well before complete cystitis, the most painful stage, has installed.

Conclusion

The present work demonstrates that hindbrain stuctures involved in pain processing can be effectively identified in behaving animals using the evoked expression of IEGs. At the present time, with careful analysis of results in terms of pain *versus* stress- or vegetative-related incidences, it would appear that hindbrain structures preferentially driven by nociceptive inputs *i.e.* those that increase and maintain their activity in parallel with the degree of nociception are both few in number and partially distinct from each other when devoted to either somatic or visceral processing. Thus, visceral pain would be processed at both levels of the nucleus of the solitary tract and the caudal part of bulbar reticular formation while somatic pain would be mostly processed in both this latter area and in the rostrodorsal portion of the lateral parabrachial complex, mostly the subnucleus superior lateralis, and closely adjacent mesencephalic areas. Other hindbrain areas which are maximally driven before the degree of nociception has reached a maximum and do not maintain their activity in parallel with it, are, in contrast, more numerous and include nucleus O and central gray pars alpha, locus coeruleus, Barrington's nucleus, caudal parabrachial area mostly in its ventral and lateral subdivisions. Although a role in pain processing cannot be excluded for these latter structures, it is quite evident that such a role would be only part of a more general function and mostly in relation to vegetative modifications that accompany stress and painful situations. In fact all these structures appear to be powerfully driven in a variety of nociception free situations [6, 17-20). Distinction between these two main sets of structures which have differential specificity in regard to nociception can only be done if consideration is given to the overall temporal evolution of slowly evolving diseases and by carefully performing experiments in parallel with paired-sham animals.

References

1. Bravo R. Growth factor inducible genes in fibroblasts. In : Habencht A, ed. *Growth factors, differenciation factors and cytokines*. Berlin : Springer, 1990 : 324-43.
2. Vogt PK, Bos TJ. Jun: oncogene and transcription factor. *Adv Cancer Res* 1990 ; 55 : 2-36.
3. Lantéri-Minet M, de Pommery J, Herdegen T, Weil-Fugazza J, Bravo R, Menétrey D. Differential time-course and spatial expression of Fos, Jun and Krox-24 proteins in spinal cord of rats undergoing subacute or chronic somatic inflammation. *J Comp Neurol* 1993 ; 333 : 223-35.
4. Lantéri-Minet M, Weil-Fugazza J, de Pommery J, Menétrey D. Hindbrain structures involved in pain processing as revealed by the expression of c-Fos and other immediate early gene proteins. *Neuroscience* 1994 ; 58 : 287-98.
5. Bon K, Lantéri-Minet M, de Pommery J, Michiels JF, Menétrey D. Cyclophosphamide cystitis as a model of visceral pain in rats. A survey of hindbrain structures involved in visceroception and nociception using the expression of c-Fos and Krox-24 proteins. *Exp Brain Res* (in press).
6. Lantéri-Minet M, Isnardon P, de Pommery J, Menétrey D. Spinal and hindbrain structures involved in viscero and visceronociception as revealed by the expression of Fos, Jun and Krox-24 proteins. *Neuroscience* 1993 ; 55 : 737-53.

7. Stein C, Millan MJ, Herz A. Unilateral inflammation of the hindpaw in rats as a model of prolonged noxious stimulation: alterations in behavior and nociceptive thresholds. *Pharmacol Biochem Behav* 1988 ; 31 : 445-51.
8. Butler SH, Godefroy F, Besson JM, Weil-Fugazza A. Limited arthritic model for chronic pain studies in the rat. *Pain* 1992 ; 48 : 73-81.
9. Calvino B, Villanueva L, Le Bars D. Dorsal horn (convergent) neurons in the intact anaesthetized arthritic rat. I. Segmental excitatory influences. *Pain* 1987 ; 28 : 81-98.
10. Menétrey D, Besson JM. Electrophysiological characteristics of dorsal horn cells in rats with cutaneous inflammation resulting from chronic arthritis. *Pain* 1982 ; 13 : 343-64.
11. Nahin RL, Hylden JLK. Peripheral inflammation is associated with increased glutamic acid decarboxylase immunoreactivity in the rat spinal cord. *Neurosci Lett* 1991 ; 128 : 226-33.
12. Schaible HG, Schmidt RF, Willis WD. Enhancement of the responses of ascending tract cells in the cat spinal cord by acute inflammation of the knee joint. *Exp Brain Res* 1987 ; 66 : 489-99.
13. Lantéri-Minet M, Bon K, de Pommery J, Michiels JF, Menétrey D. Cyclophosphamide cystitis as a model of visceral pain in rats: model elaboration and spinal structures involved as revealed by the expression of c-Fos and Krox-24 proteins. *Exp Brain Res* 1995 ; 105 : 220-32.
14. Ness TJ, Gebhart GF. Visceral pain: a review of experimental studies. *Pain* 1990 ; 41 : 167-234.
15. Brock N, Pohl J, Stekar J. Studies on the urotoxicity of oxazaphosphorine cytostatics and its prevention-I. Experimental studies on the urotoxicity of alkylating compounds. *Eur J Cancer* 1981; 17 : 595-607
16. Cox PJ. Cyclophosphamide cystitis. Identification of acrolein as the causative agent. *Biochem Pharmacol* 1979 ; 28 : 2045-9.
17. Erickson JT, Millhorn DE. Fos-like protein is induced in neurons of the medulla oblongata after stimulation of the carotid sinus nerve in awake and anaesthetized rats. *Brain Res* 1991; 567 : 11-24.
18. Krukoff TL, Morton TL, Harris KH, Jhamandas JH. Expression of c-fos protein in rat brain elicited by electrical stimulation of the pontine parabrachial nucleus. *J Neurosci* 1992 ; 12 : 3582-90.
19. Lu J, Hathaway CB, Bereiter DA. Adrenalectomy enhances Fos-like immunoreactivity within the spinal trigeminal nucleus induced by noxious thermal stimulation of the cornea. *Neuroscience* 1993 ; 54 : 809-18.
20. Rutherfurd SD, Widdop RE, Sannajust F, Louis WJ, Gundlach AL. Expression of c-fos and NGFI-A messenger RNA in the medulla oblongata of the anaesthetized rat following stimulation of vagal and cardiovascular afferents. *Mol Brain Res* 1992 ; 13 : 301-12.

12

Potential role of orbital and cingulate cortices in nociception

J.O. DOSTROVSKY, W.D. HUTCHISON, K.D. DAVIS, A. LOZANO

Department of Physiology and Division of Neurosurgery, University of Toronto, Canada.

The past twenty years have witnessed a massive research effort aimed at elucidating the mechanisms underlying pain sensation [1, 2]. However, despite major discoveries in the periphery and spinal cord, our understanding of the thalamo-cortical processing of pain has advanced much less, and many fundamental issues remain unanswered. Nevertheless, important advances utilizing anatomical tracing techniques and PET imaging are beginning to provide important clues as to the cortical regions that are involved in mediating pain sensations. This paper will review the information implicating the cingulate and VLO in pain and present new findings in support of the involvement of these regions in nociception.

The probable role of the medial thalamus in mediating the affective and motivational aspects of pain has been well accepted since the pioneering work of Head and Holmes [1-3]. Since the regions of medial thalamus that had been proposed as mediating pain have widespread and diffuse projections to cortex, the anatomy is not helpful in identifying cortical regions that might be particulary involved in pain perception. However, in 1981 Craig et al. [4, 5] described in the cat a region of medial thalamus, the nucleus submedius (Sm), that receives a major input from the spinothalamic (STT) and trigeminothalamic (TTT) tracts and which, in turn, has a very specific and reciprocal projection to the VLO. Of further interest was the finding of a descending projection from VLO to the ventrolateral periaqueductal gray (PAG), a region implicated in descending pain modulation. We and other investigators extended these anatomical studies to the rat and described the existence of a very similar pathway [6-9] (see Figures 1, 2). These findings suggest that the VLO might be involved

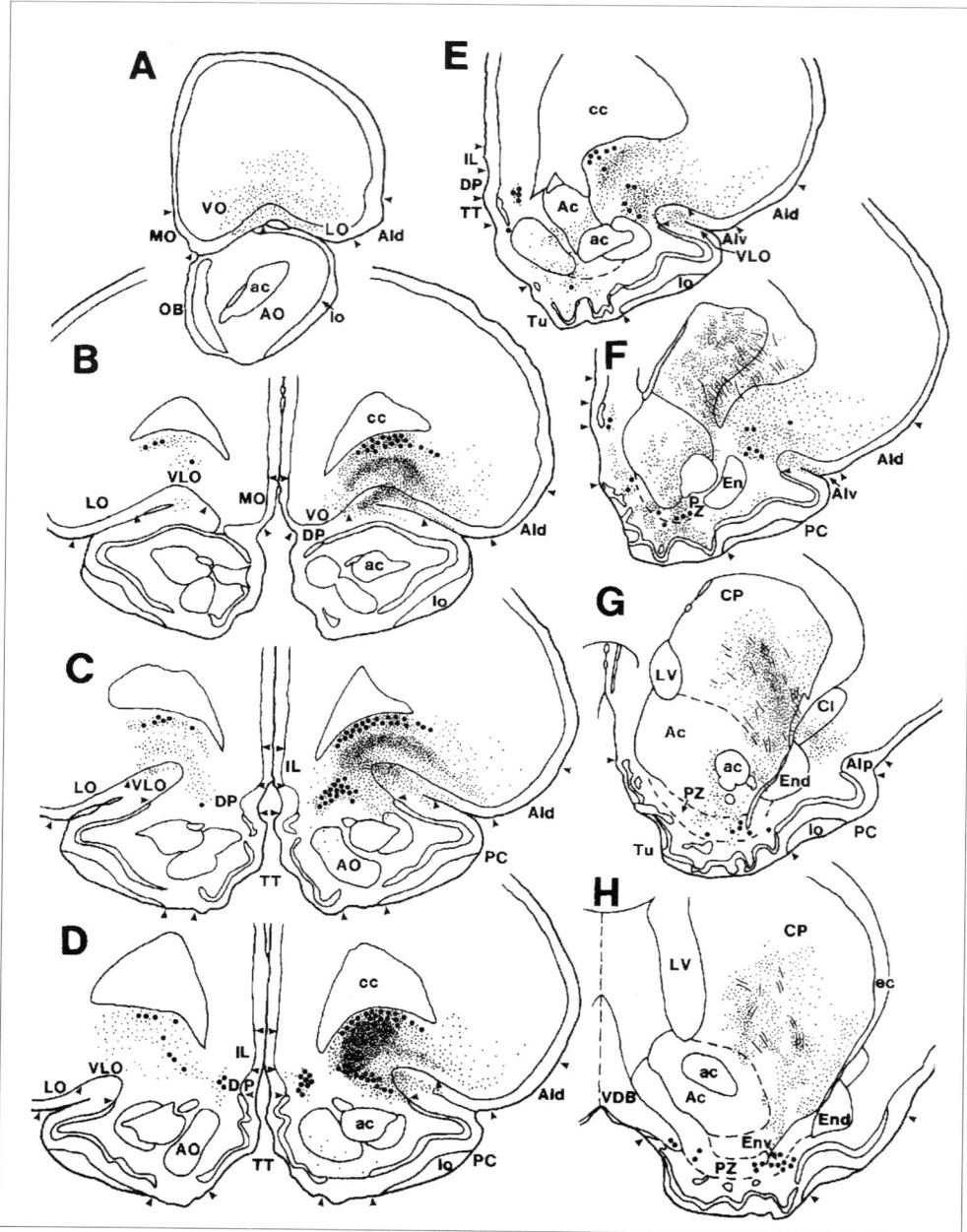

Figure 1. This figure, part of Figure 1 in Yoshida et al. [6], shows the anterograde and retrograde labelling in forebrain following an injection of WGA HRP in Sm. Note in particular the dense terminal labelling in the ipsilateral VLO in section B,C, D, and E and the presence of retrogradely labelled neurons in this same region. See original reference for additional details, injection site and abbreviations. Reprinted with permission from [6].

specifically in pain mechanisms, especially as recent electrophysiological studies have shown that many neurons in Sm respond to noxious stimuli [4, 10-12]. Our aims were therefore to determine whether neurons in rat VLO also responded to noxious stimuli and to determine the effects of stimulating VLO on subcortical pain processing and nociceptive reflexes. These results are summarized below, and have been briefly reported elsewhere [13-16].

Of particular interest is whether this same Sm to VLO pathway exists in primates. Recent anatomical studies by Craig *et al.* suggest that in the primate the ventrocaudal part of the medial dorsal nucleus (MDvc) [17, 18], a cytoarchitectonically distinct region distinguishable also in the human, receives a direct STT and TTT input from lamina I neurons and is probably anatomically homologous to Sm in rat and cat. However, in contrast to Sm in cat and rat, MDvc projects primarily to the anterior cingulate cortex, as does Sm in the rabbit [19] (Figure 2). This is particularly interesting in view of recent human PET and preliminary functional MRI studies that have shown that noxious stimuli give rise to increased blood flow in this same part of the cingulate cortex [20-24] and the many clinical observations indicating that lesions to this region can be effective in alleviating chronic pain [25]. Furthermore, recent findings in the rabbit have shown that this same region contains neurons that respond to noxious stimuli, and that these responses can be abolished by lesions of the medial thalamus [26]. Thus, these anatomical findings suggest that in the human, part of the anterior cingulate cortex (area 24) may serve similar functions as the VLO in rat and cat.

We have recently had the opportunity to record from neurons in the cingulate cortex of patients undergoing functional stereotactic surgery for alleviation of psychiatric

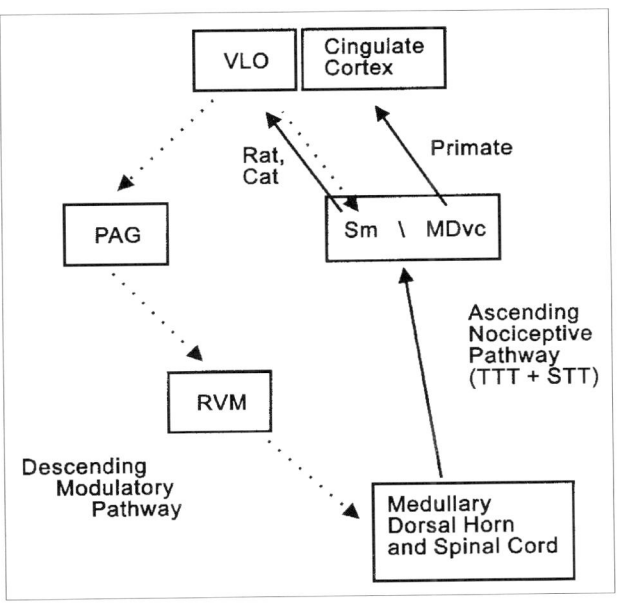

Figure 2. Schematic diagram illustrating the main pathways described in the present paper. In the cat and monkey, the ascending STT and TTT pathways terminating in Sm and MDvc respectively, originate almost exclusively from lamina I. Please note that other termination sites of the STT and TTT in thalamus are not shown.

disturbances, and to perform detailed psychophysical studies of experimental pain before and after a lesion to this region in one of these patients. These findings will be presented in the results section. Some of these findings have been reported elsewhere [27, 28].

Methods and results

Rat VLO studies

Animals were anaesthetized with chloralose/urethane. Single unit extracelluar recordings were obtained with metal microelectrodes. Stimulating electrodes were implanted in the region of Sm in order to orthodromically or antidromically activate the VLO neurons. Innocuous and noxious mechanical and thermal stimuli were delivered to the skin with hand held probes. In some experiments, stimulation electrodes were implanted in the VLO, and stimulation effects determined on neurons in Sm, PAG, and rostroventromedial medulla (RVM) and on the tail flick reflex (for further methodological details *see* [12, 29, 30])

The main aim of these studies was to determine the effect of SM stimulation on neurons in VLO and examine whether VLO neurons were activated by noxious stimuli. As predicted by the anatomical studies, many cells activated by Sm stimulation were found in VLO. One group consisted of neurons that had descending projections to Sm since Sm stimulation elicited antidromic responses. Most of these neurons had little or no spontaneous activity and only 15% were activated by skin stimulation. In these few cases, noxious stimulation elicited weak and labile responses. In contrast, another group of VLO neurons were activated orthodromically by Sm stimulation. These were usually spontaneously active and frequently (72%) activated by peripheral stimulation. The majority of the neurons were excited by noxious stimulation of the skin, usually robust slowly adapting responses, although 24% were inhibited. Innocuous skin stimulation was ineffective. In all cases, neurons excited by skin stimulation were also excited by Sm stimulation and conversely for inhibition. Receptive fields were large and, in 94% of cases, were bilateral.

Electrical stimulation of VLO produced a variety of responses on Sm neurons. The most common response was that of inhibition, although some neurons were also excited (both antidromic and orthodromic responses were observed). Stimulation at around 10Hz frequently produced an incrementing orthodromic excitatory response, that was absent at lower stimulation rates. Electrical stimulation of VLO was found to inhibit many PAG neurons, although some neurons were excited and some had both excitatory and inhibitory responses. VLO stimulation (short 200ms trains) did not affect the firing of dorsal horn neurons, although it produced a very short duration inhibition of the jaw-opening reflex [13].

VLO stimulation (10-15 sec. trains) was found to reduce the tail flick latency in lightly anesthetized rats and this was associated with an enhancement of the inhibition of OFF cells and the excitation of ON cells in the RVM.

Human cingulate cortex studies

Four patients underwent functional stereotactic cingulotomy for alleviation of psychiatric disturbances. Recordings of neuronal activity in the cingulate cortex were performed prior to making the bilateral radiofrequency lesions in order to help localize the appropriate lesion sites. In one of these patients, detailed psychophysical testing was performed prior to and after the cingulotomy.

Recordings in human cingulate

Bilateral recordings (12 trajectories) in the cingulate cortex were obtained in 6 sessions (two of the patients had repeated explorations in order to enlarge the previously performed lesions). Except for one case which was performed under general anaesthesia, the patients were awake throughout the procedure. Single unit extracellular recordings were obtained from a tungsten microelectrode as it was driven through the cortex. Innocuous and noxious mechanical and thermal stimuli were delivered with hand held probes and a Peltier thermode. The recording session was videotaped and unit and transducer recordings digitized and stored on tape for subsequent detailed analysis of neuronal responses (*see* [31, 32] for further methodological detail).

A total of 9 neurons in three of the patients was found which responded to noxious stimulation. Seven of these neurons were excited, and the remaining 2 were inhibited by noxious stimulation. Four of the neurons were excited or inhibited by noxious mechanical stimulation (usually pinpricks) and 6 by noxious heating or cooling stimuli (in most cases neurons were only tested with one of these modalities; one tested with both responded to both). It was not feasible to determine receptive field boundaries, however some neurons were only activated by contralateral stimuli and others had bilateral fields. Responses were repeatable, however, the magnitude of the response usually decreased with repeated stimulation: Innocuous cutaneous stimulation was ineffective in eliciting responses in these neurons. Figure 3 shows examples of the responses of two neurons recorded in cingulate cortex that responded to noxious thermal stimulation applied *via* a Peltier thermode to the forearm, and pinpricks to the palmar surface of the hand.

Psychophysical studies

Detailed psychophysical testing was performed on one patient before and after cingulotomy (neurons responding to noxious stimuli were recorded bilaterally in this patient in the regions lesioned). The patient was asked to rate the warm, cold, pain intensity and pain affect of cooling and warming stimuli delivered to her forearm by a computer controlled Peltier thermode. In addition, pain threshold and pain tolerance to immersion of the hand in a cold (5 °C) water bath were determined. Thresholds were

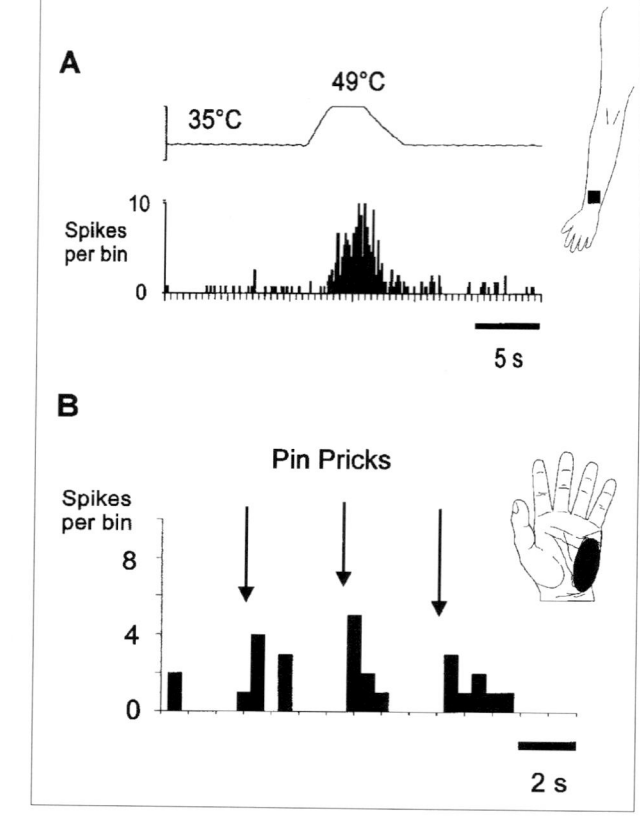

Figure 3. Ratemeter records of two neurons recorded in the cingulate cortex. Part A shows the response of a neuron to a noxious 49 °C stimulus delivered to the site on the forearm shown on the right. The patient reported this stimulus as painful. Binwidth is 100ms. Part B shows the responses of a neuron to pin pricks delivered to the palm in the area indicated on the figurine. Each arrow indicates the approximate time of application of three pin pricks delivered in close succession and reported as painful by the patient. In this case pin pricks to other regions of the body did not elicit a response. Bindwidth is 500 ms.

determined prior to the cingulotomy as well as at 3 days, and 5 and 10 weeks postoperatively. The patient also had a subsequent capsulotomy, and further ratings were obtained at 3 days and 3 months post-capsulotomy (see [28] for further details).

Compared to pre-operative levels, cingulotomy resulted in diminished warmth perception and an elevated heat pain threshold and increased ratings to suprathreshold noxious heat stimuli (see Figure 4). Prior to surgery, the patient perceived all cold stimuli as cold but not painful. However, after cingulotomy and capsulotomy cold stimuli were rated significantly colder and stimuli ≤ 12 °C evoked pain. Compared to normal control subjects, the patient's ratings of innocuous and noxious cold stimuli were reduced pre-operatively but elevated postoperatively, and cold pain tolerance was elevated pre-operatively but reduced postoperatively.

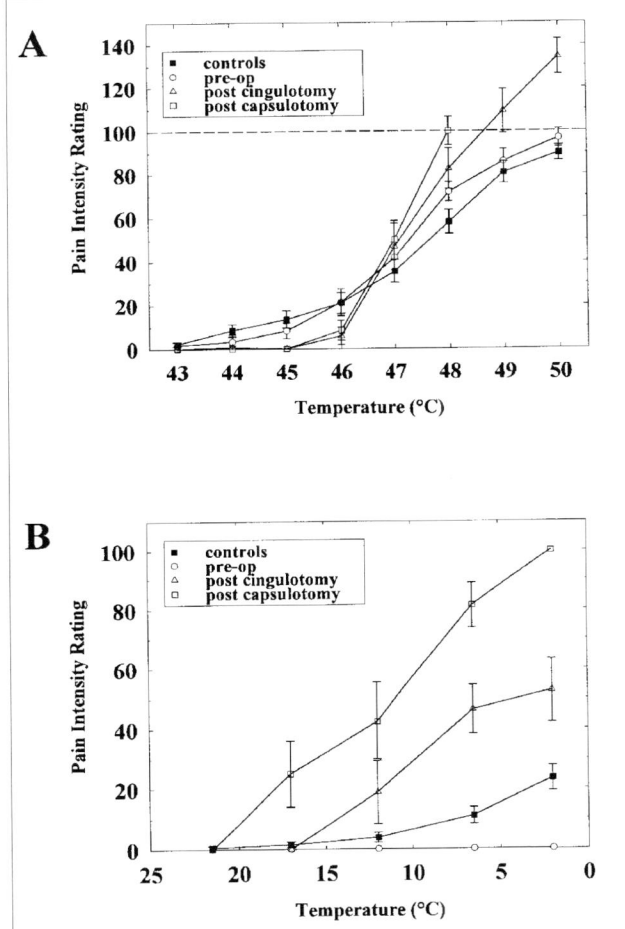

Figure 4. Ratings of heat pain and cold pain in a patient before and after cingulotomy and capsulotomy. Panel A shows the pain intensity ratings for increasing thermal stimuli pre operatively and at 10 weeks post cingulotomy and post capsulotomy, and compares these with values obtained from normal control subjects. Panel B shows the pain intensity ratings for decreasing cold thermal stimuli pre operatively and post cingulotomy and post capsulotomy, and compares these with values obtained from normal control subjects. For further details see Figures 5 and 8 in Davis et al. [28]. Modified with permission from [28].

Discussion

The data presented in this paper provide additional support for the role of limbic cortex in nociception. In particular, they have provided data for the probable involvement of rat VLO and human cingulate cortex in pain mechanisms. The data are consistent with their role in mediating, at least in part, the affective-motivational aspects of pain and possibly also in mediating descending modulation of pain. As discussed in the introduction, it is possible that these two regions serve similar functions in different species.

There have been a number of other studies that have provided evidence for a role of VLO in nociception. Electrophysiological studies in both cats and rats [33, 34] have also reported the existence in VLO of neurons responding specifically to noxious stimuli. In addition, Tsubokawa *et al.* [35] reported increased blood flow in cats in the VLO region following a noxious stimulus, which may be analogous to the increased blood flow described in cingulate cortex in humans following nociceptive stimuli [20-22]. In view of the large receptive fields of neurons in VLO, it is unlikely that it could be involved in mediating the sensory discriminatory aspects of pain. However, the findings suggest that VLO may be involved in mediating the affective-motivational aspects of pain. It could also be involved in descending modulation of pain (*see* below).

There is anatomical evidence in both rat and cat for descending projections from the VLO to the PAG [5, 36, 37], suggesting that VLO may be involved in descending modulation. Studies in our lab have confirmed, by antidromic stimulation, the existence of descending projections from the PAG, and shown that VLO stimulation inhibits or excites neurons in the PAG [16]. Since the PAG is well known to be a source of descending modulation relaying in the RVM, these findings suggest that VLO might modulate ascending nociceptive information *via* this route. Indeed our recent studies showed that VLO stimulation does alter the responses of ON and OFF cells in the RVM (*see* [38] for discussion of ON and OFF cells) in a way consistent with producing hyperalgesia, and this was confirmed by showing that VLO stimulation reduces the tail flick latency [29]. However, other findings suggest that descending modulation from VLO might produce hypalgesia. Short train stimulation produces a short lasting inhibition of the jaw opening reflex [13], and local anaesthetic block [39] or lesions of the VLO region [40] have been shown to increase pain-related behavior.

Our findings of neurons responding to noxious stimulation in the human cingulate cortex constitute the first report of such activity in the human. It is of particular interest that the location of the neurons in the region of anterior cingulate corresponds well with the location of increased blood flow in cingulate cortex as revealed in recent PET studies [20-23], and thus provides important complimentary data in support of the role of the cingulate cortex in pain. The types of responses we observed are similar to those reported by Sikes and Vogt in the cingulate cortex of the rabbit [26].

Our findings of increased thresholds to noxious stimuli in conjunction with increased perception of noxious stimuli (hyperpathia) are in general agreement with previous clinical reports of the effects of cingulotomies and leukotomies. Although such procedures have been reported to reduce or eliminate chronic pains, patients reported acute nociceptive pains as more intense. However, before general conclusions can be made, additional studies of this type must be performed, especially as the patient reported in this study had abnormal preoperative pain and temperature reports, and the surgery tended to normalize these sensations. Also, the recent study of Talbot *et al.*, although reporting some similar findings, did not obtain identical results [41]. In summary, our findings provide further support to the growing literature implicating the cingulate cortex in pain in addition to its other presumed and related roles in modulating autonomic activity, emotional responses, attention, motivation and response selection [42, 43].

Acknowledgements

The authors wish to thank Dr. Nada El-Yassir who performed the rat VLO studies, Dr. A. Yoshida who performed the anatomical studies, Dr. Zelma Kiss who assisted in some of the cingulotomy recordings and Mary Teofilo who assisted in preparation of figures. These studies were supported by grants from the US NIH and Canadian MRC.

References

1. Willis WD Jr. The pain system. The neural basis of nociceptive transmission in the mammalian nervous system. In : Gildenberg PL, ed. *Pain and headache*. Basel : S. Karger, 1985 : 1-346.
2. Price DD. *Psychological and neural mechansims of pain*. New York : Raven Press Ltd, 1988 : 1-241.
3. Head H, Holmes G. Sensory disturbances from cerebral lesions. *Brain* 1911 ; 34 : 102-254.
4. Craig AD Jr, Burton H. Spinal and medullary laminal I projection to nucleus submedius in medial thalamus: a possible pain center. *J Neurophysiol* 1981 ; 45 : 443-65.
5. Craig ADJ, Wiegand SJ, Price JL. The thalamo-cortical projection of the nucleus submedius in the cat. *J Comp Neurol* 1982 ; 206 : 28-48.
6. Yoshida A, Dostrovsky JO, Sessle BJ, Chiang CY. Trigeminal projections to the nucleus submedius of the thalamus in the rat. *J Comp Neurol* 1991 ; 307 : 609-25.
7. Yoshida A, Dostrovsky JO, Chiang CY. The afferent and efferent connections of the nucleus submedius in the rat. *J Comp Neurol* 1992 ; 324 : 115-33.
8. Coffield JA, Bowen KK, Miletic V. Retrograde tracing of projections between the nucleus submedius, the ventrolateral orbital cortex, and the midbrain in the rat. *J Comp Neurol* 1992 ; 321 : 488-99.
9. Dado RJ, Giesler GJ Jr. Afferent input to nucleus submedius in rats: retrograde labeling of neurons in the spinal cord and caudal medulla. *J Neurosci* 1990 ; 10 : 2672-86.
10. Dostrovsky JO, Guilbaud G. Noxious stimuli excite neurons in nucleus submedius of the normal and arthritic rat. *Brain Res* 1988 ; 460 : 269-80.
11. Miletic V, Coffield JA. Responses of neurons in the rat nucleus submedius to noxious and innocuous mechanical cutaneous stimulation. *Somatosens Mot Res* 1989 ; 6 : 567-87.
12. Kawakita K, Dostrovsky JO, Tang JS, Chiang CY. Responses of neurons in the rat thalamic nucleus submedius to cutaneous, muscle and visceral nociceptive stimuli. *Pain* 1993 ; 55 : 327-38.
13. Chiang CY, El-Yassir N, Moustafa EM, Dostrovsky JO, Sessle BJ. Effects of ventrolateral orbital cortex stimulation on the jaw-opening reflex and spinal cord dorsal horn neurons. *Soc Neurosci Abstr* 1989 ; 15 : 150.
14. Dostrovsky JO, Kawakita K. Effects of frontal cortex stimulation on nociceptive neurons in nucleus submedius of the anesthetized rat. *Soc Neurosci Abstr* 1988 ; 14 : 121.
15. El-Yassir N, Dostrovsky JO. Activation of neurones in the orbital region of rat cortex by noxious stimulation and by stimulation in nucleus submedius. *Soc Neurosci Abstr* 1990 ; 16 : 706.
16. El-Yassir N, Dostrovsky JO. The effect of orbital cortex stimulation on periaqueductal gray (PAG) neurons in the rat. *Pain* 1990 ; supplement 5 : s443.
17. Craig AD, Bushnell MC, Zhang E-T, Blomqvist A. A thalamic nucleus specific for pain and temperature sensation. *Nature* 1994 ; 372 : 770-3.

18. Craig AD. Spinal and supraspinal processing of specific pain and temperature. In : Boivie J, Hansson P, Lindblom U, eds. *Touch, temperature, and pain in health and disease: mechanisms and assessments.* Seattle : IASP Press, 1994 : 421-37.
19. Vogt LJ, Vogt BA, Sikes RW. Limbic thalamus in rabbit: architecture, projections to cingulate cortex and distribution of muscarinic acetylcholine, GABAA, and opioid receptors. *J Comp Neurol* 1992 ; 319 : 205-17.
20. Talbot JD, Marrett S, Evans AC, Meyer E, Bushnell MC, Duncan GH. Multiple representations of pain in human cerebral cortex. *Science* 1991 ; 251 : 1355-8.
21. Coghill RC, Talbot JD, Evans AC, Meyer E, Gjedde A, Bushnell MC, Duncan GH. Distributed processing of pain and vibration by the human brain. *J Neurosci* 1994 ; 14 : 4095-108.
22. Jones AKP, Brown WD, Friston KJ, Qi LY, Frackowiak RSJ. Cortical and subcortical localization of response to pain in man using positron emission tomography. *Proc R Soc Lond (Biol)* 1991 ; 244 : 39-44.
23. Casey KL, Minoshima S, Berger KL, Koeppe RA, Morrow TJ, Frey KA. Positron emission tomographic analysis of cerebral structures activated specifically by repetitive noxious heat stimuli. *J Neurophysiol* 1994 ; 71 : 802-7.
24. Davis KD, Wood ML, Crawley AP, Mikulis DJ. Functional magnetic resonance imaging of human somatosensory and cingulate cortex during pain and paraesthesia evoked by median nerve stimulation. *Soc Neurosci Abstr* 1995 (in press).
25. Gybels JM, Sweet WH. *Neurosurgical treatment of persistent pain. Physiological and pathological mechanisms of human pain. Pain and headache* Vol 11. Basel : Karger, 1989 : 1-442.
26. Sikes RW, Vogt BA. Nociceptive neurons in area 24 of rabbit cingulate cortex. *J Neurophysiol* 1992 ; 68 : 1720-32.
27. Hutchison WD, Dostrovsky JO, Davis KD, Lozano AM. Single unit responses and microstimulation effects in cingulate cortex of an awake patient. IASP World Congress on Pain 1993 ; 461.
28. Davis KD, Hutchison WD, Lozano AM, Dostrovsky JO. Altered pain and temperature perception following cingulotomy and capsulotomy in a patient with schizoaffective disorder. *Pain* 1994 ; 59 : 189-99.
29. Hutchison WD, Harfa L, Dostrovsky JO. Ventrolateral orbital cortex and periaqueductal gray stimulation-induced effects on ON-and OFF-cells in the rostral ventromedial medulla in the rat. *Neuroscience* 1995 (in press)
30. Chiang CY, Dostrovsky JO, Sessle BJ. Periaqueductal gray matter and nucleus raphe magnus involvement in anterior pretectal nucleus-induced inhibition of jaw-opening reflex in rats. *Brain Res* 1991 ; 544 : 71-8.
31. Tasker RR, Lenz FA, Yamashiro K, Gorecki J, Hirayama T, Dostrovsky JO. Microelectrode techniques in localization of stereotactic targets. *Neurol Res* 1987 ; 9 : 105-12.
32. Lenz FA, Dostrovsky JO, Kwan HC, Tasker RR, Yamashiro K, Murphy JT. Methods for microstimulation and recording of single neurons and evoked potentials in the human central nervous system. *J Neurosurg* 1988 ; 68 : 630-4.
33. Backonja M, Miletic V. Responses of neurons in the rat ventrolateral orbital cortex to phasic and tonic nociceptive stimulation. *Brain Res* 1991 ; 557 : 353-5.
34. Snow PJ, Lumb BM, Cervero F. The representation of prolonged and intense, noxious somatic and visceral stimuli in the ventrolateral orbital cortex of the cat. *Pain* 1992 ; 48 : 89-99.
35. Tsubokawa T, Katayama Y, Ueno Y, Moriyasu N. Evidence for involvement of the frontal cortex in pain-related cerebral events in cats: increase in local cerebral blood flow by noxious stimuli. *Brain Res* 1981 ; 217 : 179-85.

36. Hardy SGP, Leichnetz GR. Frontal cortical projections to the periaqueductal gray in the rat: a retrograde and orthograde horseradish peroxidase study. *Neurosci Lett* 1981 ; 23 : 13-7.
37. Beckstead RM. An autoradiographic examination of corticocortical and subcortical projections of the mediodorsal-projection (prefrontal) cortex in the rat. *J Comp Neurol* 1979 ; 184 : 43-62.
38. Fields HL, Heinricher MM, Mason P. Neurotransmitters in nociceptive modulatory circuits. *Annu Rev Neurosci* 1991 ; 14 : 219-45.
39. Cooper SJ. Anaesthetisation of prefrontal cortex and response to noxious stimulation. *Nature* 1975 ; 254 : 439-40.
40. Reshetniak VK, Kukushkin ML. Effects of removal of orbitofrontal cortex and the development of reflex analgesia. *Bull Exp Biol Med* 1989 ; 108 : 14-6.
41. Talbot JD, Duncan GH, Bushnell MC, Villemure J-G. Evaluation of pain perception after anterior capsulotomy: a case report. World Congress on Pain 1993 ; 7 : 464.
42. Devinsky O, Morrell MJ, Vogt BA. Contributions of anterior cingulate cortex to behaviour. *Brain* 1995 ; 118 : 279-306.
43. Vogt BA, Sikes RW, Vogt LJ. Anterior cingulate cortex and the medial pain system. In: Vogt BA, Gabriel M, eds. *Neurobiology of cingulate cortex and limbic thalamus: a comprehensive handbook*. Boston : Birkhauser, 1993 : 313-65.

13

Cortical nociceptive mechanisms. A review of neurophysiological and behavioral evidence in the primate

W.K. DONG, E.H. CHUDLER

Departments of Anesthesiology and Psychology and Multidisciplinary Pain Center, University of Washington School of Medicine, Seattle, Washington, USA.

Based on anatomic, clinical, psychophysical and physiological evidence, cortical nociception in primates appears to involve multiple and interconnected cortical sites for processing nociceptive input. Several regions of the primate cerebral cortex, especially those within the parietal lobe, have been implicated in processing nociceptive inputs from intracortical and/or thalamic sources. Each site contains neurons that can uniquely encode various features of a noxious stimulus such as its submodality (mechanical and/or thermal), location, intensity and duration. Moreover, each site may contribute a unique set of nociceptive inputs to the different dimensions of the pain experience (i.e., sensory-discriminative, cognitive-evaluative, affective-motivational). Recent studies using positron emission tomography (PET) alone or in combination with magnetic resonance imaging (MRI) generally support the conclusion that various types of painful stimulation are associated with significantly increased cerebral blood flow (CBF) or local metabolism in the parietal and cingulate cortices [1-5] (*see* also accompanying articles by Casey (chapter 15) and Jones (chapter 16)).

This review will focus on the neurophysiological and behavioral aspects of nociceptive mechanisms in the parietal cortex. An in-depth discussion of the potential role of the cingulate cortex in nociception and pain-related behavior is presented in accompanying articles by Dostrovsky (chapter 12) and Gabriel (chapter 14), and in a recent review article by Devinsky *et al.* [6]. Within the parietal cortex, regions that have been implicated in processing nociceptive input include the (1) first somatosensory area

(SI) of the postcentral gyrus, (2) second somatosensory area (SII) which occupies the parietal operculum in the sylvian (lateral) sulcus, (3) area 7b (PF) in monkey, or Brodmann's area 40 in man which occupies both the inferior parietal lobule and opercular region and (4) posterior insular areas.

SI cortex

The SI is a primary terminal site for nociceptive thalamocortical input from the ventroposterolateral (VPL) nucleus [7, 8] and possibly from the ventroposteromedial nucleus. Antidromic stimulation from the surface of SI in anesthetized monkeys can activate nociceptive somatic and visceral neurons in the thalamic VPL nucleus. Electrophysiological studies in both anaesthetized [9, 10] and unanaesthetized [11] monkeys showed that nociceptive neurons classified by their response properties to mechanical stimulation as wide dynamic range (WDR) and high threshold (HT) or nociceptive-specific (NS) were located in the SI. Although these nociceptive neurons represent a small proportion of the total somatosensory neurons with mechanical and/or thermal response properties in the SI, they appear to be organized in "aggregations" [12]. In general, SI nociceptive neurons can encode the place and intensity of noxious thermal and mechanical stimulation with high fidelity. These neurons are characterized by small contralateral, mechanical receptive fields and by their ability to grade noxious heat intensities by modulating the discharge rate. The noxious thermal threshold (43 - 44 °C) of SI nociceptive neurons in awake monkeys [11] is consistent with radiant heat pain thresholds in humans (mean 44.2 °C, [13]) and with the lowest noxious temperatures (45 - 47 °C) that elicit escape in water-restricted monkeys rewarded for not escaping [14, 15]. Moreover, the steep monotonic increase of peak discharge frequency to a continuum of noxious thermal stimuli (> 43 - 44 °C) in the majority of SI nociceptive neurons in awake monkeys [11] resembles the thermal stimulus-response functions for nociceptive neurons in the thalamic VPL nucleus [7] and in the spinal [16] and medullary [17] dorsal horn, for A-delta and C-fiber nociceptors [18], for human psychophysical pain magnitude scaling [19] and for monkey escape probabilities and latencies [14, 15]. Most SI nociceptive neurons, except those with large receptive fields, exhibit slow or no discharge adaptation at higher intensities of noxious thermal stimulation [9]. The thermal stimulus-response functions of some nociceptive WDR neurons are significantly suppressed when noxious thermal stimuli are delivered at short interstimulus intervals [10]. However, repetition of heat stimuli following prolonged, intense noxious heating can produce increased responsiveness or sensitization of thermal responses [9]. It should be noted that these characteristics of nociceptive SI neurons may underlie the reported lack of pain adaptation during noxious heat stimuli, the elevated thermal pain threshold and reduced pain sensation when thermal stimulus intervals are shortened and the hyperalgesia induced by intense noxious thermal stimulation [10, 20-22].

A large proportion of nociceptive neurons in SI are distinguished by their ability to finely encode small increases (T2 = 0.2 °C to 0.8 °C) in noxious temperature superimposed upon a steady noxious temperature (T1 = 45 °C or 46 °C) [11]. The peak discharge frequency of such cells increased monotonically as the intensity of T2 thermal shifts increased. Moreover, psychophysical experiments showed that increasing the intensity of T2 between 0.1 °C and 0.8 °C significantly increased the monkey's speed to detect such small thermal shifts [23]. Figure 1A and B, respectively, show a monkey's detection speeds and a nociceptive neuron's peak discharge frequencies to small T2 thermal shifts superimposed on T1 temperatures of 45 °C and 46 °C. Of particular importance is the demonstration that the neuronal discharge frequency is significantly correlated with the monkey's speed for detecting small increments in noxious thermal stimulation. Shown in Figure 1C is the peak discharge frequency plotted as a function of detection speed. The detection speed (1/latency) associated with these small increases in noxious thermal stimuli presumably reflects the monkey's perceived intensity of noxious thermal stimulation. This conclusion was derived from three key findings:

- the detection speed to small incremental temperature shifts superimposed on noxious levels of thermal stimulation is similar in monkey and man,
- the perceived intensity or estimated magnitude of pain sensation produced in human subjects is related, in a monotonic fashion, to T2 intensity,
- a logarithmic relationship exists between the human's detection speed and the estimated magnitude of pain [23].

The neurophysiological data from monkeys combined with psychophysical evidence from both monkey and man provide strong inference that SI nociceptive neurons, WDR neurons in particular, participate in the encoding process by which monkeys perceive the intensity of noxious thermal stimulation.

Another line of evidence that supports SI cortex as an important component in the sensory-discriminative aspect of pain comes from the behavioral consequence of ablating the SI cortex. Kenshalo *et al.* [24] showed that bilateral ablation of the SI in monkeys resulted in deficits related to the detection speed of T2 and to the frequency and speed for discriminating intense noxious temperatures from both an innocuous warm baseline temperature and a lower noxious temperature (T1) used iteratively in antecedent presentations. It is important to note that these impairments were not due to motor or attentional deficits because the post-ablation detection of skin cooling and of visual stimuli was unchanged and that detection and discrimination speeds gradually improved over several months but did not return to pre-ablation levels. These observations suggest that SI constitutes at least part of the neural substrate underlying detection of noxious thermal intensities. Kenshalo and Willis [12] suggested that SI may be necessary for the "pain sensing system" to operate at maximum efficiency.

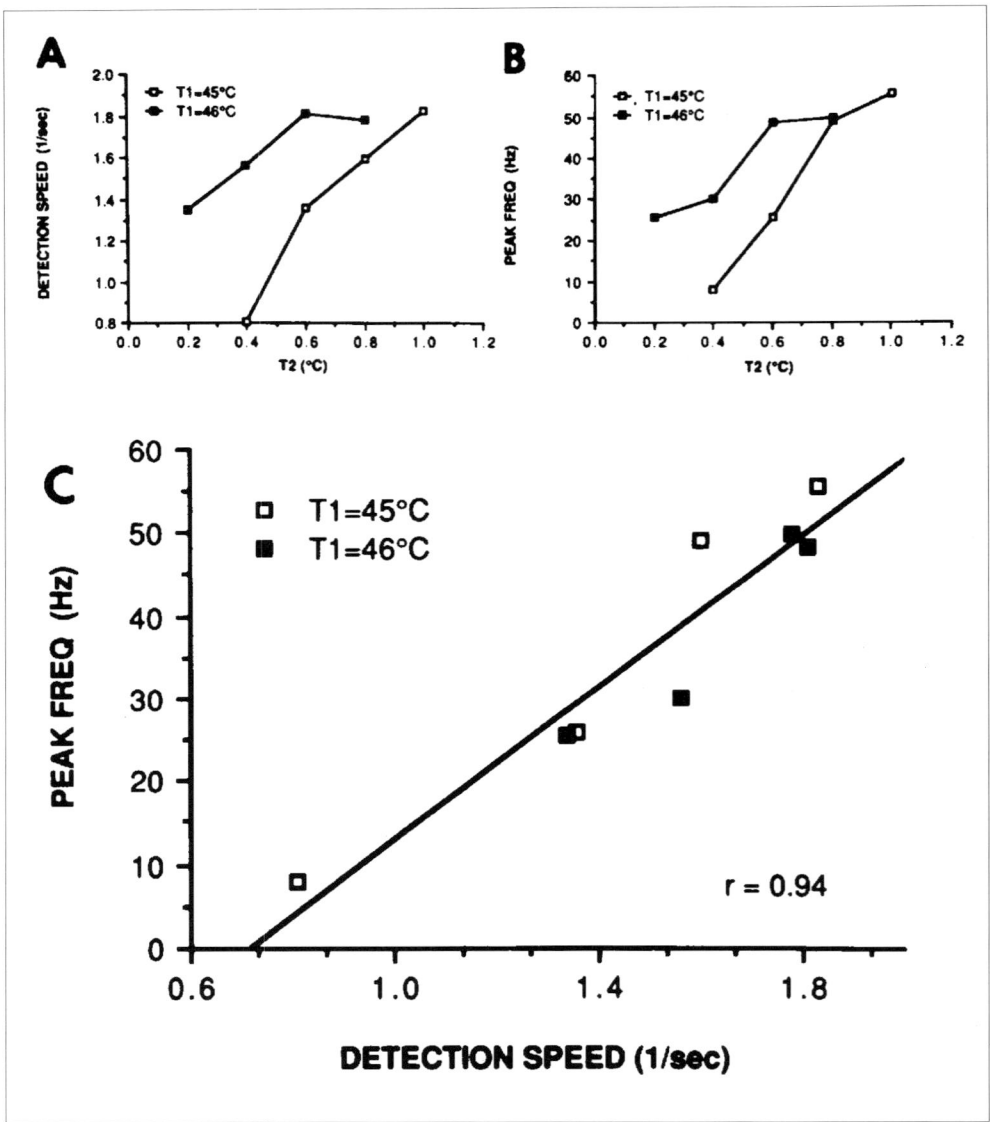

Figure 1. Relationships of small thermal shifts to detection speed and to neuronal discharge frequency and of detection speed to discharge frequency. A: average detection speed plotted as a function of T2 stimulus intensity from a T1 of either 45 or 46 °C. B: peak frequency of neuronal discharge plotted as a function of T2 intensity for either a 45 or 46 °C T1. The peak frequency was determined from peristimulus time histograms (200 ms bin width) after the onset of T2 and before the monkey released the response button. Each point represents the average of 4 trials. C: peak frequency plotted as a function of detection speed for all T2 stimuli. Solid line represents the linear regression of the equation fit to the scatter plot. (r), regression coefficient. (From Kenshalo et al., [11].)

Posterior parietal cortex

The experimental evidence presented in the preceding discussion clearly suggests that the SI cortex plays a crucial role in signaling the spatial, temporal and intensive features of noxious cutaneous stimulation and in contributing to the sensory-discriminative aspects of the pain experience. However, it is evident, from experimental and clinical data, that injury to SI alone does not abolish nociception and pain (*see* Kenshalo and Willis [12]), and that other brain sites must contribute to the pain experience. Sensory discrimination and other dimensions of the pain experience (i.e., affective-motivational, cognitive-evaluative) may require processing of nociceptive information along with related sensory and motor signals at multiple sites beyond the confines of SI. Brain injury confined primarily to the rostral inferior parietal lobule and parietal operculum which include area 7b and SII cortex and to the insular regions can alter pain sensibility [25-29]. Patients with damage to these posterior parietal regions reported aberrations of pain sensation that include hyp(o)algesia, analgesia, pain asymbolia and even spontaneous pain. Experimental evidence from human studies of CBF using PET alone or in combination with MRI and appropriate control procedures showed that various types of painful stimulation significantly increased local metabolism in the parietal operculum and insula [1-3, 5]. Serial connectivity between SI and SII and between SI and area 7b *via* SII in primates may be potentially important to nociception and pain, given the fact that ablation of SI severely impacts the serial processing of tactual information in SII [30-33]. The serial cortical processing of nociceptive information from SI to area 7b may also be possible through a direct corticocortical connection [34, 35]. Processing of nociceptive information through parallel thalamocortical pathways is also suggested from the observation that bilateral removal of the SI cortices does not abolish nociception and pain. This notion is supported by anatomic evidence that putative nociceptive regions in posterior parietal cortex (i.e., SII, area 7b, insula) receive their own unique set of thalamocortical afferents and intracortical afferents that are not serially connected to SI (*see* below and reviews by Dong *et al.* [29] and Coghill *et al.* [2]).

Although direct evidence for projection of nociceptive thalamocortical afferents to various regions of the posterior parietal cortex has not been reported, thalamic sites such as the intralaminar nuclei [36], VPM [37-39], ventral medial nucleus [40], ventral posterior inferior nucleus [41], pulvinar-lateral posterior nuclei and suprageniculate-limitans nuclei [42], and posterior nucleus [41, 42] contain nociceptive neurons and send dense fiber projections into the SII cortex, area 7b and insula [43, 44]. The SII cortex, area 7b and insula are also interconnected to each other [30, 35, 45]. Whether these interconnections in the posterior parietal cortex form a hierarchical functional organization for processing nociceptive and related information is uncertain.

Electrophysiological surveys of SII, area 7b and insula indicate that each site contains nociceptive neurons that represent a small proportion of the total somatosensory neurons sampled [29, 46-48]. Detailed study of area 7b has revealed nociceptive neurons with highly complex response properties attributed to spatial, multimodal and multisensory convergence. In contrast to nociceptive neurons in SI, those in area 7b do not encode the location and intensity of noxious thermal and mechanical stimulation with the same high fidelity. The cutaneous receptive fields of area 7b nociceptive neurons are often large and bilateral. Moreover, the somatotopic map is relatively crude. For example, the trigeminal nerve is represented in the rostral portion of area 7b, but the somatotopic representation of its subdivisions is not evident. Nociceptive WDR and NS neurons, whose classifications are based on mechanical response properties, and low threshold mechanoreceptive neurons are found in area 7b. Many of these neurons are multimodal that respond exclusively to noxious thermal stimuli (high threshold thermoreceptive, HTT) or differentially to both nonnoxious and noxious thermal stimuli (wide-range thermoreceptive, WRT) [29]. Multimodal neurons with similar thermal and mechanical response properties are found in the thalamic VPM of monkeys [38]. Multimodal somesthetic output from VPM may project directly to area 7b [43] or indirectly to area 7b *via* SII [30, 44]. We determined that thermal nociceptive neurons are functionally differentiated by statistical analysis into subpopulations that do encode (HTT-EN, WRT-EN) and do not encode (HTT-NE, WRT-NE) the magnitude of noxious thermal stimulus intensities [29]. It is noteworthy that WDR neurons in SI are also comprised of two subpopulations that do and do not grade noxious thermal intensities [10], and these may contribute inputs to the EN and NE subpopulations of thermal nociceptive neurons in area 7b. We also identified multisensory nociceptive neurons with visuosensory properties that respond to either an

Figure 2. Response properties of a multisensory WRT neuron that graded noxious thermal intensities (WRT-EN). A: visuosensory responses. Peristimulus time histograms show maximal responses obtained by the approach of a novel or threatening object toward the maxillary region of the face. Responses were inconsistently evoked by the experimenter's finger (A_1) when it approached the contralateral face (motion in depth) and was held ~1 cm from the maxillary skin surface for a few seconds. No additional response was obtained by applying pressure or pinch to the skin (not shown). Responses were consistently evoked by novel stimuli such as a tube (A_2) or hex wrench (A_3, B) that were moved toward or held close to the contralateral or ipsilateral maxillary skin region. No additional response was elicited by touching the novel objects on the skin, or withdrawing these visual targets from the face. B: graded thermoreceptive responses. Poststimulus time (PST) histograms show the responses evoked by graded thermal shifts applied to the skin on the contralateral maxillary region of the face. Each PST histogram is an accumulation of activity from the presentation of 5 completed trials of the same thermal shift that were not associated with escapes. Indicated below the histogram time base are the operant responses (BP, button press; BR, button release) and stimulus events (T, temperature onset; Sd2, light-tone discriminative cue; ITI, reward and intertrial interaval). In each block of 5 trials, one of the following conditions was implemented: 1) heating from a baseline temperature of 32 °C to temperatures ranging from 34 to 50 °C (left column), 2) cooling from an adapting temperature of 38 to 33 °C (top of right column), or 3) no thermal shift from an adapting temperature of 38 °C or heating from 38 °C to temperatures ranging from 40 to 50 °C (right column). Thermal shifts were applied at a rate of 10 °C/s. Horizontal bar above each histogram: temperature rise or fall (open segment) and final plateau temperature (filled segment). C: thermal S-R functions. Abscissa: plateau temperatures for thermal shifts from a basline temperature of 32 °C (open circles) or 38 °C (filled circles). Ordinate: discharge frequency (mean (SE) during the plateau temperature. D: recording site in cortical area 7b (filled circle). The approximate locus of the neuron was marked by an electrolytic lesion and determined histologically. A1, 1st auditory area; CS, central sulcus; Ig, granular insular cortex; IPS, intraparietal sulcus; LS, lateral sulcus; Pi, parainsular area; S2, second somatosensory area; T1 and T2, temporal areas; 1, 2, 3a, and 3b, first somatosensory area; 4, primary motor area; 5, superior parietal lobule; 7b, inferior parietal lobule. (From [29]).

approaching visual target whose trajectory is aligned with the cutaneous receptive field or a stationary visual target held in close proximity to but not touching the skin receptive field. A visuotopic organization is not apparent in area 7b. Figure 2 illustrates the multisensory response properties of a WRT-EN neuron. The regression coefficients (r2) for the two thermal stimulus-response functions are 0.79 (34 °C - 50 °C) and 0.91 (40 °C - 50 °C). WRT neurons may be dependent on convergence of multimodal input from warm and cold receptors as well as A- thermal nociceptors and/or C polymodal

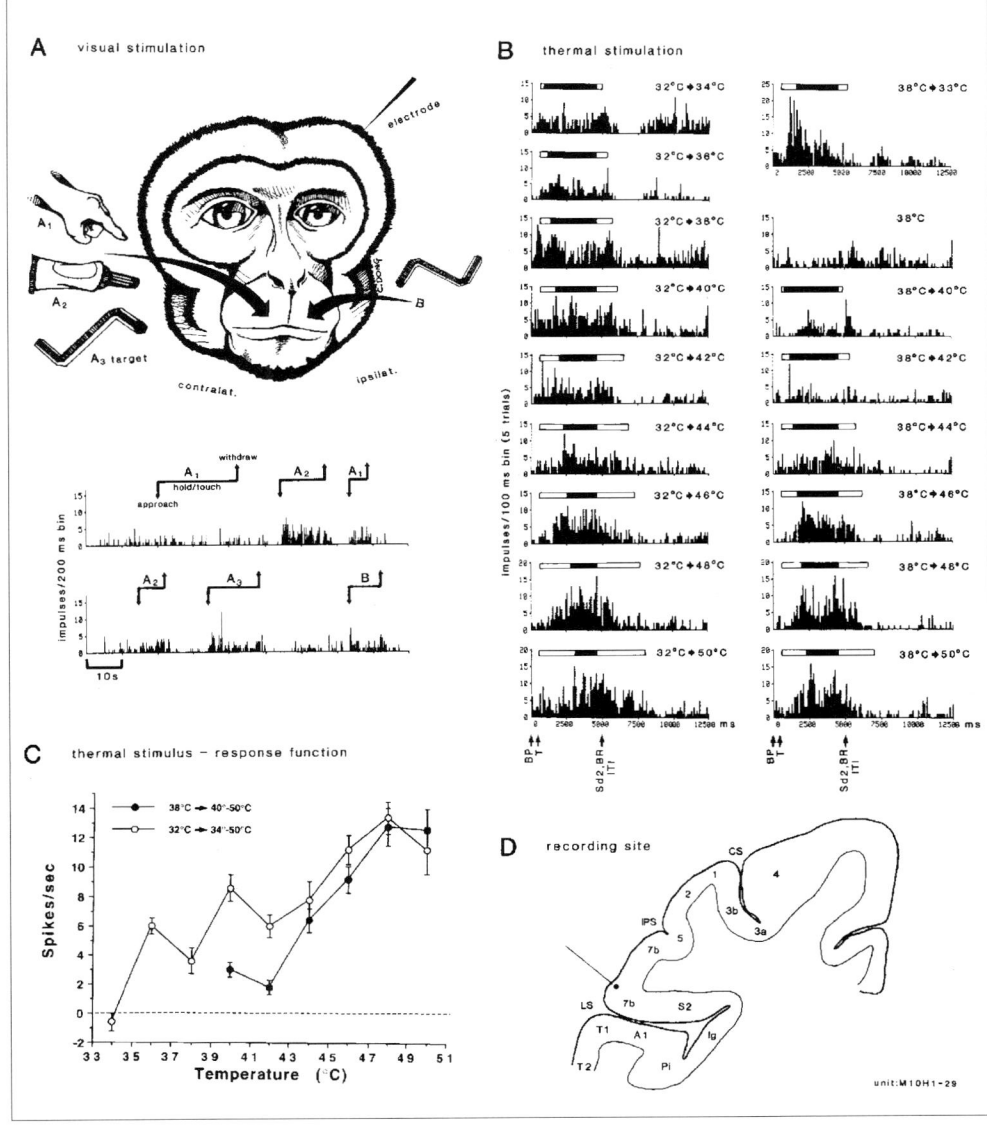

nociceptors. The capacity of nociceptive HTT-EN and WRT-EN neurons in area 7b to contribute to the sensory-discriminative component of thermal pain is suggested by the functions for stimulus intensity *versus* discharge frequency and stimulus intensity *versus* escape frequency shown in Figure 3. The median Spearman rank correlation coefficients (rs) between the S-R function for each neuronal population and behavioral S-R function were as follows: WRT-EN, 0.90; WRT-NE, -1.00; HTT-EN, 0.90; HTT-NE, -0.20. Whether WRT-EN and HTT-EN neurons play a role in the encoding process by which monkeys perceive the intensity of noxious thermal stimulation or engage in other aspects of the pain experience will require further study.

Our laboratory is attempting to understand the functional and behavioral significance of multisensory input convergence onto area 7b nociceptive neurons. Such neurons are likely engaged in amodal coding of multisensory input because their output signals are not differentiated for a particular modality by either response magnitude (*see* Figure 3) or temporally modulated spike trains. Despite the ambiguity of the response signal for sensory modality, these signals do provide information about multisensory response magnitude and duration as well as coordinates of events in spatially aligned cutaneous and visual receptive fields. We speculate that such information is transmitted faster to subcortical and other cortical sites, and is processed faster at the same sites when coding and decoding for modality are precluded from multisensory pathways. The spatial congruence between visual and cutaneous receptive fields is a distinguishing feature of these multisensory neurons; the location and size of the cutaneous receptive field appear to complement those of the visual receptive field. The visual receptive field appears to be immediately adjacent to the somatic receptive field and to subtend solid angles in both the vertical and horizontal visual planes that extend out from the body. Graziano and Gross [49] have hypothesized that multisensory somatic-visual neurons code the location of visual stimuli in somatocentric or body-centered coordinates rather than in retinocentric or eye-centered coordinates. Accordingly, if a somatic-visual neuron's somatic receptive field moved to a new position in 3-dimensional space, the adjacent visual receptive field would synchronously move with respect to the somatic receptive field. Preliminary evidence suggests that multisensory nociceptive neurons in area 7b have spatial selectivity within visual receptive fields especially with respect to target distance from the somatic receptive field, and direction of target motion toward the same point on the somatic receptive field.

Our recent observations of multisensory integrative processes in area 7b provide a clue to the functional significance of multisensory convergence onto nociceptive neurons. We determined that visuosensory input evokes activity that enhances the neural responses to weak somatosensory input. For example, the response magnitude of nociceptive WRT and HTT neurons to thermal shifts from warm to near-noxious (43 °C - 44 °C) or mildly noxious (44 °C - 45 °C) heat are enhanced by antecedent or concurrent visual stimuli. The enhanced responses evoked by near- or mildly noxious heat are not significantly different from responses evoked by frankly noxious heat (e.g., 47 °C) alone. This integrative process is dependent on several critical factors that include the 1) target location or direction of motion within a visual receptive field that

CORTICAL NOCICEPTIVE MECHANISMS 191

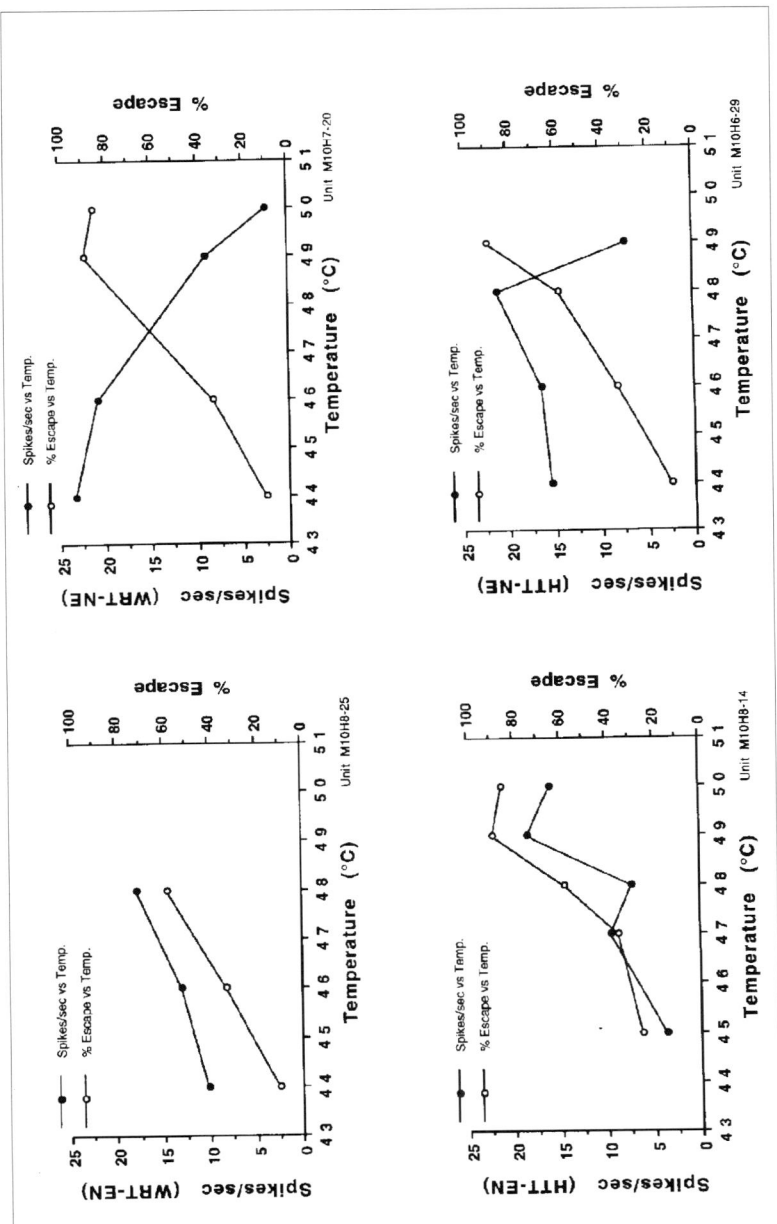

Figure 3. Relationships of noxious thermal stimulus intensity to the discharge frequency of WRT and HTT neurons and to escape frequency. All electrophysiological and behavioral data illustrated were obtained from the same monkey. The mean discharge frequencies evoked during noxious plateau temperatures are plotted for individual WRT and HTT neurons that did grade noxious thermal intensities (WRT-EN and HTT-EN) and did not grade noxious thermal intensities (WRT-NE and HTT-NE). For each type of neuron the mean discharge frequencies and mean escape frequencies (percent) that were associated with the same thermal shifts are plotted. In these representative examples, note that the slopes of the stimulus intensity-discharge frequency function and stimulus intensity-percent escape function for WRT-EN and HTT-EN neurons are more alike than the slopes of the same functions for WRT-NE and HTT-NE neurons. (From [29]).

is spatially aligned to a cutaneous receptive field, 2) time interval between presentation of each sensory modality and, 3) behavioral relevance of the visual stimuli (e.g., threatening *versus* non-threatening). A degradation of the response enhancement occurs if one or more of these critical factors are less than optimal. However, if the response magnitudes of nociceptive WRT and HTT neurons to frankly noxious heat are near or at maximum, their responses to such noxious stimuli are not significantly enhanced by relevant visuosensory input. The behavioral significance associated with enhancement of weak somatosensory responses by spatially congruent, appropriately timed and relevant visuosensory stimuli is uncertain. Our hypothesis is that such a facilitatory mechanism in area 7b may be related to enhanced detection of near- or mildly noxious stimuli when the spatial-temporal parameters and relevance of the visual stimuli are optimal. While an overtly noxious somatic stimulus that produces or threatens to produce tissue damage represents a clear and present danger to which a primate must immediately detect, attend and orient toward, a near- or even mildly noxious somatic stimulus would be less detectable and less likely to provoke attentive and orientation behaviors. However, enhanced detection of near- or mildly noxious stimuli under certain circumstances may be an important behavioral adaptation for survival if the outcome is greater reward or less pain and tissue injury. A primate is likely to use other available sensory cues, especially visual ones, to enhance detection of minimally effective somatic stimuli. Human psychophysical studies have suggested that detection thresholds of one sensory modality can be altered by activation of another modality [50, 51]. Enhancement of weak somatosensory responses by integration of multisensory inputs in area 7b and enhanced detection of weak somatosensory stimuli following multisensory interaction may subserve animal attention and orientation. The related physiological and behavioral events may be necessary to engage and direct spatially oriented movements toward or away from relevant somatic and/or visual stimuli. The magnitude and duration of multisensory neuronal responses may be important for initiating and sustaining "awareness" of multisensory stimuli as well as purposeful (goal-directed) exploratory or avoidance movements. In addition, the somatocentric coordinates provided by the responding multisensory cells may be information needed to locate multisensory stimulation on an internal map of personal and near-extrapersonal space and to select the appropriate spatial direction of exploratory movements toward multisensory stimuli or avoidance movements away from multisensory stimuli. Conceivably, somatomotor and visuomotor neurons operate from a motor coordinate system that relies on the transformation of a multisensory spatial coordinate system provided in part by area 7b. We are in accord with Graziano and Gross [49] who have speculated that purposeful, spatially directed movements such as reaching toward objects, saccading to targets and avoidance of threatening and looming stimuli may rely on information from multisensory (somatic-visual) neurons found in interconnected regions like area 7b, ventral intraparietal area, areas 6 and 5 and putamen.

Acknowledgements

This work was supported by the National Institute of Neurological Disorders and Stoke Grant NS-29459.

References

1. Casey KL, Minoshima S, Berger KL, Koeppe RA, Morrow TJ, Frey KA. Positron emission tomographic analysis of cerebral structures activated specifically by repetitive noxious heat stimuli. *J Neurophysiol* 1994 ; 71 : 802-7.
2. Coghill RC, Talbot JD, Evans AC, Meyer E, Gjedde A, Bushnell MC, Duncan GH. Distributed processing of pain and vibration by the human brain. *J Neurosci* 1994 ; 14 : 4095-108.
3. Derbyshire SWG, Jones AKP, Devani P, Firston KJ, Feinmann C, Harris M, Pearce S, Watson JDG, Frackowiak RSJ. Cerebral responses to pain in patients with atypical facial pain measured by positron emission tomography. *J Neurol Neurosurg Psychiat* 1994 ; 57 : 1166-72.
4. Iadarola MJ, Berman KF, Byas-Smith M, Gracely RH, Max M, Zeffiro T, Bennett GJ. Positron emission tomography (PET) studies of pain and allodynia in normals and patients with chronic neuropathic pain. *Soc Neuroci Abstr* 1992 ; 19 : 1074.
5. Talbot JD, Marrett S, Evans AC, Meyer E, Bushnell MC, Duncan GH. Multiple representations of pain in human cerebral cortex. *Science* 1991 ; 251 : 1355-8.
6. Devinsky O, Morrell MJ, Vogt BA. Contributions of anterior cingulate cortex to behaviour. *Brain* 1995 ; 118 : 279-306.
7. Kenshalo DR Jr, Giesler G JrJ, Leonard RB, Willis WD. Responses of neurons in primate ventral posterior lateral nucleus to noxious stimuli. *J Neurophysiol* 1980 ; 43 : 1594-614.
8. Chandler MJ, Hobbs SF, Fu Q-G, Kenshalo DR Jr, Blair RW, Foreman RD. Responses of neurons in ventroposterolateral nucleus of primate thalamus to urinary bladder distension. *Brain Res* 1992 ; 571 : 26-34.
9. Kenshalo DR Jr, Isensee O. Responses of primate SI cortical neurons to noxious stimuli. *J Neurophysiol* 1983 ; 50 : 1479-96.
10. Chudler EH, Anton F, Dubner R, Kenshalo DR Jr. Responses of nociceptive SI neurons in monkeys and pain sensation in humans elicited by noxious thermal stimulation: effect of interstimulus interval. *J Neurophysiol* 1990 ; 63 : 559-69.
11. Kenshalo DR Jr, Chudler EH, Anton F, Dubner R. SI nociceptive neurons participate in the encoding process by which monkeys perceive the intensity of noxious thermal stimulation. *Brain Res* 1988 ; 454 : 378-82.
12. Kenshalo DR Jr, Willis WD Jr. The role of the cerebral cortex in pain sensation. In : Peters A, ed. *Cerebral cortex*. New York : Plenum, 1991 : 153-212.
13. Hardy JD, Wolff HG, Goodell H. *Pain sensations and reactions*. New York : Hafner, 1967.
14. Dubner R, Beitel RE, Brown FJ. A behavioral animal model for the study of pain mechanisms in primates. In : Weisenberg M, Tursky B, eds. *Pain: new perspectives in therapy and research*. New York : Plenum, 1976 : 155-70.
15. Dubner R, Price DD, Beitel RE, Hu JW. Peripheral neural correlates of behavior in monkey and human related to sensory-discriminative aspects of pain. In: Anderson DJ, Matthews B, eds. *Pain in the trigeminal region*. Amsterdam : Elsevier, 1977 : 57-66.
16. Kenshalo DR Jr, Leonard RB, Chung JM, Willis WD. Responses of primate spinothalamic neurons to graded and to repeated noxious heat stimuli. *J Neurophysiol* 1979 ; 42 : 1370-89.

17. Price DD, Dubner R, Hu JW. Trigeminothalamic neurons in nucleus caudalis responsive to tactile, thermal, and nociceptive stimulation of monkey's face. *J Neurophysiol* 1976 ; 39 : 936-53.
18. Dubner R. Specialization of nociceptive pathways: sensory discrimination, sensory modulation and neural connectivity. In : Fields HL *et al.*, eds. *Advances in pain research and therapy.* New York : Raven, 1985 : 111-37.
19. Price DD. *Psychological and neural mechanisms of pain.* New York : Raven, 1988.
20. Greene LC, Hardy JD. Adaptation of thermal pain in the skin. *J Appl Physiol* 1962 ; 17 : 693-6.
21. LaMotte RH, Campbell JN. Comparison of responses of warm and nociceptive C-fiber afferents in monkey with human judgements of thermal pain. *J Neurophyiol* 1978 ; 41 : 509-28.
22. LaMotte RH, Torebjork HE, Robinson CJ, Thalhammer JG. Time-intensity profiles of cutaneous pain in normal and hyperalgesic skin: a comparison of C-fiber nociceptive activities in monkey and human. *J Neurophysiol* 1984 ; 51 : 1434-50.
23. Kenshalo DR Jr, Anton F, Dubner R. The detection and perceived intensity of noxious thermal stimuli in monkey and in human. *J Neurophysiol* 1989 ; 62 : 429-36.
24. Kenshalo DR Jr, Thomas DA, Dubner R. Somatosensory cortex lesions change the monkey's reaction to noxious stimulation. *J Dent Res Abstr* 1989 ; 68 : 897.
25. Berthier M, Starkstein S, Leiguarda R. Asymbolia for pain: a sensory-limbic disconnection syndrome. *Ann Neurol* 1988 ; 24 : 41-9.
26. Greenspan JD, Winfield JA. Reversible pain and tactile deficits associated with a cerebral tumor compressing the posterior insula and parietal operculum. *Pain* 1992 ; 50 : 29-39.
27. Schmahmann JD, Leifer D. Parietal pseudothalamic pain syndrome. *Arch Neurol* 1992 ; 49 : 1032-7.
28. Dong WK, Roberts VJ, Hayashi T, Fusco BM, Chudler EH. Thermoreceptive neurons and behavioral outcome of injury in area 7b cortex in monkeys. *Soc Neurosci Abstr* 1992 ; 18 : 834.
29. Dong WK, Chudler EH, Sugiyama K, Roberts VJ, Hayashi T. Somatosensory, multisensory, and task-related neurons in cortical area 7b (PF) of unanesthetized monkeys. *J Neurophysiol* 1994 ; 72 : 542-64.
30. Friedman DP, Murray EA, O'Neill JB, Mishkin M. Cortical connections of the somatosensory fields of the lateral sulcus of macaques: evidence for a corticolimbic pathway for touch. *J Comp Neurol* 1986 ; 252 : 323-47.
31. Burton H, Sathian K, Dian-Hua S. Altered responses to cutaneous stimuli in the second somatosensory cortex following lesions of the postcentral gyrus in infant and juvenile macaques. *J Comp Neurol* 1990 ; 291 : 395-414.
32. Pons TP, Garraghty PE, Mishkin M. Serial and parallel processing of tactual information in somatosensory cortex of rhesus monkeys. *J Neurophysiol* 1992 ; 68 : 518-27.
33. Sinclair RJ, Burton H. Neuronal activity in the second somatosensory cortex of monkeys (*Macaca mulatta*) during active touch of gratings. *J Neurophysiol* 1993 ; 70 : 331-50.
34. Vogt BA, Pandya DN. Cortico-cortical connections of somatic sensory cortex (areas 3, 1 and 2) in the rhesus monkey. *J Comp Neurol* 1978 ; 177 : 179-92.
35. Cavada C, Goldman-Rakic PS. Posterior parietal cortex in rhesus monkey. I. Parcellation of areas based on distinctive limbic and sensory corticocortical connections. *J Comp Neurol* 1989 ; 287 : 393-421.
36. Bushnell MC, Duncan GH. Sensory and affective aspects of pain perception: is medial thalamus restricted to emotional issues? *Exp Brain Res* 1989 ; 78 : 415-8.
37. Bushnell MC, Duncan GH. Mechanical response properties of ventroposterior medial thalamic neurons in the alert monkey. *Exp Brain Res* 1987 ; 67 : 603-14.
38. Bushnell MC, Duncan GH, Tremblay N. Thalamic VPM nucleus in the behaving monkey. I. Multimodal and discriminative properties of thermosensitive neurons. *J Neurophysiol* 1993 ; 69 : 739-52.

39. Yokota T, Nishikawa Y, Koyama N. Distribution of trigeminal nociceptive neurons in nucleus ventralis posteromedialis of primates. In : Dubner R, ed. *Pain research and clinical management.* Amsterdam : Elsevier, 1988 : 555-66.
40. Craig AD Jr, Bushnell MC, Zhang E-T, Blomqvist A. A thalamic nucleus specific for pain and temperature sensation. *Nature* 1994 ; 372 : 770-3.
41. Apkarian AV, Shi T. Squirrel monkey lateral thalamus. I. Somatic nocirespive neurons and their relation to spinothalamic terminals. *J Neurosci* 1994 ; 14 : 6779-95.
42. Casey KL. Unit analysis of nociceptive mechanisms in the thalamus of awake squirrel monkey. *J Neurophysiol* 1966 ; 29 : 727-50.
43. Schmahmann JD, Pandya DN. Anatomical investigation of projections from the posterior parietal cortex in the rhesus monkey: a WGA-HRP and fluorescent tracer study. *J Comp Neurol* 1990 ; 295 : 299-326.
44. Friedman DP, Murray EA. Thalamic connectivity of the second somatosensory area and neighboring somatosensory fields of the lateral sulcus of the macaque. *J Comp Neurol* 1986 ; 252 : 348-73.
45. Neal JW, Pearson RCA, Powell TPS. The ipsilateral cortico-cortical connections of the area 7b, PF, in the parietal and temporal lobes of the monkey. *Brain Res* 1990 ; 524 : 119-32.
46. Whitsel BL, Petrucelli LM, Werner G. Symmetry and connectivity in the map of the body surface in somatosensory area II of primates. *J Neurophysiol* 1969 ; 32 : 170-83.
47. Robinson CJ, Burton H. Somatic submodality distribution within the second somatosensory (SII), 7b, retroinsular, postauditory, and granular insular cortical areas of *M. fascicularis*. *J Comp Neurol* 1980 ; 192 : 93-108.
48. Dong WK, Salonen LD, Kawakami Y, Shiwaku T, Kaukoranta EM, Martin RF. Nociceptive responses of trigeminal neurons in SII-7b cortex of awake monkeys. *Brain Res* 1989 ; 484 : 314-24.
49. Graziano MSA, Gross CG. The representation of extrapersonal space: a possible role for bimodal, visual-tactile neurons. In: Gazzaniga MS, ed. *The cognitive neurosciences.* Cambridge : MIT Press, 1995 : 1021-43.
50. Walk RD, Pick HL. *Intersensory perception and sensory integration.* New York : Plenumi, 1981.
51. Welch RB, Warren OH. Intersensory interactions. In : Bott KR, Kaufman L, Thomas JP, eds. *Handbook of perception and human performance.* New York : Wiley, 1986 : 1-36.

14

The role of pain in cingulate cortical and limbic thalamic mediation of avoidance learning

M. GABRIEL, A. POREMBA

Beckman Institute for Advanced Science and Technology, University of Illinois, Urbana, USA.

This chapter presents the current status of a long-term program of research on the neural mediation of learned behavior and memory.

The research to be described represents an application of what has been termed the "model system" strategy, wherein the neural substrates of learning in a particular species are analyzed in relation to a particular learning paradigm. In the case reviewed here, the species is the rabbit, and the task is discriminative avoidance learning. A special emphasis is given in this paper to the role of aversive stimulation in the production of learning-related neural changes.

A great deal of the research on brain substrata of learning and memory attempts to discover the functional role of particular brain structures (e.g., the hippocampus). Typically, the effects of lesions in the target structure are examined. Our project is based on the conviction that individual structures do not influence behavior in isolation from other structures. Rather, adaptive functions emerge from the interactions among interconnected structures that form functional circuits. To analyze circuits, we use, in conjunction with lesions, recordings of neuronal ensemble activity simultaneously in multiple brain areas, during learning in the behaving animal. This approach provides information, not obtainable with lesions, about the dynamic flow of information in learning-relevant brain circuitry.

In one experimental situation, rabbits learn to take a step in an activity wheel in response to a 5-second tone conditional stimulus (CS+), in order to prevent a brief, mild but startling foot-shock scheduled 5 seconds after tone onset. A second tone (CS-) is never followed by shock and the rabbits learn that no response is necessary. Rabbits reach asymptotic discriminative performance after about three days of training whereupon they avoid shock on about 85% of CS+ trials and they respond on fewer than 8% of the CS- trials. A few years ago, we implemented an appetitive analog of the avoidance task wherein contact with a drinking tube presented 5 seconds after the CS+ earns water but contact after CS- presentation does not. The same rabbits/neurons can be studied concurrently in both tasks using the same, reversed or different CSs.

Some advantages of these paradigms are:
- they are under excellent stimulus control, and are rapidly and uniformly acquired by nearly all rabbits;
- brain neuronal activity is relatively easily recorded as the subjects remain motionless (important for the recording of low-level brain signals) during cue reception and processing;
- we now know that this learning depends on the brain's limbic system, which is also importantly involved in human memory.

A working model

Our studies of the neural circuitry and dynamic events underlying discriminative avoidance learning began in 1970. The findings have provided the basis of a theoretical working model, first published in 1980 [1] and frequently updated since then [2-5]. The chapter published in 1993 illustrates and provides citations for the results discussed here. Citations are given below for items not cited in the chapter.

The working model is illustrated in Figure 1. Posited as a key dynamic substratum of learning is the development of excitatory and discriminative training-induced neuronal activity (TIA) in the anterior and posterior cingulate cortex, and in neurons of the reciprocally interconnected nuclei of limbic thalamus (the anterior and medial dorsal [MD] thalamic nuclei). Discriminative TIA refers to development during training of distinctive neuronal firing patterns in response to the danger signal (CS+) compared to firing elicited by the safety signal (CS-). Excitatory TIA is increased firing to the CS+ during training, compared to firing elicited before training. Excitatory and discriminative TIA occur in response to the conditional stimuli as early as 15 milliseconds after stimulus onset and, depending on the recording site, may persist for the full duration of sampling, to 700 milliseconds after tone onset. The two forms of TIA have different brain origins, as indicated below.

It is proposed that excitatory and discriminative TIA elicited by the CS give rise, in cingulate cortex, to a "command volley" (neuronal firing that precedes the output of the learned behavior), which is projected from cingulate cortex *via* pathway 5 (Figure 1) to

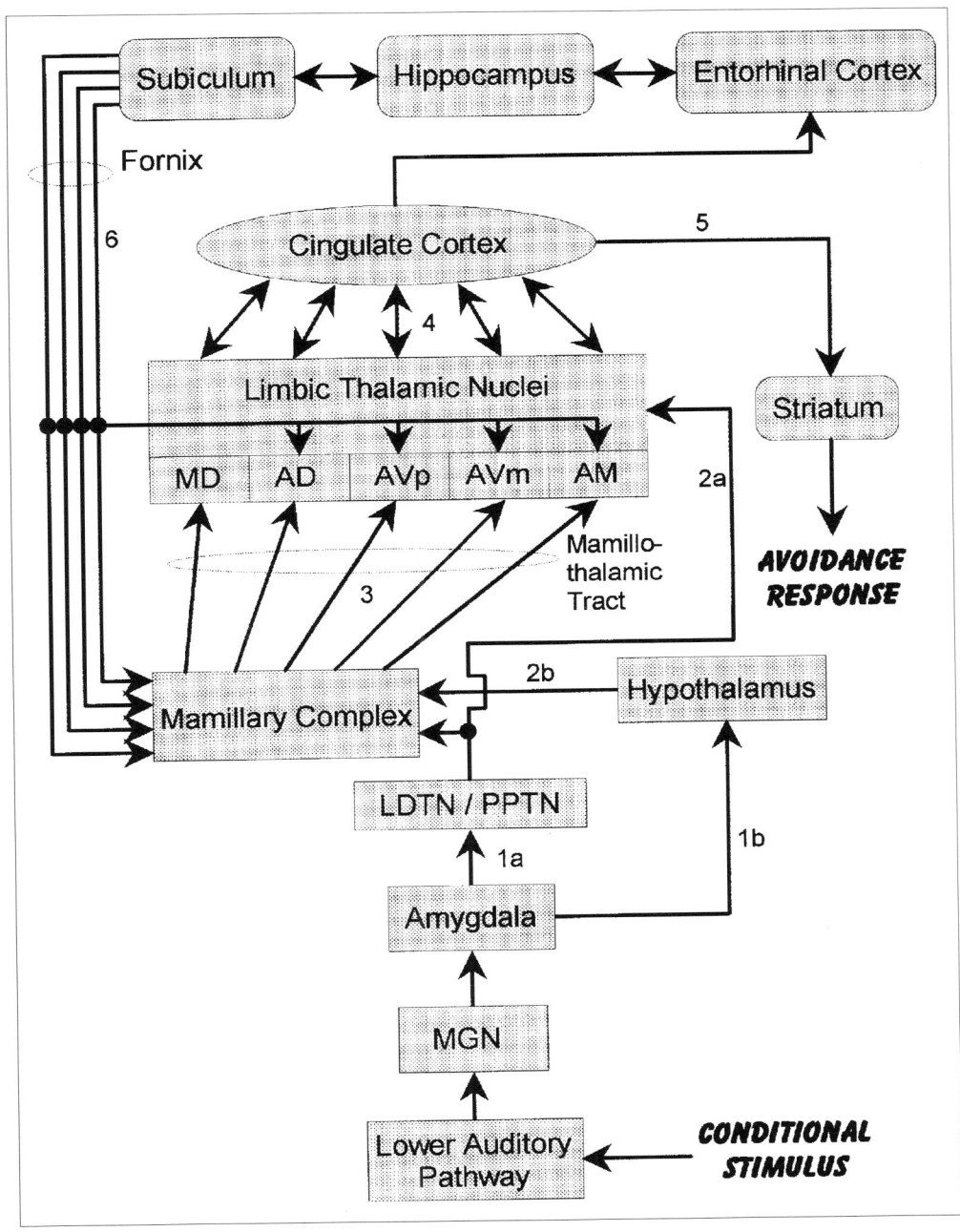

Figure 1. Working model of neural circuitry involved in the mediation of discriminative instrumental learning (details in text).

a motor system structure, the striatum, to initiate response output. The cuedriven discriminative activity, and the occurrence of single-cell "command volleys" in cingulate cortex, have been extensively documented by these studies since the late 1970's.

One might imagine from the foregoing that cingulate cortex and limbic thalamus are essential structures for avoidance learning, a proposition also well-documented by lesion studies.

In addition to plasticity of the neuronal activity in the limbic thalamic nuclei, the model also posits conditioning-induced plasticity in the motor system, which allows the appropriate action (locomotion) to be primed (made ready) when the rabbit enters the learning situation. That is, contextual stimuli of the experimental environment evoke priming of the learned response. Given that cingulate cortical neurons send axons extensively to the neostriatum, and that neostriatal lesions block avoidance learning, we hypothesized that the striatal areas of the brain are the sites of motor priming.

Thus, the basic thrust of the model is that limbic system neurons "learn" to respond to significant events in the outside world, i.e., events which call for action. The striatal motor system prepares the action or actions likely to be required in a particular environment. Communication from the limbic to the striatal system is responsible for the output of required actions at the right time, i.e., in coordination with specific events in the environment such as CS+ presentation. Here, I will refer to the functions of the limbic and motor systems, respectively, as Spatio-Temporal Modelling (SM) and Action Priming (AP).

The limbic SM system receives perceptual data (the event stream) as input. The outputs of the SM system are command volleys, i.e., nerve impulse volleys of cingulate cortical neurons that send axonal projections to the striatal AP system. The command volleys represent neural information flows which tell the AP system when to execute a primed action. To accomplish this, the SM system must encode the event stream temporally and spatially, and learn inductively to issue command volleys when the animal encounters key nodes in spatio-temporal event space. To accomplish these things, the limbic SM system thus must be (and is) a massively plastic neural system.

It is important to note that limbic SM system command volleys do not specify the nature of the action to be performed. Such specification is the domain of the neostriatal AP system, which associatively primes certain actions and sees to the details of their execution. On the other hand, the AP system does not have the vaguest idea when to do things, as it cannot perform a real-time, high-resolution analysis of the event stream. All it can do is to prime associatively certain actions and execute those actions when it receives well-timed command volleys from the SM system.

Pain and the learning circuitry

Two major considerations relate our model and findings to the issue of pain. First, neurological analyses of avoidance learning necessarily address the role of painful stimulation in the elaboration of learning-related neuronal change. Second, cingulate cortex and limbic thalamus are centrally involved in the mediation of discriminative avoidance learning, and these areas have also been implicated in the processing of painful stimuli (reviewed by [6]).

The essential question regarding avoidance learning and pain processing is, how does the aversive unconditional stimulus (US) used for avoidance training act to induce neural circuit changes that bring about behavioral learning? In other words, how does the painful US induce excitatory and discriminative TIA in the SM system, and priming of the avoidance response in the AP system?

In general, afferent streams of neuronal activity specific to the US must converge with sensory (e.g., CS driven) neuronal information flow. This convergence gives rise to synaptic plasticity (e.g., associative long-term potentiation, activity-dependent facilitation [7, 8], which then facilitates transmission of the CS driven activity at the site of plasticity. In order to apply this general model to the circuitry of discriminative avoidance learning, it is necessary to consider what is known about the origins of learning-relevant TIA. By origins of TIA, we mean the sites of convergence at which synaptic plasticities develop that give rise to TIA.

Origins of discriminative TIA

Discriminative TIA represents an important form of dynamic neuronal plasticity that is involved in determining which stimuli will be responded to. Combined lesion and unit recording studies have demonstrated that neither excitatory nor discriminative TIA in limbic thalamus requires input from the cingulate cortex or from the subiculum, areas of the cerebral cortex that project directly to limbic thalamus. However, TIA in cingulate cortex does require the integrity of projecting limbic thalamic neurons. Therefore, the events which give rise to limbic thalamic and cingulate cortical excitatory and discriminative TIA are subcortical events.

The projection of norepinephrine (NE) to the limbic thalamus from the brainstem locus coeruleus is not responsible for TIA in thalamus (although this pathway is involved in mechanisms whereby novel and unexpected stimuli modulate thalamic TIA). Thus, TIA production is not a product of noradrenergic subcortical circuit interactions.

We now know that three distinct subcortical circuits are involved in the production of the discriminative TIA. The circuits differ primarily in terms of when, during the course of learning, the discriminative TIA is exhibited and they account for "early developing" and "late-developing" TIA found in cingulate cortex and limbic thalamus.

A very early discriminative TIA develops in the medial division of the medial geniculate nucleus (MGm), the auditory thalamic relay for hearing (Figure 2, top row), [9]. This TIA reaches maximal magnitude in the first session of conditioning, and declines in magnitude in subsequent training sessions. Damage induced in this system blocks learning and TIA development in limbic thalamus and cingulate cortex [10], suggesting that the very early TIA in the MGm is a necessary precursor of the TIA in

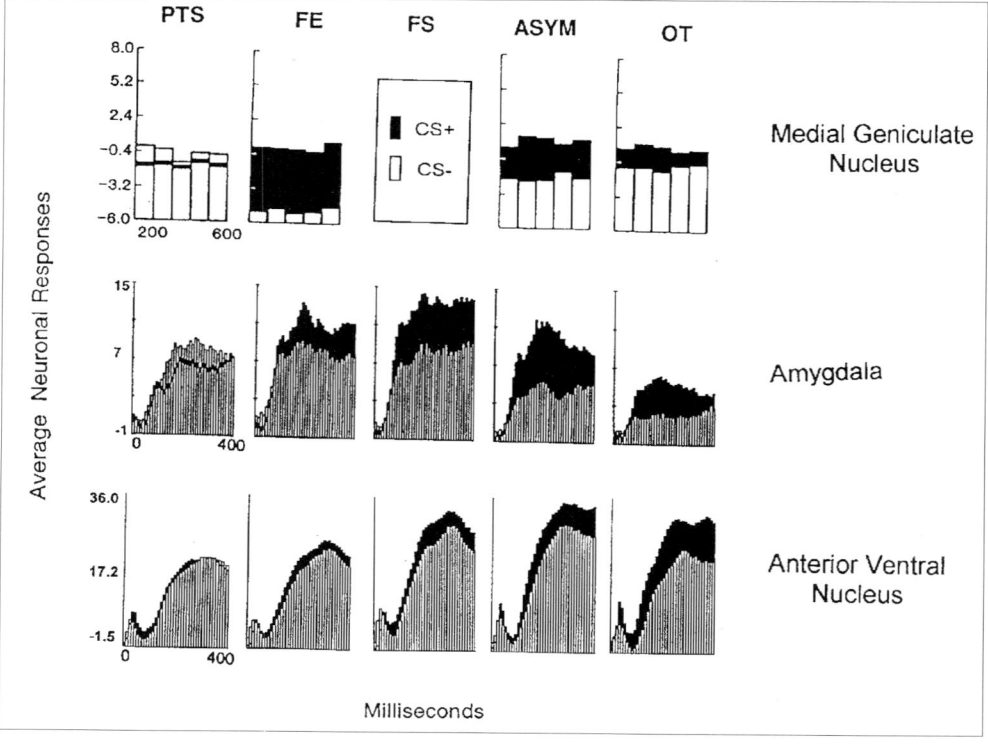

Figure 2. Multi-unit neuronal activity of the medial division of the medial geniculate nucleus (MGm), the basolateral nucleus of the amygdala and in the anterior ventral thalamic nucleus, following presentation of the positive and negative conditional stimuli (CS+ and CS-) during discriminative avoidance learning in rabbits. Each panel shows the average magnitude for, 5 - 20 neuronal records, of the neuronal discharge in consecutive intervals or "bins" following CS+ and CS- onset. The plotted values are z-scores indicating discharge magnitude normalized relative to a 300 millisecond pre-stimulus baseline period. The columns of the figure represent training sessions as follows: PTS, a "pretraining" session (given before training) in which the CS+, CS- and shock US were presented in an explicitly unpaired manner; FE, the "first exposure" to the conditioning procedure, wherein the CS+ predicted the US and US avoidance could be earned by responding to the CS+; FS, the session in which a given rabbit first exhibited significant discriminative behavior, defined as avoidance on 25% more of the CS+ than CS- trials; ASYM, the session in which a given rabbit first performed asymptotic discriminative behavior, defined as avoidance on 60% more of the CS+ than CS- trials. and; OT, the third session of "overtraining" following the attainment of performance asymptote.

limbic thalamus and cingulate cortex. However, very early TIA as found in the MGm is not found in cingulate cortex or limbic thalamus.

An intermediate-term discriminative TIA develops in the basolateral nucleus of the amygdala (Figure 2, second row), [11]. This TIA occurs robustly in the first conditioning session, but reaches maximal magnitude in the session in which the first behavioral discrimination is performed (typically the second or third training session). It declines in magnitude thereafter as the rabbits reach asymptotic performance levels. Therefore, this TIA is somewhat slower to develop and it is more persistent than the TIA in the MGm. Dependency of the TIA in the amygdala on the very early MGm TIA is indicated by the fact that lesions in the medial geniculate nucleus block learning and the development of the amygdaloid TIA [12]. It is very likely that this dependency is based on axonal projections of MGm neurons to amygdaloid and periamygdaloid regions [13]. Finally, intermediate-term discriminative TIA, essentially identical to the amygdaloid TIA, can be recorded in the anterior cingulate cortex (Brodman's area 24b) and in layer V of the posterior cingulate cortex (Brodman's area 29). Lesions of the amygdala block learning and they eliminate the development of all excitatory and discriminative TIA in cingulate cortex and limbic thalamus [14].

A third, late-developing variety of discriminative TIA occurs in the mamillary nuclei of the hypothalamus, the anterior and MD thalamic nuclei, and in layer IV of the posterior cingulate cortex [15, 16]. This TIA develops gradually during the course of behavioral learning and attains maximal magnitude as the rabbits' performance reaches the criterion (Figure 2, bottom row). This TIA declines gradually during the course of extended post-asymptotic overtraining. It should be noted that the discriminative TIA in the MD nucleus is actually hybrid, as it is evident robustly in the first and intermediate training sessions. However, it does not decline but rather increments as training is continued, and it reaches maximal magnitude as the rabbits reach behavioral criterion. It declines subsequently as training is continued beyond criterion.

Note that the intermediate and late forms of discriminative TIA are both dependent on the integrity of the amygdala. We propose that intermediate-term TIA is triggered in the MD nucleus and in the anterior cingulate cortex as a result of amygdaloid efferent flow of intermediate-term amygdaloid TIA *via* documented direct axonal projections [17]. The intermediate-term amygdaloid TIA may also be projected *via* pathway 1b and 2b to the mamillary nuclei wherein it initiates the development of late-developing discriminative TIA as found in the mamillary and anterior thalamic nuclei (Figure 1).

As indicated above, lesions in the MGm and amygdala induced before training eliminate learning and block the development of TIA in cingulate cortex and limbic thalamus. Also, lesions of the entire cingulate cortex or limbic thalamus block learning. However, more subtle deficits are revealed by lesions restricted to either the intermediate or late circuit elements. Remarkably, the nature of the behavioral deficits is predicted by the rate of TIA development.

Briefly, as reviewed above, discriminative TIA develops more rapidly in the anterior cingulate cortex than in the posterior cingulate cortex, and discrimination in the MD nucleus develops more rapidly than in the anterior thalamic nuclei. In correspondence with these neuronal differences, lesions in the former circuit at either the cortical or thalamic level retard behavioral acquisition, but allow it to occur, eventually, to normal performance levels. Lesions in the late circuit at either the cortical or thalamic level allow acquisition to occur at a normal rate, but significantly reduce the efficiency of avoidance response performance after asymptotic performance is attained. In both instances the performance impairments are due to a reduced level of performance, not to an inability to withhold responding to the CS-.

These results suggest, in accord with the different rates of discriminative TIA development in these systems, that the anterior cingulate cortex and MD nucleus form a circuit that is involved preferentially in mediating original acquisition, but this circuit makes a lessened contribution to performance, as training is continued after criterion. The more gradual acquisition of discriminative TIA in the posterior cingulate and anterior thalamic nuclei is completed as the anterior system contribution begins to decline. This circuit is thus the principal mediator of the behavior during asymptotic and post-asymptotic task performance.

These more subtle effects of the lesions have been replicated often (*see* [5]). Most recently the behavioral contribution of the "late" circuit was indicated in a study which showed that lesions of the mamillothalamic tract (MTT) which eliminated discriminative TIA in the anterior thalamus impaired asymptotic performance of the avoidance response, but not its rate of original acquisition [18].

Pain and discriminative TIA

We offer the suggestion that sites of CS and US convergence likely to be involved in the production of synaptic plasticity underlying TIA are sites that first exhibit a particular variety of TIA. Here, the term "first" refers to the position of a given site in the afferent stream.

On this principle, neurons of the inferior colliculus relay auditory afferents to the MGm, but do not themselves exhibit discriminative TIA [9]. Thus, the MGm may be the first station in the auditory afferent pathway to exhibit discriminative TIA and may thus put forward as a candidate site of convergence which gives rise to the early TIA described above. US information could reach the MGm *via* somatosensory and other projections [19, 20].

It is unlikely that the discriminative TIA in the MGm is relayed directly to the basolateral nucleus of the amygdala, as the latter TIA reaches its maximal magnitude in the intermediate training stage, and remains ample as asymptotic performance is attained, whereas the TIA in the MGm is lost as asymptotic performance is reached. We would thus argue that the basolateral amygdala may be the site of convergence for intermediate-term discriminative TIA. This idea is supported by the studies reviewed above which showed that intermediate-term TIA is blocked in all "downstream" circuit elements after amygdala lesions. Moreover, synaptic plasticity can be induced in the amygdala by stimulation of convergent afferents. We assume that CS information reaches the amygdala from the MGm. The fact that this activity is already discriminative provides a boost to the amygdala's plasticity coding mechanism. The source of US-driven afferents that may give rise to TIA development in the amygdala is unknown, but biogenic amine and basal forebrain cholinergic afferents are possibilities.

By a similar line of reasoning, neurons of the medial and lateral mamillary nuclei are likely to be sites of convergence involved in the production of late-developing discriminative TIA. Medial mamillary neurons themselves exhibit late TIA [16] and they supply afferent input to the anterior thalamic and posterior cingulate cortical neurons that also exhibit late TIA. Lesions of the mamillothalamic tract block the late developing TIA in these downstream structures. Information about the CS could be relayed from the basolateral amygdala to the mamillary nuclei *via* relays in the bed nucleus of the stria terminalis, the tuberomamillary nucleus and lateral hypothalamic area [21, 22]. Again brainstem biogenic amine projections and acetylcholine projections from the lateral dorsal tegmentum could supply US information to the mamillary nuclei.

Origins of excitatory TIA

Excitatory TIA has enhanced neuronal firing in response to the conditional stimuli during training, relative to firing levels before training when the CS and US were presented non-contingently. There is abundant evidence that the mechanisms which control excitatory TIA are distinct from those which control discriminative TIA and that the modulation of excitatory TIA has a functional significance different from that of discriminative TIA.

An indication of the dissociability of excitatory and discriminative TIA is afforded by the finding of dramatic cytoarchitecturally-specific modulation of excitatory TIA in the anterior thalamic nuclei during learning. The excitatory TIA elicited by the CS+ in different nuclei (the anterior dorsal, parvocellular anterior ventral, magnocellular anterior ventral, anterior medial and lateral dorsal nuclei) attains a maximum (peak) amplitude in a particular stage of behavioral acquisition. The various nuclei exhibit peak excitatory TIA either in the first conditioning session, the session of the first discriminative behavior, or in the session of criterion attainment (Figure 3). The peaks in each nucleus decline with further training. Similar distinct peaks of excitation occur in different posterior cingulate cortical layers to which the thalamic nuclei project. As indicated above, no such modulation of discriminative TIA occurs. Discriminative TIA is gradually acquired during learning, reaching maximal magnitude in all anterior thalamic nuclei when the behavioral criterion is met.

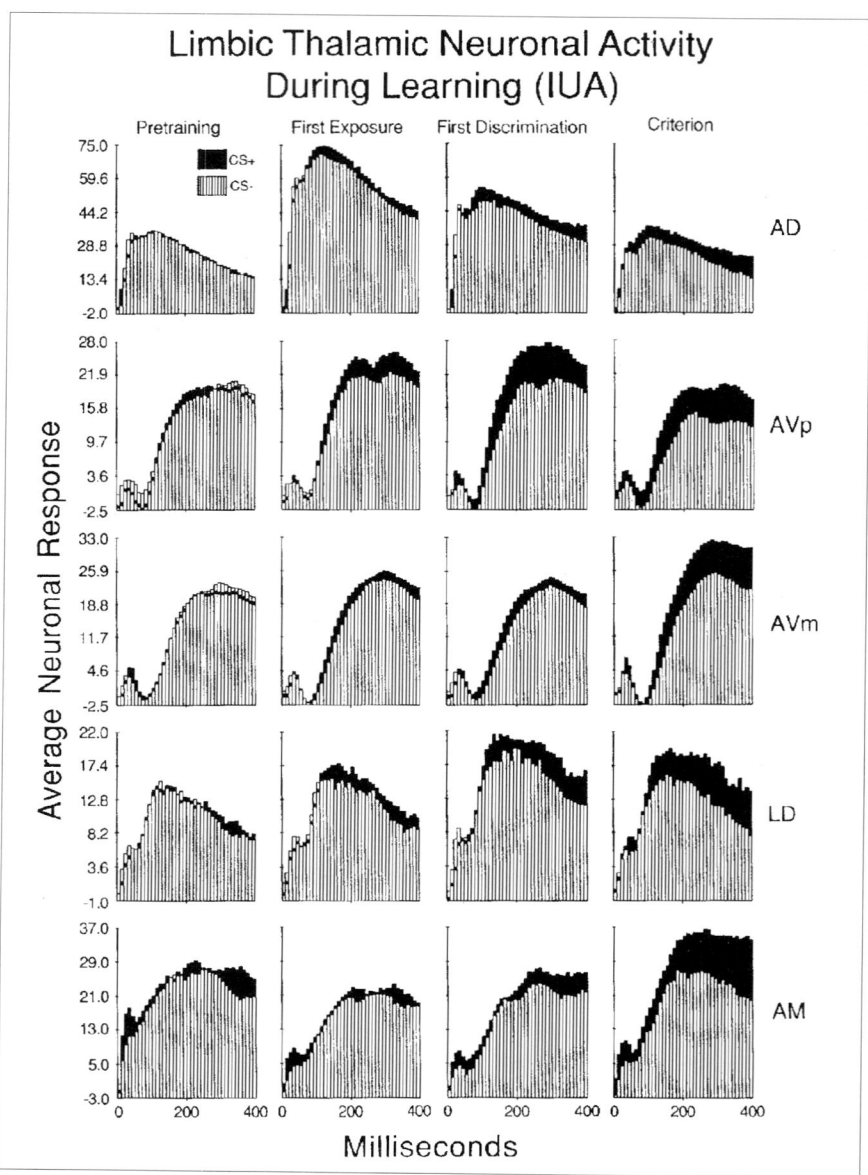

Figure 3. Average multi-unit neuronal discharge to CS+ and CS- in 40 consecutive 10 millisecond intervals after CS onset during four stages of acquisition. PT: Pretraining with unpaired CS/US presentations; FE, the first exposure to conditioning with paired CS+ - US presentations; FS, first discrimination, the first session in which significantly more avoidance responses were performed to the CS+ than to the CS-; CRIT, criterion, the session in which the criterion of behavioral discrimination was attained. Data are shown for the anterior dorsal (AD), parvocellular anterior ventral (AVp), magnocellular anterior ventral (AVm), lateral dorsal (LD) and anterior medial (AM) nuclei. The plotted values are standard scores normalized relative to a 300-millisecond pre-CS baseline. These results illustrate training-stage-related peaks of TIA.

The excitatory TIA at any given training stage comprises a distinctive trans-cytoarchitectural topography of tone-elicited excitation. The topography changes systematically as learning progresses, as different nuclei and layers are maximally activated in different stages of acquisition. These topographic patterns of excitatory TIA appear to require input to the anterior nuclei from posterior cingulate cortex and from the hippocampal formation. Moreover, ongoing analyses indicate that the patterns serve as a neural code representing the spatio-temporal context that defines the learning situation. This code is important for the rabbits' ability to exhibit context-appropriate memory retrieval, an ability which is especially handy when more than one discriminative habit is being learned concurrently [23], thus raising the possibility of confusion and inter-task interference. These functions of the patterns of excitatory TIA are not realizable on the basis of discriminative TIA alone.

Pain and excitatory TIA

Neurochemical blockade of muscarinic acetylcholine receptors using systemically injected scopolamine hydrobromide (SH) blocked avoidance responding and excitatory TIA in limbic thalamus, but these injections did not block thalamic discriminative TIA [24]. This finding supports the dissociability of the two forms of TIA and it suggests that the expression of excitatory TIA in limbic thalamus depends on inputs from brainstem areas such as the lateral dorsal tegmental (LDT) and the pedunculopontine tegmental (PPT) nuclei which are rich in acetylcholine-containing neurons (*see* Figure 1). Yasuo Kubota has shown that a 1-microliter injection of SH into the anterior thalamus also blocks the expression of the avoidance behavior and excitatory TIA, while leaving discriminative TIA intact [25]. These results indicate that the effect of the systemically injected scopolamine is localized in limbic thalamus. Additional work has shown that M_2 muscarinic acetylcholine receptors on mamillothalamic tract axon terminals in anterior thalamus are up-regulated during training in correspondence with the TIA peaks in each thalamic nucleus [26]. That is, the receptor numbers in a given nucleus rise and fall just as do the TIA peaks, in the early, intermediate or late stage of behavioral acquisition. Because these modulations of excitatory TIA in limbic thalamus do not occur either in the mamillary nuclei or in the dorsal tegmental cholinergic nuclei, they are likely to be products of convergences that occur either in posterior cingulate cortex, in the anterior thalamic nuclei, or in both areas.

The foregoing information suggests that convergent US driven information from the LDT nucleus and CS driven information from the MTT in the anterior thalamus may bring about excitatory TIA *via* activity dependent synaptic facilitation of anterior thalamic neurons [27, 28]. The facilitation could be based on up-regulation of muscarinic M_2 acetylcholine receptors. Specific gating of MTT excitation controlled by hippocampal formation influences articulated among the various "channels" of the MTT [29, 30] is responsible for the training-stage-dependent topographic patterns of excitatory TIA which occur in the anterior thalamic nuclei and layers of posterior cingulate cortex.

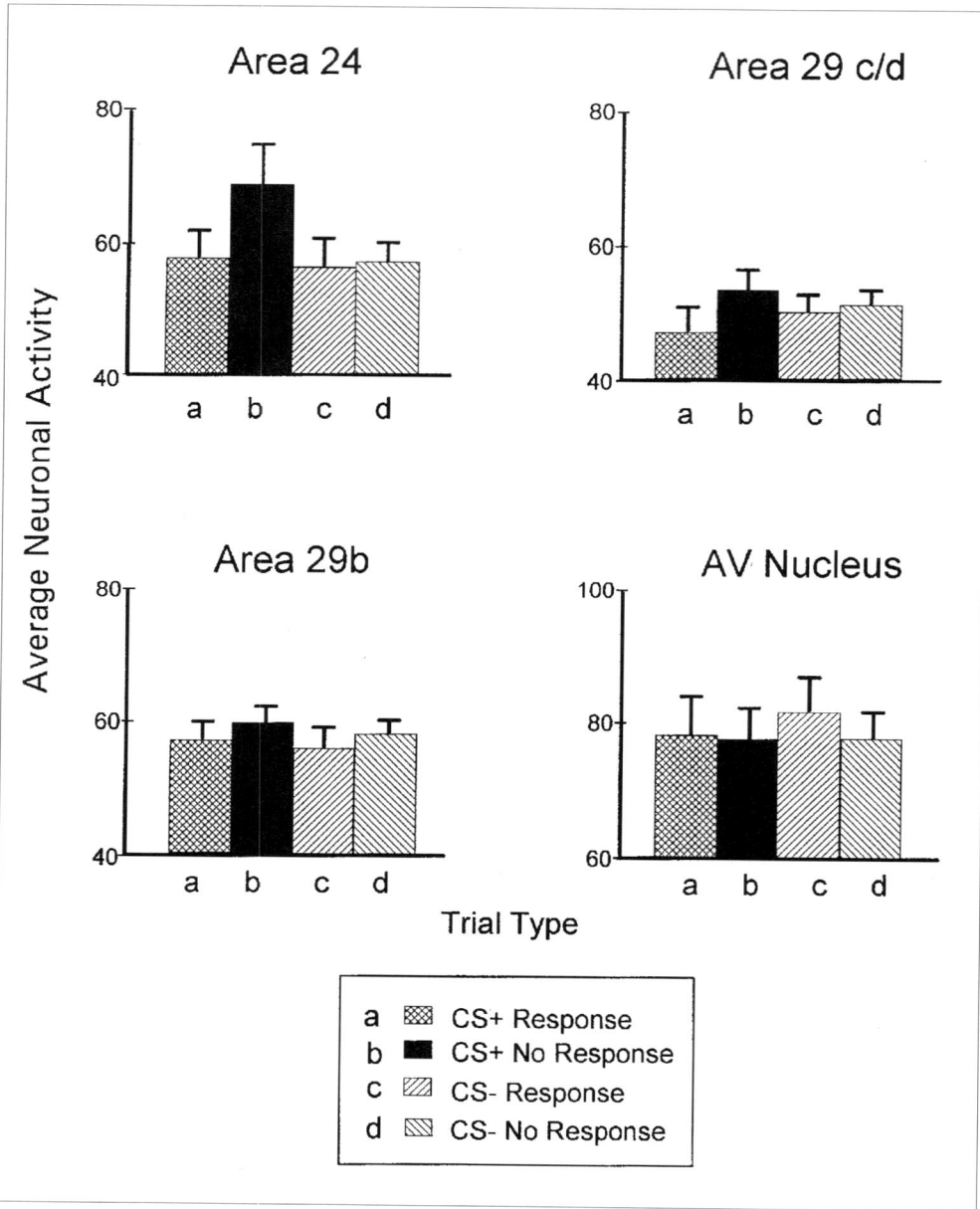

Figure 4. Average multi-unit activity recorded in posterior cingulate cortical areas 29c/d, 29b and 24, and in the anterior ventral (AV) thalamic nucleus, during a 1second interval, following the completion of four different types of avoidance conditioning trials (trial types a - d as described in the text).

Direct neuronal coding of pain in the anterior cingulate cortex during avoidance learning

It has been evident from casual observation that the presentation of the US very often elicits a dramatic increase in the firing of anterior cingulate cortical neurons, but this effect is not seen in other areas.

In order systematically to investigate this possibility, we have routinely recorded a one-second sample of the baseline neuronal activity after the completion of each avoidance training trial. These data in a subset of rabbits were analyzed recently, for the first time, because of their possible relevance to this volume. The post-trial neuronal firing levels were examined in anterior cingulate cortical area 24b, posterior cingulate cortical areas 29c/d and 29b, and in the anterior ventral (AV) thalamic nucleus, after each of four different trial types:
 a) CS+ followed by an avoidance response;
 b) CS+ followed by no avoidance response;
 c) CS- followed by a response;
 d) CS- followed by no response.

In all cases, the data were sampled after the end of each trial (cessation of post-trial locomotion or 5 seconds after CS onset) and the rabbit was resting quietly for at least 3 seconds. Thus, the sample typically was taken 5 to 15 seconds after the presentation of the US (trial type "b"). The results showed unequivocally a significant elevation of firing in the anterior cingulate cortex following trial type "b", the only one of the four trial types in which the US was presented ($P<.0005$; Figure 4). This effect was present in all of the training stages, and no significant effects of the "trial type" factor were found for any of the other areas. These results indicate that the shock US elicited a rather prolonged enhancement of neuronal activity, and that this enhancement was specific to the anterior cingulate cortex. These findings agree with other data indicating pain-specific activation of anterior cingulate cortex in animals and in humans (*see* [6]) and they afford future means to analyze the neurological bases and functional significance of this effect.

Acknowledgements

The research reported here was supported by the National Institute of Neurological Disorders and Stroke.

References

1. Gabriel M, Foster K, Orona E, Saltwick SE, Stanton M. Neuronal activity of cingulate cortex, anteroventral thalamus and hippocampal formation in discriminative conditioning: encoding and extraction of the significance of conditional stimuli. In : Sprague J, Epstein AN, eds. *Progress in physiological psychology and psychobiology*. Vol 9. New York : Academic Press, 1980 : 126-223.
2. Gabriel M, Sparenborg S, Stolar N. Hippocampal control of cingulate cortical and anterior thalamic information processing during learning. *Exp Brain Res* 1987 ; 67 : 131-52.
3. Gabriel M. Functions of the anterior and posterior cingulate cortex during learning in rabbits. *Prog Brain Res* 1990 ; 85 : 457-73.
4. Gabriel M, Schmajuk N. Neural and computational models of avoidance learning. In : Gabriel M, Moore J, eds. *Learning and computational neuroscience: foundations of adaptive networks*. Cambridge MA : Bradford Division of MIT press, 1990 : 143-71.
5. Gabriel M. Discriminative avoidance learning: a model system. In : Vogt BA, Gabriel M, eds. *Neurobiology of cingulate cortex and limbic thalamus: a comprehensive handbook*. Boston : Birkhauser, 1993 : 478-526.
6. Vogt BA, Sikes RW, Vogt LJ. Anterior cingulate cortex and the medial pain system. In : Vogt BA, Gabriel M, eds. *Neurobiology of cingulate cortex and limbic thalamus: a comprehensive handbook*. Boston : Birkhauser, 1993 : 313-44.
7. Madison DV, Malenka RC, Nicoll RA. Mechanisms underlying longterm potentiation of synaptic transmission. *Ann Rev Neurosci* 1991 ; 14 : 379-97.
8. Colley PA, Routtenberg A. Long-term potentiation as synaptic dialogue *Brain Res Rev* 1993 ; 18 : 115-22.
9. Gabriel M, Poremba A, Ellison-Perrine C, Miller JD. Brainstem mediation of learning and memory. In : Klemm WR, Vertes RP, eds. *Brainstem mechanisms of behavior*. New York : John Wiley and Sons Inc, 1990 : 269-313.
10. Poremba A, Gabriel M. Lesions of the medial geniculate nucleus impair avoidance learning, limbic thalamic and cingulate cortical training-induced neuronal activity in rabbits. *Soc Neurosci Abstr* 1993 ; 19 : 802.
11. Maren S, Poremba A, Gabriel M. Basolateral amygdaloid multi-unit neuronal correlates of discriminative avoidance learning in rabbits. *Brain Res* 1991 ; 549 : 311-6.
12. Poremba A, Gabriel M. Lesions of the medial geniculate nucleus impair avoidance learning, limbic thalamic and cingulate cortical training-induced neuronal activity in rabbits. *Soc Neurosci Abstr* 1993 ; 19 : 802.
13. LeDoux JE, Ruggiero DA, Reis DJ. Projections to the subcortical forebrain from anatomically defined regions of the medial geniculate body in the rat. *J Comp Neurol* 1985 ; 242 : 182-213.
14. Poremba A, Gabriel M. Amygdala lesions, avoidance learning and training-induced neuronal activity of limbic thalamus in rabbits (manuscript in preparation).
15. Gabriel M, Vogt VA, Kubota Y, Poremba A, Kang E. Training-stage related neuronal plasticity in limbic thalamus and cingulate cortex during learning. A possible key to mnemonic retrieval. *Behav Brain Res* 1991 ; 46 : 175-85.
16. Kubota Y, Burkybile C, Gabriel M. Training-related neuronal activity in the mamillary complex and brainstem cholinergic nuclei during avoidance learning in rabbits. *Soc Neurosci Abstr* 1994 ; 20 : 797.
17. Krettek JE, Price JL. Amygdaloid projections to subcortical structures within the basal forebrain and brainstem in the rat and cat. *J Comp Neurol* 1978 ; 178 : 225-54.

18. Gabriel M, Cuppernell C, Shenker Jl, Kubota Y, Henzi V, Swanson D. Mamillothalamic tract transection blocks anterior thalamic training induced neuronal plasticity and impairs discriminative avoidance behavior in rabbits. *J Neurosci* 1995 ; 15 : 1437-45.
19. Jones EG, Burton H. Cytoarchitecture and somatic sensory connectivity of thalamic nucleis other than the ventrobasal complex in the cat. *J Comp Neurol* 1974 ; 154 : 395-432.
20. Ledoux JE, Ruggiero DA, Forrest R, Stornetta R, Reis DJ. Topographic organization of convergent projections to the thalamus from the inferior colliculus and spinal cord in the rat. *J Comp Neurol* 1987 ; 264 : 123-46.
21. Canteras NS, Simerly RB, Swanson LW. Connections of the posterior nucleus of the amygdala. *J Comp Neurol* 1992 ; 324 : 143-79.
22. Price JL, Amaral DG. An autoradiographic study of the projections of the central nucleus of the monkey amygdala. *J Neurosci* 1981 ; 1 : 1242-59.
23. Freeman JH Jr, Cuppernell C, Flannery K, Gabriel M. Contextspecific multi-site limbic neuronal activity during concurrent discriminative approach and avoidance training (manuscript in preparation).
24. Henzi V, Kubota Y, Gabriel M. Scopolamine but not haloperidol disrupts training-induced neuronal activity in cingulate cortex and limbic thalamus during learning in rabbits. *Brain Res* 1990 ; 518 : 107-14.
25. Kubota Y, Mayo J, Gabriel M. Brainstem cholinergic projections and limbic thalamic training-related neuronal activity during avoidance learning in rabbits. *Soc Neurosci Abstr* 1993 ; 19 : 802.
26. Vogt BA, Gabriel M, Vogt LJ, Poremba A, Jensen EL, Kubota Y, Kang E. Muscarinic receptor binding increases in anterior thalamus and cingulate cortex during discriminative avoidance learning. *J Neurosci* 1991 ; 11 : 1508-14.
27. Carew TJ, Hawkins RD, Abrams TW, Kandel ER. A test of Hebb's postulate at identified synapses which mediate classical conditioning in Aplysia. *J Neurosci* 1984 ; 4 : 1217-24.
28. Hawkins RD, Kandel ER, Siegelbaum SA. Learning to modulate transmitter release: themes and variations in synaptic plasticity. *Ann Rev Neurosci* 1993 ; 16 : 625-65.
29. Seki M, Zyo K. Anterior thalamic afferents from the mamillary body and the limbic cortex in the rat. *J Comp Neurol* 1984 ; 229 : 242-56.
30. Shibata H. Ascending projections to the mamillary nuclei in the rat: a study using retrograde and anterograde transport of wheat germ agglutinin conjugated to horseradish peroxidase. *J Comp Neurol* 1987 ; 264 : 205-15.
31. Gabriel M, Moore J. *Learning and computational neuroscience: foundations of adaptive networks*. Cambridge MA : Bradford Division of the MIT Press, 1990.
32. Madison DV, Malenka RC, Nicoll RA. Mechanisms underlying longterm potentiation of synaptic transmission. *Annu Rev Neurosci* 1991 ; 14 : 379-97.
33. Poremba A, Gabriel M. Amygdala lesions block acquisition of discriminative active avoidance learning in rabbits. *Soc Neurosci Abstr* 1991 ; 17 : 325.
34. Poremba A, Gabriel M. The nomadic engram: distinct brain circuits for learning and maintenance of avoidance behavior. *PNAS* 1995 (submitted).

15

The forebrain network for pain: an emerging image

K.L. CASEY [1,2,4], S. MINOSHIMA [3]

*Departments of Neurology [1], Physiology[2],
and Internal Medicine (Division of Nuclear Medicine) [3], University of Michigan,
Neurology Research Laboratories, Veteran's Affairs Medical Center [4],
Ann Arbor, Michigan, USA.*

Positron emission tomography (PET) is a method for examining *in vivo* the metabolic function of the human brain. Only within the latter half of this decade has the method of identifying functionally induced increases in regional cerebral blood flow (rCBF) been developed to the extent that it is now applicable for humans in a variety of experimental and clinical conditions. PET studies of rCBF complement the more recently developed functional magnetic resonance imaging (fMRI) technique. Both methods depend on metabolically activated increases in rCBF, but PET currently allows simultaneous monitoring of rCBF changes throughout the brain, from the cortex through the brainstem, whereas fMRI is currently limited in humans to one or a few planes of monitoring, primarily in the cerebral cortex. In addition, the statistical procedures for identifying sites of significant rCBF changes are well developed in PET, although the standards for analysis are still undergoing revision and refinement. Nonetheless, the speed and anatomical precision of fMRI currently far exceeds that of PET. Together, these two methods provide a window on the neurobiology of human experience.

Several studies have now been published in which PET has been used with human subjects to investigate rCBF responses to noxious stimuli. Different forms of stimulation were used in each of these studies. Noxious heat was common to some of these investigations, but the parameters of stimulation differed in many instances. Slight variations in the methods of analysis may also have been present. These sources of variance may contribute to some of the differences in the results. At this stage in the development of this new line of investigation, it may be helpful to review briefly the current state of the technology, some of the sources of variance, the results thus far, and to offer some tentative guidelines for interpretation. This will be far from a complete review of this field, however. It is intended primarily for those less familiar with the conduct of PET activation studies, but who are interested in following the results of these and related studies. We will focus primarily on PET rCBF studies of pain, primarily in normal subjects, and will emphasize comparisons with work from our own facility where similar methods have been used in different studies. The rationale for this exercise is that we, as a clinical and research community interested in pain mechanisms, are just beginning to develop some concepts of how forebrain activity results in the pain experience. As part of this development, we must learn about how to use this new tool and how to analyze and interpret the results. This is a continuing process, which will evolve as more information appears and as we gain experience.

How pet rCBF studies are done

Physiological basis

There is substantial evidence that regional CBF is highly positively coupled to synaptic activity [1], although the degree of this coupling shows some regional variation [2]. One major factor controlling regional CBF is the local production of nitric oxide (NO) [3, 4]. This, in turn, is produced in neurons by calcium-calmodulin activated NO synthase [5]. Calcium influx is the triggering event for presynaptic neurotransmitter release, so NO production reflects predominantly the activity within the synaptic neuropil. However, NO synthase is not evenly distributed among neurons [5]; therefore, the absence of a CBF increase may not mean synaptic inactivity. Recently, evidence has been presented that NO may not be the link between neuronal activity and regional CBF in the rat somatosensory system [6, 7] and that adenosine may be important in mediating this effect [8].

Data acquisition

In PET, CBF is computed from the coincidental counts of gamma rays emitted by the annihilation of positrons from a radioactive compound in the blood and electrons within the surrounding media. In most current studies, water (as $H_2{}^{15}O$) is injected intravenously, or carbon dioxide (as $C^{15}O_2$) is inhaled and converted in the lungs to $H_2{}^{15}O$. The ^{15}O has a half-life of 122 sec. This is sufficient for CBF measurements because, at the CBF levels being measured in human studies, a bolus injection (*e.g.*: 50mCi) of this compound is nearly completely diffused into brain tissue on the first arterial pass [9]. The counts of emissions from a given volume of brain tissue is therefore a good estimate of the amount of blood within that brain region during the counting period. The difference in the number of counts between sequential counting periods provides an estimate of CBF within that volume of brain tissue. The location of that volume (a voxel) within the brain is computed from the intersection of the radial lines formed by the set of opposing (180°) detectors that have registered the gamma emissions from that site.

The volume within which counts are made is the voxel. With the analytical methods used in our facility, there are approximately 95,000 voxels in the gray matter of the average human brain. However, the spatial resolution of PET is limited by the ability of the radiation detectors to differentiate the radiation emitted from two separate point sources. Because the radioemissions spread outward from each point source, there is a spatial limitation on the detectable distance between them. For PET, this distance is the width of the distribution of radioactivity at one-half of the maximum counting rate, called the "full width at half maximum" (FWHM). The FWHM defines the spatial resolution for PET scanners; for a typical scanner today, this is between 6 and 9 mm. However, the spatial resolution can be increased considerably (to less than half the FWHM) when subtraction images are made.

Each image set is then normalized to whole brain counts [10] and mean radioactivity concentration images are created estimating regional cerebral blood flow across all subjects by stereotactic anatomical standardization techniques, which may differ somewhat among facilities. We align CBF images onto the coordinates of a standard stereotactic atlas [11], using anatomical landmarks identified within the PET images of each individual so that the CBF differences are compared within the same brain regions [12-14]. Other facilities use each subject's brain MRI images, which are then transformed onto a standard MRI for localization [15, 16]. To determine whether a task or a stimulus has produced an increase in regional CBF, the rCBF computed during a control condition is subtracted from that computed during the test condition. Areas of significant CBF changes and the locations of volumes of interest (VOI) are determined stereotaxically. The resulting subtraction image, then, shows those brain regions with differences in CBF between the two conditions.

Data analysis

A voxel-by-voxel statistical subtraction analysis (Z-score) with adjustment for multiple comparisons is performed by estimating the smoothness of subtraction images [17] following 3 dimensional Gaussian filtering (FWHM = 9 mm currently in our facility) to enhance signal-to-noise ratio and compensate for anatomical variance. Voxels showing a significantly increased CBF compared to the average noise variance computed across all voxels (pooled variance) are identified [18]. The critical level of significance is determined by adjusting $p = 0.05$ using this information [18, 19]. Typically, only those voxels with normalized CBF values larger than 60% of the global value are analyzed because these represent the gray matter of the brain.

In addition, volumes of interest (VOI) may be established within brain structures selected because of *a priori* hypotheses and the results of previously published PET studies [15, 16, 20, 21]. The size and shape of each VOI may be standardized across studies or determined separately according to functional criteria. We presently use a method similar to that described by Burton *et al.* [22] in which voxels showing significant peak increases in CBF between comparison conditions are identified within the brain structure of interest and progressively expanded in 3 dimensions to include contiguous voxels that meet the statistical criterion established by the voxel-by-voxel Z-score analysis. To determine the statistical significance of rCBF increases, a paired t statistic is computed for each VOI from the average percentage increase in CBF across all subjects. Levels of significance are established based on the Bonferroni correction for multiple comparisons among VOI.

Interpretation

A statistically significant increase in rCBF can reasonably be assumed to be due to increased synaptic activity. Thus, it is the synaptic neuropil, rather than the neuronal cell bodies, that generates the measured response. There is currently no method for distinguishing between increased inhibitory and excitatory synaptic activity with PET CBF studies. Increases in local metabolism are seen during increased inhibitory synaptic activity [23], so increases in regional CBF would be expected during the activity of either excitatory or inhibitory synapses. The neurophysiological significance of decreases in regional CBF is less clear; presumably, this could reflect a decrease in synaptic activity induced by active synaptic inhibition elsewhere. This has not been established firmly in PET CBF studies, although Seitz and Roland [24] have shown that both increases and decreases in rCBF are tightly coupled to regional cerebral oxygen metabolism.

One would like to establish a mathematical relationship between rCBF increases and the amount of synaptic activity. Unfortunately, quantitative measures of synaptic activity are technically difficult to obtain and may be impossible to correlate with changes in rCBF. Some approximations have been attempted, however, using sensory stimulus parameters, evoked potentials, and single unit recording to estimate changes in synaptic activity [25-27]. At present, however, it is not possible to be certain of more than a non-parametric ordinal relationship between rCBF and measures of neuronal activity.

Interpreting the functional significance of increases in rCBF in any single region or in a pattern of brain regions depends upon prior information obtained from other studies (lesions, stimulation, anatomy) and from correlation with performance measures obtained at the time of PET data acquisition. In the case of studies of sensory function, including pain, it is essential to obtain measures of the sensory experience, so that this may be correlated with the observed pattern of rCBF. It is likely that some behavioral performance measures may not be related to the rCBF in one or a few regions, but will correlate better with measures of the activity within all or part of the inter-regional network of activated areas. Put in another way, the function of any given brain region may be best defined in terms of its function within the inter-regional network. Network function, then, becomes the important unit of measurement in establishing brain-behavior relationships. Finally, it must be kept in mind that we may be detecting only part of the network of activity evoked by the stimulation. There are obvious technical limitations, as with any technique, and these limit the volume and intensity of activity that can be detected with PET rCBF studies.

The results thus far

Studies by others

Talbot et al. [16] applied 12 cutaneous contact heat pulses (5 sec duration) repetitively and sequentially to 6 different forearm sites of 8 normal male subjects during PET $H_2^{15}O$ scans. The onset of the stimulation period with respect to the onset of the scan was not otherwise specified. The field of view was restricted to the cerebral cortex. Subjects were instructed to rate the intensities of the stimuli, which were warm (41 - 42 °C) or painful "double pulses" increasing from 47 °C to 48 °C or from 48 °C to 49 °C. After subtracting the warm from the heat pain scans, significant activation was found in the contralateral S1, S2, and anterior cingulate cortices.

Jones et al. [21] used a wider field of view in studying 6 normal subjects receiving approximately 12 ramps of contact heat pulses (5 sec peak duration) [28] applied repetitively to the same site during 3 min PET scans. The PET acquisition technique used inhaled $^{15}CO_2$ and a combination of dynamic and integral methods [29]. Three different temperatures were applied during a total of 6 scans in each subject: 36.3 °C (warm), 41.3 °C (non-painful hot), and 46.4 °C (heat pain). When the scans taken during non-painful hot and warm stimulation were compared, no regions of activation were found. However, a subtraction of the scans taken during the 41.3 °C stimulation from those acquired during the 46.4 °C stimulation revealed significant rCBF increases in the contralateral thalamus, lenticular nucleus, and anterior cingulate cortex. There was no response in the S1 somatosensory cortex, but the prefrontal cortex showed increases that were just below the threshold for statistical significance.

Coghill et al. [15] used PET with $H_2^{15}O$ as a tracer in a study of 9 normal right-handed subjects, each of whom received innocuous vibratory (110 Hz.), mild warm (34 °C), and heat pain (47-48 °C) stimulation of the left forearm. Heat pulses of 6 sec duration were delivered every 4 sec, thus allowing a maximum of 6 stimuli during the scan. Psychophysical ratings showed that the vibration was perceived as more intense than the warm stimulus, and that the heat pain was the most intense. When compared with the warm sensation, heat pain was shown to increase rCBF in the contralateral S1, S2, anterior insula, anterior cingulate, and supplementary motor (SMA) cortices. The ipsilateral anterior insula showed a response just below the statistical threshold.

Subcortical pain-related activation was seen in the contralateral thalamus and ipsilateral lenticular nucleus (putamen). Although the anterior cingulate cortex, SMA, insula, and thalamus also responded during vibration (compared to warm), the rCBF increases were below statistical threshold. A direct comparison of pain and vibration revealed that the contralateral anterior insular cortex was the only structure activated uniquely during heat pain stimulation.

Apkarian et al. [30] used single photon emission computed tomography (SPECT) and Tc99m-hexamethyl propylene amine oxime (Tc99m-HMPAO) as a tracer to study rCBF increases in 3 normal subjects while each held the left hand in 46.2 °C water (rated as moderately painful) for 3 minutes during a single scan. The same hand was held in warm (36 °C) water during control scans. Response localization was performed by superimposing SPECT and MRI scans from the same subject. Change distribution images were formed by subtracting counts in individual pixels obtained during control scans from those obtained during heat pain. The results showed a decrease in rCBF in the region of the contralateral S1 cortex. Two of the same subjects showed an increased rCBF in the same region during vibratory stimulation or during finger movements.

Two studies performed in patients are mentioned here because of their relevance to pain mechanisms. Cesaro et al. [31] used SPECT with the metabolic marker ^{123}I N-isopropyl-iodoamphetamine (IMP) to demonstrate hyperactivity in the thalamus contralateral to a region of post-stroke hyperpathia in 2 patients. Di Piero et al. (1991) used PET with inhaled $^{15}CO_2$ in 5 patients with unilateral, severe cancer pain. Compared to normal control subjects, the patients, who were maintained on morphine throughout the study, had decreased thalamic blood flow contralateral to the pain; this returned to normal following successful percutaneous anterolateral cordotomy.

Studies from our facility

These are summarized in Table I, which shows the average, (not the peak) rCBF increases within the volume of tissue that contains contiguous voxels that met the statistical threshold for response. Our PET acquisition and analysis methods are described above. In the heat pain studies, we stimulated the non-dominant forearm with 5 seconds applications of either 40 °C (warm) or 50 °C (heat pain) delivered with contact thermodes pre-set to the stimulus temperature. This assured that the skin reached the stimulus temperature as quickly as possible. The thermode was moved among the 6 stimulus sites as quickly as possible to minimize interstimulus time while assuring that at least 25 seconds elapsed between stimuli delivered to the same site. Approximately 12 stimuli were delivered during each scan. In the study of cold pain, the non-dominant hand was immersed in a 6 °C water bath approximately 30 sec before the injection of tracer and throughout the 60 seconds scan period. Hand temperature was 17-15 °C during the scans. Psychophysical measures of stimulus intensity were performed in all studies.

Two features of the studies we performed provide an interesting basis for comparison. The first is the use of cold water immersion as a noxious stimulus [32]. This method, which has been used in the "cold pressor" test of cardiovascular reactivity, produces an intense pain that is perceived as deep, rather than cutaneous, and continuous, rather than phasic, as in the repetitive contact heat stimulation we applied. The second notable comparison is in the timing of the scans during the repetitive contact heat stimulation. As previously reported [33], for 4 of the 8 scans in each subject, we began stimulation only when the radioactive bolus arrived in the brain. For the remaining 4 scans, stimulation started approximately 45 seconds earlier. In both cases, the scans were 60 seconds in duration.

In comparing the results of two repetitive heat pain studies with the single study of continuous cold pain, we find considerable overlap of activated regions (Table I, Figure 1). This suggests that there may be a pattern of activation that is common to different forms of pain. The common pattern may include the contralateral premotor, sensorimotor, anterior cingulate and insular cortices, the contralateral ventral posterior thalamus and lenticular nucleus, the ipsilateral insular cortex and medial thalamus, and the cerebellar vermis. However, there are notable differences between the cerebral responses to repetitive, cutaneous heat pain, and continuous, deep cold pain. Some regions that responded during heat pain were not active during deep cold pain. This includes the contralateral S2 cortex, ventral posterior thalamus, and dorsomedial midbrain.

Table I. Average percent rCBF increases in structures activated by noxious thermal stimuli.

Structure	Heat Pain (skin, early)	Heat Pain (skin, late)	Cold Pain (deep, late)
Contralateral			
premotor cortex		3.29	3.43
sensorimotor cortex	1.71	2.88	3.78
anterior cingulate cortex	2.08	2.89	3.35
insula / lenticular nucleus		3.50	4.07
S2/posterior insula		2.74	
ventral posterior thalamus	1.61	2.86	(3.21)
Ipsilateral			
lateral prefrontal cortex			3.03
anterior cingulate cortex			3.26
insula / precentral operculum		3.03	3.30
v.p./ medial thalamus		2.90	3.24
Midline			
cerebellar vermis		2.76	3.08
dorsomedial midbrain		3.46	

The structures listed were activated, as determined by VOI or independent voxel-by-voxel statistical analysis, in at least one of the 3 studies of repetitive cutaneous heat or in the single study of pain during immersion of one hand in 6 °C water. The contralateral thalamus showed an increase in rCBF during deep cold pain ( ), but the variability of intersubject responses lowered the significance of this response to just below statistical threshold on VOI analysis.

Conversely, the ipsilateral prefrontal and anterior cingulate cortices were active during deep cold, but not cutaneous heat pain. Additional studies will be necessary to determine whether these differences are consistently observed in comparing these two conditions and, if so, what their physiological function might be.

Another salient difference between these two response patterns is that, among each of the 7 regions activated in both conditions, the increase in rCBF is greater during deep cold pain. Across all regions, the average % rCBF increase during deep cold pain (3.46 ± 0.13 s.e.) is significantly greater than during cutaneous heat pain (3.04 ± 0.10; $t_{12} = 2.62$, p = 0.022). This difference cannot be attributed to differences in global blood flow because global blood flow responses are normalized between conditions in each subject [10]. Although the functional significance of these differences in cerebral response patterns cannot be specified with our current level of analysis, there are some

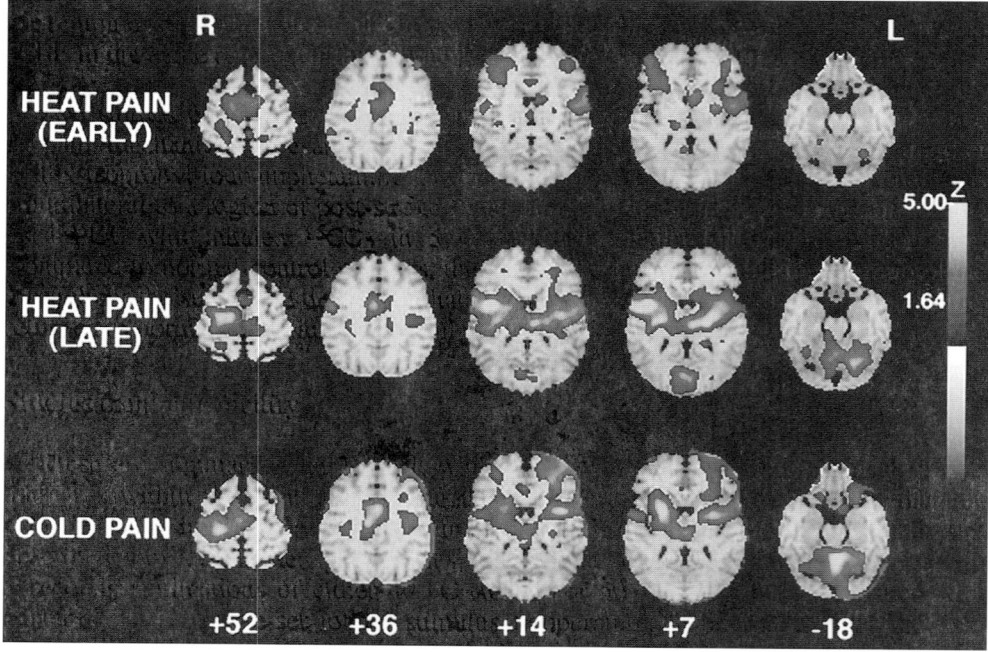

Figure 1. Statistical maps of brain regions activated during the early phase (top row; first 60 seconds) or the later phase (middle row; last 55 seconds) of 100 seconds of repetitive cutaneous heat stimulation of the left forearm, or during the last 60 seconds of immersion of the left hand in 6 °C water for approximately 90 seconds (bottom row). Color bar at right encodes the statistical Z-score of the activation. Regions responding at a p = 0.05 level of significance (uncorrected for multiple comparisons) or greater on independent voxel-by-voxel analysis are displayed on a standardized MRI scan at stereotactic coordinates [11]. The right hemisphere is on the left. The level, in mm, above a plane intersecting the anterior and posterior commissures is shown below each column. The peak activation of all regions listed in Table I is not shown in this display because a limited number of images were chosen for comparison. Although the average increase in rCBF was greater during cold immersion pain than during cutaneous heat pain (*see* text), this difference may not be reflected in these maps because of the relatively greater variance of reponses obtained during cold pain. (See appendix for colour figures.)

obvious differences between these conditions that deserve consideration. Compared with the heat stimulus, the cold stimulation is continuous, tonic, and excites a different set of thermosensitive afferents [34-36]. Noxious cold immersion stimulation at the intensity we used also produces marked sympathetic autonomic responses that are not seen during stimulation with phasic cutaneous heat [37-41]. Finally, there are striking differences between the subjective experiences associated with these stimuli. The heat stimulus is felt as phasic, burning and cutaneous, whereas the cold immersion stimulus is described by all subjects as constant, aching, and deep rather than cutaneous. Psychophysical studies have also shown that the pain of cold immersion has a much higher degree of perceived unpleasantness than phasic cutaneous heat pain [42]. Subsequent PET experiments should attempt to control some of these stimulus and response variables and relate them more specifically to the differences in the pattern and intensity of rCBF responses.

In comparing the activation pattern of the scans taken during the early part of the noxious heat stimulation period with the pattern obtained during the later scans, we found that the number of activated regions increased dramatically as the stimulation progressed (Table I, Figure 1). During the first 60 seconds of cutaneous heat pain, significant responses were seen only in the contralateral sensorimotor and anterior cingulate cortices and the contralateral ventral posterior thalamus. When stimulation proceeded for another 40-45 sec, 7 additional regions responded. These included the contralateral premotor, S2 and insular cortices, the ipsilateral insular and premotor cortices, ipsilateral thalamus, and the medial midbrain and cerebellum. In addition, the regions activated during the early phase showed an increased response. Across the 3 regions that responded during both phases, the average increase was greater during the late period (2.88 ± 0.01 s.e.) than during the early phase (1.80 ± 0.14 s.e.; $t_4 = 7.52$, $p = 0.002$). As originally reported [33], psychophysical studies showed that these differences in forebrain response could reflect significant increases in perceived intensity and unpleasantness as the repetitive stimulation continued.

Comparison of the results

Table II summarizes a comparison of the results of PET studies of normal subjects experiencing heat pain. There is complete agreement that the contralateral, but not the ipsilateral anterior cingulate gyrus responds, and that no response is detected within the ipsilateral S1 cortex. Three of the 4 studies agree that the contralateral sensorimotor (S1/M1) and S2 cortices respond. Among the 3 studies that examined subcortical structures, there is complete agreement that there is a contralateral response in the thalamus. Two of these studies also detected responses in the contralateral lenticular nucleus. Responses were detected in the contralateral insula in 2 of the 4 studies. This analysis suggests that present methods of functional imaging can reveal a basic pattern of cerebral activity that identifies an experience of pain. If one were to be presented with the results of a PET rCBF study that showed, within one hemisphere, activity in the sensorimotor, insular, S2, and anterior cingulate cortices, accompanied by subcortical activation in the ventral posterior thalamus and lenticular nucleus, there would be a good chance of correctly predicting the presence of contralateral pain. It is possible that the same prediction would be correct most of the time if only the ventral posterior thalamus and anterior cingulate gyrus of the same hemisphere were active.

What about the discrepancies among the studies summarized in Table II ? If we set aside structures that have not been examined by others, such as the midbrain and cerebellum, the major difference is in the activation of regions ipsilateral to the noxious stimulus. The studies from our facility are unique in showing pain-related activation of both the ipsilateral and contralateral thalamus, S2 and insular cortices. Although there are modest differences in the PET technique and analysis methods used among these studies, these are not likely to account for the additional ipsilateral activity seen in our investigations. Differences in PET acquisition methods, stereotactic localization, analysis methods, and in the statistical criteria used to identify active regions, should contribute to variations in the identification of structures within both hemispheres. Technical factors are not likely to account for a systematic and consistent difference primarily in the identification of activity ipsilateral to the stimulus.

Table II. Regions showing significant increases in rCBF in pet studies of normal subjects experiencing heat pain

Structure	study #1	study #2	study #3	study #4
Contralateral				
premotor cortex	0	0	+	0
S1/(M1)	+	0	+	+
S2	+	0	+	+
insula	0	0	+	+
ant. cingulate/sma	+	+	+	+
thalamus	n.a.	+	+	+
lenticular/putamen	n.a.	+	+	0
Ipsilateral				
S1	0	0	0	0
S2	0	0	+	0
insula	0	0	+	0
ant. cingulate/sma	0	0	0	0
thalamus	n.a.	0	+	0
lenticular/putamen	n.a.	0	0	+
Midline				
cerebellum	n.a.	n.a.	+	n.a.
midbrain	n.a.	n.a.	+	n.a.

Structures activated during cutaneous heat pain in 4 different PET rCBF studies. Study #1, Talbot et al. [16]; study #2, Jones et al. [21]; study #3, Casey et al. (1994a,b); study #4, Coghill et al. [15]. The summary of study #3 includes the late phase of heat stimulation (see text). + = response detected; 0 = response not detected; n.a.= not examined.

We suggest that the most significant factor contributing to the identification of ipsilateral activity in our studies is the intensity and frequency of noxious stimulation. These stimulation characteristics distinguish our studies from the others; in every instance, the stimuli we applied were more intense and frequent during the scans. The importance of these stimulus variables is shown in Table I. During the early phase of heat pain, only the contralateral thalamus and the sensorimotor and anterior cingulate cortices are active. It is only during the last half of the approximately 100 seconds of stimulation that additional structures, including those in the ipsilateral hemisphere and posterior fossa, become active. Because the intensity and frequency of the stimulation remained constant throughout this period, it appears that the total amount of noxious stimulation, rather that simply the intensity or frequency of stimulation, may be the critical variable. Similarly, in comparing constant, deep cold pain with phasic cutaneous heat pain, activity in the ipsilateral prefrontal and anterior cingulate cortices joins the ongoing activity within the ipsilateral insula/precentral operculum and medial thalamus. Psychophysical measurements showed that stimulus intensity and unpleasantness increased as the noxious stimulation continued, suggesting a perceptual correlate of this increased activation pattern [32, 33]. Overall, the results of this comparison suggest that the total amount of noxious stimulation delivered and, hence, the total amount of pain experienced is a very important determinant of the pattern and intensity of cerebral activity.

Interpreting the results: now and in the future

For decades, we have known that the stimulation of nociceptive afferents could activate large areas of the brain. We could predict, with some precision, which regions of the brain these would be — and approximately the order in which they might become active. We knew that this activity was under the dynamic control of multiple neuronal systems throughout the neuraxis. But, in attempting to understand the physiology and pathophysiology of pain through experiment and observation, we were forced to ignore this network as an object for study and analysis because we had almost no means of studying it directly in humans — or even in animals. That is no longer true. Now we are in the era of functional imaging of the brains of conscious humans and animals. We are beginning to see the dynamics of the network that is activated by nociceptive stimulation and that can be related directly to the perception of pain. In the past, neuroscientists were expected to acknowledge only a small fraction of a larger problem like pain. It was not necessary, or even possible, to consider the problem of relating one's own data to the functioning of a larger network. Now, however, the function of each component of this network may soon be defined as much in terms of its role in the network as in terms of pain-related behavior or response.

We may be approaching the ability to recognize critical features of the spatial pattern of cerebral activity that identify the experience of pain. It seems possible that the intensity of the experience may be represented, perhaps in some systematic way, by the distribution and intensity of the neuronal response as reflected by increased rCBF. In addition, we are beginning to learn that this pattern may have unique temporal, as well as spatial, characteristics. These temporal features may turn out to be at least as important as the spatial pattern, not only because they may uniquely identify some aspects of the experience, but because of what the sequence of pattern development may tell us about the function of each region in the development of the full network. For example, the activation of the contralateral thalamus, sensorimotor cortex, and anterior cingulate cortex early in the course of the pain experience suggests the possibility that one or more of these structures is responsible for the subsequent activity in the contralateral insula, lenticular nucleus, and S2 cortex. An alternative possibility is that this sequence of events is due to independent, parallel activation with polysynaptic delays in one pathway. These hypotheses are not readily testable in human studies today, but an animal model that permits the analysis of nociceptively induced rCBF patterns could reveal the behavioral and physiological effects of selective surgical or pharmacological interruptions within the network of activated regions. Fortunately, Morrow [43] has developed the appropriate animal model in our laboratory so that the relevant analyses of the dynamics of the nociceptive network can proceed. Invasive studies in the animal model promise to provide an essential complement to future PET studies in normal subjects and patients. Their limitations notwithstanding, human studies will always be critical because of the opportunity to correlate drug or lesion-induced changes in the rCBF pattern with psychophysical measures of the pain experience.

The functional significance of each of the structures or regions comprising the cerebral network for pain may have to be determined both in terms of its role in the network and in separate physiological or behavioral experiments. For example, numerous clinical and experimental observations have shown that the S1 cortex and the thalamo-cortical projection neurons innervating it are essential for the capacity to recognize the spatial, temporal, and intensive characteristics of somatic stimuli. However, it is not clear how this activity is influenced by the activity of other components of the network, such as the cingulate cortex, and how this interaction may affect pain or pain-related behaviors. Lesions within the anterior cingulate cortex are known to attenuate pain-related behaviors in humans [44-48], and we have recently demonstrated that medial frontal and cingulate lesions produce a selective, apparently apraxic, impairment of the hot plate response in the rat [49]. Anatomical, physiological, and behavioral studies lend support to the speculation that the cingulate portion of the medial frontal cortex, in addition to other functions, may serve as an integrative center for nociceptive responses. The cingulate cortex is part of a complex network that makes extensive connections with limbic, sensory, and motor structures (for review, *see* [50]). How lesions within the anterior cingulate cortex also affect the activation of the sensorimotor cortex or thalamus — or of other components of the pain-activated network — is not known.

There is little doubt that much will be learned in the future about pain mechanisms because of questions, like those above, posed by the results of imaging studies in humans and animals. In these studies, certain aspects of the activity of the whole brain, or large components of it, will be studied with increasingly quantitative precision. These activities will be related directly to changes in pain behavior or experience, which will also be measured and manipulated with some precision. This will lead to the identification of critical components of the cerebral network and to an understanding of how the activity within these regions affects the experience of pain and the many levels of response to pain. Attention will then be focused on the cellular and molecular physiology and pathophysiology of these critical network elements, leading to greatly improved opportunities to manipulate the function of the whole network for therapeutic benefit. Then we may hope to achieve more effective and specific relief for intractable chronic pain conditions, such as those produced by diseases of the central and peripheral nervous system.

Acknowledgements

Supported in part by the Department of Veteran's Affairs (K.L.C.) and by a grant from the Department of Energy (S.M.; David E. Kuhl, Principal Investigator). The authors gratefully acknowledge the support, advice, and encouragement of David E. Kuhl, M.D. The expert technical assistance of Jill Rothley, Todd Hauser, Paul Kison, Edward McKenna, Andrew Weeden, and Laura Pastoriza was essential for the conduct of the studies discussed here, and is greatly appreciated.

References

1. Sokoloff L. Relationship between functional activity and energy metabolism in the nervous system: whether, where and why? In : Lassen NA, Ingvar DH, Raichle ME, Friberg L, eds. *Brain work and mental activity*. Copenhagen : Munksgaard, 1991 : 52-64.
2. Raichle ME. Circulatory and metabolic correlates of brain function in normal humans. In : Plum F, ed. *Handbook of physiology. Section 1: The nervous system, Vol 5. Higher functions of the brain, Part 2*. Bethesda : American Physiological Society, 1987 : 643-74.
3. Dirnagl U, Lindauer U, Villringer A. Role of nitric oxide in the coupling of cerebral blood flow to neuronal activation in rats. *Neurosci Lett* 1993 ; 149 : 43-6.
4. Iadecola C. Regulation of the cerebral microcirculation during neural activity: is nitric oxide the missing link? *Trends Neurosci* 1993 ; 16 : 206-14.
5. Vincent SR, Hope BT. Neurons that say NO. *Trends Neurosci* 1992 ; 15 : 108-13.
6. Adachi K, Takahashi S, Melzer P, Campos KL, Nelson T, Kennedy C, Sokoloff L. Increases in local cerebral blood flow associated with somatosensory activation are not mediated by NO. *Am J Physiol Heart Circ Physiol* 1994 ; 267 : H2155-162.
7. Wang Q, Kjaer T, Jorgensen MB, Paulson OB, Lassen NA, Diemer NH, Lou HC. Nitric oxide does not act as a mediator coupling cerebral blood flow to neural activity following somatosensory stimuli in rats. *Neurol Res* 1993 ; 15 : 33-6.
8. Dirnagl U, Niwa K, Lindauer U, Villringer A. Coupling of cerebral blood flow to neuronal activation: role of adenosine and nitric oxide. *Am J Physiol Heart Circ Physiol* 1994 ; 267 : H296-301.

9. Ter-Pogossian MM, Eichling JO, Davis DO. The determination of regional cerebral blood flow by means of water labeled with radioactive oxygen. *Radiology* 1969 ; 93 : 31-40.
10. Fox PT, Raichle ME. Stimulus rate dependence of regional cerebral blood flow in human striate cortex, demonstrated by positron emission tomography. *J Neurophysiol* 1984 ; 51 : 1109-20.
11. Talairach J, Tournoux A. *A coplanar stereotaxic atlas of the human brain.* New York : Thieme Medical Publishers Inc, 1988.
12. Minoshima S, Berger KL, Lee KS, Mintun MA. An automated method for rotational correction and centering of three-dimensional functional brain images. *J Nucl Med* 1992 ; 33 : 1579-85.
13. Minoshima S, Koeppe RA, Frey KA, Kuhl DE. Anatomic standardization: linear scaling and nonlinear warping of functional brain images. *J Nucl Med* 1994 ; 35 : 1528-36.
14. Minoshima S, Koeppe RA, Mintun MA, Berger KL, Taylor SF, Frey KA, Kuhl DE. Automated detection of the intercommissural line for stereotactic localization of functional brain images. *J Nucl Med 1993* ; 34 : 322-9.
15. Coghill RC, Talbot JD, Evans AC, Meyer E, Gjedde A, Bushnell MC, Duncan GH. Distributed processing of pain and vibration by the human brain. *J Neurosci* 1994 ; 14 : 4095-108.
16. Talbot JD, Marrett S, Evans AC, Meyer E, Bushnell MC, Duncan GH. Multiple representations of pain in human cerebral cortex. *Science* 1991 ; 251 : 1355-8.
17. Friston KJ, Frith CD, Liddle PF, Frackowiak RS. Comparing functional (PET) images: the assessment of significant change. *J Cereb Blood Flow Metab* 1991 ; 11 : 690-9.
18. Worsley KJ, Evans AC, Marrett S, Neelin P A three-dimensional statistical analysis for CBF activation studies in human brain. *J Cereb Blood Flow Metab* 1992 ; 12 : 900-18.
19. Adler RJ, Hasofer AM. Level crossings for random fields. *Ann Probabil* 1976 ; 4 : 1-12.
20. Casey KL, Minoshima S, Berger KL, Koeppe RA, Morrow TJ, Frey KA. Positron emission tomographic analysis of cerebral structures activated specifically by repetitive noxious heat stimuli. *J Neurophysiol* 1994 ; 71 : 802-7.
21. Jones AKP, Brown WD, Friston KJ, Qi LY, Frackowiak RSJ. Cortical and subcortical localization of response to pain in man using positron emission tomography. *Proc R Soc Lond (Biol)* 1991 ; 244 : 39-44.
22. Burton H, Videen TO, Raichle ME. Tactile-vibration-activated foci in insular and parietal-opercular cortex studied with positron emission tomography: mapping the second somatosensory area in humans. *Somatosens Mot Res* 1993 ; 10 : 297-308.
23. Ackerman RF, Finch DM, Babb TL, Engel J Jr. Increased glucose metabolism during long-duration recurrent inhibition of hippocampal pyramidal cells. *J Neurosci* 1984 ; 4 : 251-64.
24. Seitz RJ, Roland PE. Vibratory stimulation increases and decreases the regional cerebral blood flow and oxidative metabolism: a positron emission tomography (PET) study. *Acta Neurol Scand* 1992 ; 86 : 60-7.
25. Celesia GG, Polcyn RD, Holden JE, Nickles RJ, Gatley JS, Koeppe RA. Visual evoked potentials and positron emission tomographic mapping of regional cerebral blood flow and cerebral metabolism: can the neuronal potential generators be visualized? *Electroencephalogr Clin Neurophysiol* 1982 ; 54 : 243-56.
26. Fox PT, Raichle ME. Stimulus rate determines regional brain blood flow in striate cortex. *Ann Neurol* 1985 ; 17 : 303-5.
27. Tsubokawa T, Katayama Y, Kondo T, Ueno Y, Hayashi N, Moriyasu N. Changes in local cerebral blood flow and neuronal activity during sensory stimulation in normal and sympathectomized cats. *Brain Res* 1980 ; 190 : 51-64.
28. Fruhstorfer H, Lindblom U, Schmidt WG. Method for quantitative estimation of thermal thresholds in patients. *J Neurol Neurosurg Psychiat* 1976 ; 39 : 1071-5.

29. Lammertsma AA, Cunningham VJ, Deiber MP, Heather JD, Bloomfield PM, Nutt JG, Frackowiack RSJ, Jones T. Combination of dynamic and integral methods for generating reproducible functional CBF images. *J Cereb Blood Flow Metab* 1990 ; 10 : 675-86.
30. Apkarian AV, Stea RA, Manglos SH, Szeverenyi NM, King RB, Thomas FD. Persistent pain inhibits contralateral somatosensory cortical activity in humans. *Neurosci Lett* 1992 ; 140 : 141-7.
31. Cesaro P, Mann MW, Moretti JL, Defer G, Roualdès B, Nguyen JP, Degos JD. Central pain and thalamic hyperactivity: a single photon emission computerized tomographic study. *Pain* 1991 ; 47 : 329-36.
32. Casey KL, Minoshima S, Koeppe RA, Morrow TJ, Frey KA. Differences in cortical and subcortical responses to noxious heat and cold stimuli in humans. *Soc Neurosci Abstr* 1993 ; 19 : 1074.
33. Casey KL, Minoshima S, Koeppe RA, Weeder J, Morrow TJ. Temporo-spatial dynamics of human forebrain activity during noxious heat stimulation. *Soc Neurosci* 1994 ; 20 : 1573 (abstract).
34. Darian-Smith I. Thermal sensibility. In : Darian-Smith I, ed. *Handbook of physiology. Section 1: The nervous system*. Bethesda : American Physiological Society, 1984 : 879-914.
35. Klement W, Arndt JO. The role of nociceptors of cutaneous veins in the mediation of cold pain in man. *J Physiol (Lond)* 1992 ; 449 : 73-83.
36. Yarnitsky D, Ochoa JL. Warm and cold specific somatosensory systems. Psychophysical thresholds, reaction times and peripheral conduction velocities. *Brain* 1991 ; 114 : 1819-26.
37. Fagius J, Karhuvaara S, Sundlof G. The cold pressor test: effects on sympathetic nerve activity in human muscle and skin nerve fascicles. *Acta Physiol Scand* 1989 ; 137 : 325-34.
38. Hampf G. Influence of cold pain in the hand on skin impedance, heart rate and skin temperature. *Physiol Behav* 1990 ; 47 : 217-8.
39. Kregel KC, Seals DR, Callister R. Sympathetic nervous system activity during skin cooling in humans: relationship to stimulus intensity and pain sensation. *J Physiol (Lond)* 1992 ; 454 : 359-71.
40. Peckerman A, Hurwitz BE, Saab PG, Llabre MM, McCabe PM, Schneiderman N. Stimulus dimensions of the cold pressor test and the associated patterns of cardiovascular response. *Psychophysiol* 1994 ; 31 : 282-90.
41. Victor RG, Leimbach WN Jr, Seals DR, Wallin BG, Mark AL. Effects of the cold pressor test on muscle sympathetic nerve activity in humans. *Hypertension* 1987 ; 9 : 429-36.
42. Rainville P, Feine JS, Bushnell MC, Duncan GH. A psychophysical comparison of sensory and affective responses to four modalities of experimental pain. *Somatosens Mot Res* 1992 ; 9 : 265-77.
43. Morrow TJ, Danneman PJ, Frey KA, Casey KL. Regional cerebral blood flow (rCBF) changes during pain: an animal model. *Soc Neurosci* 1994 ; 20 : 1573 (abstract).
44. Devinsky O, Luciano D. The contributions of cingulate cortex to human behavior. In : Vogt BA, Gabriel M, eds. *Neurobiology of cingulate cortex and limbic thalamus: a comprehensive handbook*. Boston : Birkhauser, 1993.
45. Foltz EL, White LE. Pain "relief" by frontal cingulumotomy. *J Neurosurg* 1962 ; 19 : 89-100.
46. Hurt RW, Ballantine HT. Stereotactic anterior cingulate lesions for persistent pain: a report on 68 cases. *Clin Neurosurg* 1973 ; 21 : 334-51.
47. Sweet WH. Treatment of medically intractable mental disease by limited frontal leucotomy-justifiable? *N Engl J Med* 1973 ; 289 : 1117-25.
48. Sweet WH. Cerebral localization of pain. In : Thompson RA, Green JR, eds. *New perspectives in cerebral localization*. New York : Raven Press, 1982 : 205-42.

49. Pastoriza LN, Morrow TJ, Casey KL. Medial frontal cortex lesions selectively attenuate the hot plate response: possible nocifensive apraxia in the rat. *Pain* 1995 (in press).
50. Vogt BA, Sikes RW, Vogt LJ. Anterior cingulate cortex and the medial pain system. In : Vogt BA, Gabriel M, eds. *Neurobiology of cingulate cortex and limbic thalamus: a comprehensive handbook*. Boston : Birkhauser, 1993.

16

Cortical and thalamic imaging in normal volunteers and patients with chronic pain

A.K.P. JONES [1,2], S.W.G. DERBYSHIRE [2]

[1] *University of Manchester Rheumatic Diseases Centre, Clinical Sciences Building, Hope Hospital, Salford, UK.*
[2] *MRC Cyclotron Unit, Hammersmith Hospital, London, UK.*

The purpose of this chapter is to briefly review our functional imaging studies using positron emission tomography (PET) and more recently functional magnetic resonance (fMRI) studies. Many of these results have been extensively reviewed elsewhere [1] and therefore the authors will confine themselves to a discussion of the main findings and the hypotheses generated by these findings.

Two types of PET studies will be described:
- So called "activation" studies where changes in regional cerebral blood flow (rCBF) are measured in response to standardised painful and nonpainful experimental heat stimuli or to just a change in the ongoing pain state. The close relationship between neuronal activity and changes in rCBF allows this technique to be used to monitor changes in neuronal activity in response to different components of cerebral pain processing. Both inhalation of $C^{15}O_2$ and i.v. injection $H_2^{15}O$ have been used as tracers to measure rCBF.
- I.v. injection of [^{11}C]-diprenorphine, which is a non-selective μ, δ and κ antagonist, is used as a tracer to quantitate available *in vivo* opioid receptor binding sites. This technique cannot differentiate between changes in occupation of receptors by endogenous peptides, changes in total receptor number (B_{max}) or changes in affinity (k_D). However, in context of animal experiments some reasonable assumptions can be made.

Responses to acute phasic thermal pain in normal volunteers will be considered first. We designed these experiments specifically to exclude the sensory discriminative components of these responses. The experiments consisted of the application of a Somedic thermal probe to the back of the right hand to deliver phasic and highly reproducible ramps of increasing heat, the peak of which were either painfully hot or non-painfully hot. These were delivered every 15 seconds for a two minute period during which time regional rCBF was measured using PET. Most of the data described was acquired in 2D, although 3D acquired data will also be described. In all the 2D studies six measurements were made in each subject in response to either non-painful (X3) or painful (X3) stimulation with six subjects in each group. The significant responses to the non-discriminative components or the "suffering components" of the pain are obtained by subtracting the rCBF responses to non-painful from the painful heat stimuli to generate a significance map of significant response for the whole group. These group responses can then be compared to other experimental groups. The steps including stereotactic normalisation to standardised Talairach coordinates as has been extensively described elsewhere [1].

The non-discriminatory components of an acute thermal pain stimulus activate predominantly the contralateral thalamus, anterior insula, lentiform nucleus and anterior cingulate cortex, ipsilateral dorsolateral prefrontal cortex (Brodman areas 9, 10, 44 and 46) and inferior parietal cortex (areas 39 and 40) [2, 3] (Table I). Subsignificant activations have also been seen in region of the periaqueductal gray in the brain stem. A similar pattern of activation has been observed in normal volunteers subjected to a tonic heat stimulus to the back of the right hand [4]. Confirmation of these areas being activated by acute pain has come from a number of different laboratories including the Ann Arbor [5], Montreal [6], Stockholm [7] and Rome (SPECT) [8] groups. However, there are some important additional observations. Casey *et al.* [9] activated the thalamus bilaterally but did not show prefrontal cortical activation.

Table I. Within group comparison of painful hot *vs* non-painful hot indicating significant pain-related foci of activation. Coordinates of peak activation are expressed with reference to the atlas of Talairach and Tournoux (1988). Statistical magnitudes are expressed as Z scores significant at $p < 0.001$.

Region	Coordinates			Z-score
	x	y	z	
Pooled controls - left rCBF increases				
Thalamus/insula	-24	-10	8	3.887
Anterior cingulate (BA 24)	-8	-10	40	3.818
Pooled controls - right rCBF increases				
Thalamus/lentiform nucleus	22	6	8	3.843
Prefrontal cortex (BA 44)	42	10	16	3.401
Inf. parietal cortex (BA 40)	56	-42	28	3.380

The latter may be a numbers problem, as our group initially only showed subsignificant activation of the prefrontal cortex [2], which in a pooled group of twelve volunteers became significant [3, 4]. Although insula cortical responses have mostly been reported contralateral to the side of the acute pain stimulus there is evidence for ipsilateral [10] and bilateral responses [11] The latter study also described bilateral thalamic responses and two main areas of increased blood flow in the anterior cingulate cortex. In addition to the mid-cingulate area previously described there was an additional highly significant area at the peri-genual cingulate.

The possibility arises that there may be a bilateral component to thalamic, insula and basal ganglia processing although the contralateral component may well be quantitatively more important. Bilateral activation of these structures is consistent with what is known about the nociceptive inputs to these regions of the brain. Nociceptive

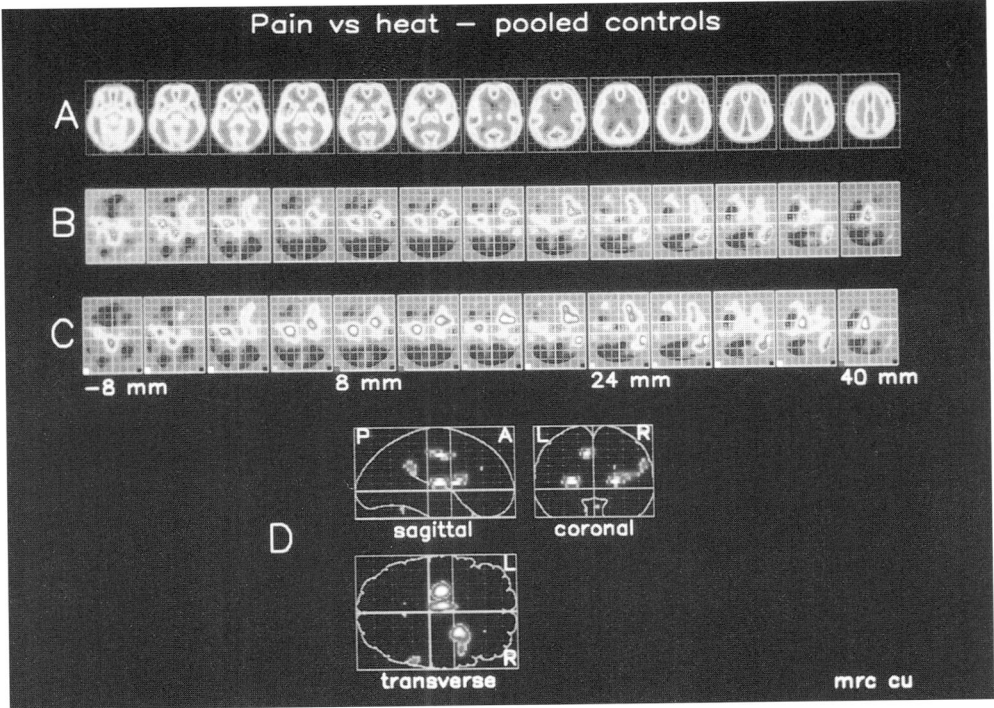

Figure 1. Data averaged from the combined group of twelve subjects. At the top are transverse images of the brain after stereotaxic normalization, with the distances from the AC-PC plane indicated. A: Anatomical features obtained by averaging all blood flow scans from the twelve subjects. B: The arithmetical difference between adjusted mean blood flows for painful hot and nonpainful hot phasic stimuli. C: The SPM{t} values derived from the formal pixel by pixel comparison of the adjusted mean blood flows and variances for each of the two conditions. The colour scale is arbitrary, threshold significance is indicated by the lower left pixel for each plane. D: The orthogonal projections of the statistical comparison at a P < 0.001 (Z threshold 3.09). The areas showing significant increases in blood flow are thalamus, insula, lentiform nucleus, frontal area 44, inferior parietal area 40 and anterior cingulate cortex. (See appendix for colour figures.)

responses in units in area 24 of anterior cingulate often exhibit whole body receptive fields. Some bilaterality of response might therefore be expected in this region. Although PET studies suggest that acute pain responses are mainly contralateral, chronic neurogenic pain appears to be processed ipsilaterally [12]. It has to be remembered that the effective spatial resolution of activation studies is about 16 mm and therefore there always remains some uncertainty about the distinction between structures either side of the midline. Functional magnetic resonance studies suggest that there is bilateral anterior cingulate activation in response to tonic cold pain [13]. There is also some variability of responses in the somatosensory cortex. Our group have been unable to elicit consistent responses in SI with PET with both increases and decreases in flow in this area in responses to phasic heat pain of the contralateral hand. Apkarian *et al.* have also found decreases in flow in response to tonic pain in SI/SII [14]. Both the Montreal and Ann Arbor group have documented responses in SI.

Contralateral responses in S2 to phasic pain [5, 6] and tonic pain [4, 15] have been more consistently documented. The explanation for these inconsistencies is likely to be mainly due to the differences in experimental design. All the groups except our own group moved a heat probe at a given temperature from one location to another on the forearm in order to minimise habituation. This is likely to increase attention to the discriminatory components of the stimulus which is unlikely to be matched in the control condition. In the authors opinion there is little doubt that SI is involved in the sensory discriminatory components of pain processing as has been clearly shown by recent PET studies. However, the presence or absence of pain is unlikely to be the main determinant of whether there is an increase in flow in this area.

It would therefore appear that the non-discriminatory components of acute pain are mainly processed in the region of the periaqueductal gray, thalamus and subsequently in structures which may be the principle subcortical and cortical projections structures related to the medial pain system, *i.e.* anterior insula cortex, lentiform nucleus, mid- and peri-genual cingulate cortex, inferior parietal cortex and prefrontal cortex (DLPF areas 9, 10 and 46). The anterior insula has rather sparse connections with the perigenual cingulate cortex and is thought to be associated with affective responses and learning, whereas the posterior insula is more concerned with integration of multisensory inputs. It is possible that the anterior insula is involved in a parallel distributed network that is involved in affective responses to pain.

The cingulate cortex is involved in a number of integrated tasks including cognition, affect and response selection [16]. It is likely that the mid- and peri-genual cingulate cortical areas are involved in the experience of pain. Although local anaesthetic injection into the cingulum bundle induces analgesia in animals [17], removal or deafferentation of anterior cingulate cortex in patients with severe intractable pain did not abolish the pain, but the patients reported that the pain was no longer bothersome [18]. This suggests that the cingulate cortex is not necessary for the registration of pain which may take place in the thalamus, but may be responsible for the attentional and affective responses to pain. In the conscious appreciation of any sensory experience, the brain has to prioritise the components of a stream of sensory information with subsequent selection of appropriateness and timing of response. This ability is generally called attention. Based on the study of patients with neglect syndromes, it has been proposed that there is a network of three main structures concerned with directing attention comprising a motivational map within the anterior cingulate which includes response/target selection, a schema for exploratory movements in the frontal cortex, which has also been implicated in the supervision of attention [19], a schema for exploratory movements in the frontal cortex and a sensory representation in the posterior parietal cortex [20]. In addition a subsystem responsible for alerting/vigilance is located in the right anterior hemisphere has been proposed by Posner et al. [21].

Cognitive tasks which make severe attentional demands such as the Stroop conflict task commonly activate the anterior cingulate cortex. The task consists of asking subjects to read the ink colour of colour words (such as "red", "green", "yellow", etc.) printed in ink colours which are either congruent or not with the reading of the word. PET studies suggest that attention to sensory stimuli is processed in the right parietal and right anterior cingulate cortex, regardless of side of stimulus [22]. However, the precise conditions of the attentional task are critical in determining which aspects of the "attention network" are activated [23].

To what extent the anterior cingulate responses to pain involve the "attentional network" is not established. A series of experiments to establish whether similar areas of cingulate cortex are activated by an attentionally demanding task (Stroop) and pain in the same individuals has been performed. This suggests that both activate structures within mid cingulate cortex but only pain activates the more anterior peri-genual cingulate cortex [24, 25]. Although a possibility, it is not feasible to establish whether the same networks within the mid cingulate are involved in both tasks. However, what is clear from this is that the anterior cingulate responses to pain are more than just attentional processing. There is some evidence that the peri-genual cingulate is involved in affective, vocalisation and autonomic responses to pain [26]. It is likely but so far difficult to prove that the anterior cingulate responses comprise a linked attentional and affective network concerned with response selection. It is also possible that the contralateral component of the mid cingulate response is more concerned with motor response selection than the passive attentional and affective components of the response. There are important connections between mid cingulate cortex and dorsolateral prefrontal cortex (DLPF) area 46. The latter region has been associated with the generation of willed actions but may also be concerned with response inhibition [27]. The inferior parietal cortical involvement in the pain response may be either concerned with the posterior attentional system which Posner has suggested is involved in directed spatial attention [28]. However, with its connections to the posterior cingulate cortex, where substantial reductions in flow in responses to pain have been recorded, it is possibly more likely that this is related to an inhibition of the nociceptive visual orientation response that has been demonstrated in inferior parietal cortex in animals [29], as the subjects were in a darkened room and were not specifically asked to look at the stimulus.

The reason for discussing the acute experimental pain results in some detail is that there is still some considerable support for the idea originally suggested by Albe-Fessard [30], that as pain becomes less acute it is processed by more medial structures in the brain. Our studies suggest that both acute phasic and tonic heat pain are processed by very similar structures and that neither result in increases in rCBF in SI, although tonic pain causes increases in SII. However, the size of the signal changes during tonic pain would appear to much less than for phasic pain. Increases in rCBF have been observed in very similar areas during acute phasic experimental and chronic neurogenic pain. Hsieh *et al.* [31] have demonstrated increases in rCBF in bilateral anterior insula, posterior parietal, lateral inferior prefrontal and unilateral right midcingulate cortex (BA 24) during ongoing neurogenic pain compared to after nerve block. The right cingulate response was irrespective of the side of the pain. There was no significant change in SI.

Interestingly there was a decrease in thalamic flow contralateral to the side of the pain. The absence of a response in SI has been interpreted by some to indicate that acute experimental and chronic clinical pain are processed by different brain regions [32]. We think this is highly unlikely for the reasons stated above. In addition in a series of single pain activation studies acquired in 3D mode, we found considerable variability of both extent and location of activation sites within the cingulate cortex and prefrontal cortex [11]. Variability of the size, precise location and extent of pain processing within the network of structures processing pain may be influenced by attentional, affective, motivational (response selection) states in addition to arousal during experiments. Anticipation has been shown to have a profound effect on the direction of rCBF changes in the frontal cortex in response to experimental pain. It also is difficult to imagine what advantages a structural division of acute and chronic pain processing might have in terms of economy and integration of signal processing. It seems much more likely that both acute and chronic pain are processed by a similar network of structures proposed above, and that these are subject to very different neuropharmacological modulation during different types of acute and chronic pain. Some evidence for this concept comes from the following experiments.

We have performed a series of experiments during which a group of patients with different types of acute and clinical pain were exposed to the same standardised experimental heat pain stimulus to the back of the right hand. A group of six patients were scanned 4-6 hours after routine molar extraction from the left jaw (opposite site of experimental pain). The same pain activation protocol as described previously was implemented. Significant contralateral activation of the thalamus and lentiform nucleus was observed in response to experimental pain but not in the prefrontal cortex or anterior cingulate. The latter was seen clearly activated when all conditions were compared between the two groups (*i.e.* the presence of dental pain being the main difference). This experiment suggests that the influences on cingulate responses to pain are not strictly contralateralised, otherwise pain on one side of the body would not influence responses to pain on the other. This is consistent with the finding of whole body nociceptive fields in the anterior cingulate. It also suggests that the pain registration may occur at least at the level of the thalamus and that if the anterior cingulate cortex is involved in the attentional and affective components of pain response then these may have been fully activated during the relatively intense dental pain.

By contrast when a group of patients with atypical facial pain were subjected to exactly the same protocol with poorly localised severe chronic pain on the same side of the face as the acute dental pain, very different results were obtained. These are female patients with underlying depression and chronic poorly defined unilateral facial pain. No nociceptive source for this type of pain has ever been identified and it is considered that the very persistent pain in this group is likely to be perseverated and reinforced by abnormal psychological mechanisms, the central basis for which has been unclear. The pattern of structures activated is similar qualitatively to those of the painfree controls. However, quantitatively the pattern is very different with substantially greater anterior cingulate response and reduced prefrontal responses [33]. The exaggerated anterior cingulate responses are thought to reflect abnormal attentional and affective responses to pain. It is suggested that such amplified responses and the failure to adequately supervise them, possibly by the prefrontal cortex, may be responsible for the perseveration of their ongoing clinical pain.

These latter responses are in sharp contrast to the responses seen during severe dental pain on the same side of the face and also to responses seen in patients suffering from inflammatory arthritic pain. A group of patients with active polyarthritic rheumatoid disease were studied using the same experimental pain protocol with the thermal probe being applied co-segmental but not overlying any inflamed joints. This group of patients demonstrated quite remarkable cortical and subcortical damping of their responses to experimental pain. Although the perceived intensity of the pain sensation was lower in the patient group, the difference was not significant, and the physical intensities of stimulation were similar in the patient and control group. This is the only patient group in whom we have seen this kind of generalised damping of cerebral responses to experimental pain. It is not possible to define the level at which pain responses are modified in this group, but it is clear that there are some important adaptive responses operating during inflammatory pain, the consequences of which are very different to those operating in acute dental and psychogenic facial pain. It is possible that the recruitment of coping strategies may alter at least some of these frontal responses. The effect of psychological state on frontal responses has already been discussed. However, further sequential studies are required to identify the main behavioural correlates of these altered responses. The neuropharmacological basis of such adaptive changes is not known but there is evidence from both human and animal studies that during established inflammatory arthritis there is an increased production of endogenous opioid peptides in the brain [34, 35]. Animal studies suggest that these may only occur during more established disease. The evidence in man comes from studies of patients during and subsequently out of inflammatory pain as a result of natural remission of their disease or injection of locally acting intra-articular steroids. Substantial increases in the volume of distribution of *in vivo* opioid receptor binding, using [^{11}C]diprenorphine and PET, were measured in response to relief of pain. In addition to the generalised changes there were region specific changes in the prefrontal, anterior cingulate and temporal cortices. It is interesting that the acute changes in rCBF in response to morphine induced analgesia in a patient with cancer pain were demonstrated mainly in the prefrontal, anterior cingulate and insula cortices without any effect on SI or SII. It is therefore possible that opiates may preferentially modify areas of the brain related to projections of the medial pain system.

On the basis of these studies we propose that there is a specific network of structures involved in the processing of non-discriminatory components of pain as described above and that the quantitative pattern of response of this network to experimental pain is critically dependent on the types of ongoing pain. Such modulation of cortical and subcortical responses may in part be opiate mediated, with early modulation of the cingulate and prefrontal responses. It is possible that opiates may act to reinforce such coping and other positive psychological strategies that may be implemented during inflammatory pain. However, the activation of opiates could also be a consequence of such coping strategies acting downline to modify affect. Subsequently more extensive modulation *via* descending opiate receptor bearing long efferents may operate. Such efferents exist from the deeper layers of the cingulate cortex to medial thalamus and brain stem structures. Structures such as periaqueductal gray might be expected to mediate more generalised changes in cortical and subcortical responses to pain. Careful sequential studies on cohorts of patients in different inflammatory pain states will be required to substantiate these hypotheses.

References

1. Jones AKP, Derbyshire SWG. Positron emission tomography (PET) as a tool for understanding the cerebral processing of pain. In : Boivie J, Hansen P, Lindblom U, eds. *Touch, temperature and pain in health and disease. Progress in pain research and management*, Vol 3. Seattle : IASP Press, 1994 : 491-520.
2. Jones AKP, Friston KJ, Brown D, Qi L, Frackowiak RSJ. Cortical and subcortical localisation of response to pain in man using positron emission tomography. *Proc Roy Soc B* 1991 ; 244 : 39-44.
3. Derbyshire SWG, Jones AKP, Brown WD, Devani P, Friston KJ, Qi LY, Pearce S, Frackowiak RSJ, Jones T. *Cortical and subcortical responses to pain in male and female volunteers*. IASP Publications, 7th World Congress on Pain 1993 : 500.
4. Derbyshire SWG, Jones AKP, Apkarian AV, Jones T. Cerebral responses to a continuous tonic pain stimulus measured by positron emission tomography. 1995 (submitted).
5. Casey KL, Monoshima S, Berger KL, Koeppe RA, Morrow TJ, Frey KA. Positron emission tomographic analysis of cerebral structures activated specifically by repetitive noxious heat stimuli. *J Neurophysiol* 1994 ; 2 : 802-7.
6. Talbot JD, Marrett S, Evans AC, Meyer E, Bushnell MC, Duncan GH. Multiple representations of pain in human cerebral cortex. *Science* 1991 ; 251 : 1355-8.

7. Hsieh JC, Stahle M, Hagermark O, Srone-Elander S, Rosenquist G, Ingvar M. Traumatic nociceptive pain activates the hypothalamus and the periaqueductal gray: a positron emission tomography study. *Pain* 1995 (in press).
8. Di Piero V, Ferracuti S, Sabatini, Pantano P, Crucci G, Lenzi GL. A cerebral blood flow study on tonic pain activation in man. *Pain* 1994 ; 56 : 167-73.
9. Casey KL, Monoshima S, Berger KL, Koeppe RA, Morrow TJ, Frey KA. Positron emission tomographic analysis of cerebral structures activated specifically by repetitive noxious heat stimuli. *J Neurophysiol* 1994 ; 2 : 802-7.
10. Hsieh JC, Stahle M, HagermarkO, Srone-Elander S, Rosenquist G, Ingvar M. Traumatic nociceptive pain activates the hypothalamus and the periaqueductal gray: a positron emission tomography study. *Pain* 1995 (in press).
11. Vogt BA, Derbyshire SWG, Jones AKP. Pain processing in four regions of the human cingulate cortex localised with coregistered PET and MR imaging. *Eur J Neurosci* 1995 (in press).
12. Hsieh JC, Belfrage M, Stone-Elander S, Hansson P, Ingvar M. Central representation of chronic ongoing neuropathic pain studied by positron emission tomography. *Pain* 1995 (in press).
13. Jones AP, Jones AKP, Hughes DG, Robinson L, Sykes JR, Derbyshire SWG, Chen ACN. Functional magnetic resonance imaging at 1 Tesla in the study of pain. Proceedings of SMR 3rd scientific meeting. Nice, SMR Berkeley. *Proc Soc Mag Res* 1995 : 149.
14. Apkarian VA, Stea RA, Manglos SH, Szevemyi NM, King RB, Thomas FD. Persistent pain inhibits contralateral somatosensory cortical activity in humans. *Neurosci Lett* 1992 ; 140 : 141-7.
15. Jones AKP, Derbyshire SWG, Apkarian AV, Jones T. Cerebral responses to a continuous tonic pain stimulus measured by positron emission tomography. *J Cereb Blood Flow Metabol* 1985 ; 15(S1) : S860.
16. Devinsky O, Morrell MJ, Vogt BA. Contributions of anterior cingulate cortex to behaviour. *Brain* 1995 ; 118 : 279-306.
17. Vaccarino AL, Melzack R. Analgesia produced by injection of lidocaine into the anterior cingulum bundle of the rat. *Pain* 1989 ; 39 : 213-9.
18. Foltz EL, White LEJ. Pain relief by frontal cingulotomy. *Neurosurg* 1962 ; 19 : 89-100.
19. Shallice T. The allocation of processing resources. In : *From neuropsychology to mental structure*. Cambridge : Cambridge University Press, 1988.
20. Mesulam MM. A cortical network for directed attention and unilateral neglect. *Ann Neurol* 1981 ; 10 : 309-25.
21. Posner MI, Petersen SE. The attention system of the human brain. *Ann Rev Neurosci* 1990 ; 13 : 25-42.
22. Pardo JV, Fox PT, Raichle ME. Localisation of a human system for sustained attention by positron emission tomography. *Nature* 1991 ; 349 : 61-4.
23. Bench CJ, Frith CD, Grasby PM, Friston KJ, Paulescu E, Frackowiak RSJ, Dolan RJ. Investigations of the functional anatomy of attention using the stroop test. *Neuropsychol* 1993 ; 9 : 907-22.
24. Derbyshire SWG, Jones AKP, Vogt BA, Frackowiak RSJ. An investigation of central processing with stroop task and pain using positron emission tomography. A within subject design. *J Cereb Blood Flow Metabol* 1985 ; 15(S1) : S45.
25. Vogt BA, Derbyshire S, Jones AKP. Pain processing in four regions of the human cingulate cortex localised with coregistered PET and MR imaging. *Eur J Neurosci* 1995 (in press).
26. Vogt BA, Sikes RW, Vogt LJ. Anterior cingulate cortex and the medial pain system. In : Vogt BA, Birkhauser GM, eds. *Neurobiology of cingulate cortex and limbic thalamus*. Boston, Basel, Berlin 1993 : 313-44.

27. Goldman-Rakic PS. Circuitry of the prefrontal cortex and the regulation of behaviour by representational memory. In : *Handbook of physiology* : 373-417.
28. Posner MI, Petersen SE. The attentional system of the human brain. *Ann Rev Neurosci* 1990 ; 13 : 25-42.
29. Dong WK, Chudler EH, Sugiyama K, Roberts VJ, Hayashi T. Somatosensory, multisensory and task-related neurons in cortical area 7b (PF) of unanaesthetised monkeys. *J Neurophysiol* ; 72 : 542-64
30. Albe-Fessard D, Berkely KJ, Kruger L, Ralston HJ, Willis WD. Diencephalic mechanisms of pain sensation. *Brain Res Rev* 1985 ; 9 : 217-96.
31. Hsieh J-C, Belfrage MO, Stone-Elander S, Hansson P, Ingvar M. Central representation of chronic ongoing neuropathic pain studied by positron emission tomography. *Pain* 1995 (in press).
32. Apkarian VA. Functional imaging of pain: new insights regarding the role of the cerebral cortex in human pain perception. *Neuroscience* 1995 ; 7 : 279-93.
33. Derbyshire SWG, Jones AKP, Devani, P, Friston KJ, Feinman C, Harris M, Pearce S, Watson JDG, Frackowiack RSJ. Cerebral responses to pain in patients with atypical facial pain measured by positron emission tomography. *J Neurol Neurosurg Psychiatry* 1994 ; 57 : 1166-72.
34. Jones AKP, Cunningham VJ, Ha-Kawa S, FujiwaraT, Luthra SK, Jones T. Changes in central opioid receptor binding in relation to inflammation and pain in patients with rheumatoid arthritis. *Br J Rheumatol* 1994 ; 33 : 909-16.
35. Panerai AE, Sacerdote P, Bianchi M, Brini A, Mantergazza P. Brain and spinal cord neuropeptides in adjuvant induced arthritis in rats. *Life Sci* 1987 ; 41 : 1297-303.

17

Central pain syndromes

J. BOIVIE [1], A. ÖSTERBERG [1,2]

1. Department of Neurology, University Hospital, Linköping Sweden.
2. Department of Geriatrics and Rehabilitation, Motala Hospital, Motala, Sweden.

The early history of central pain syndromes (CPS) is heavily linked to French neurology around 1900-1910. Dejerine and Roussy´s original description from 1906 of the thalamic syndrome with thalamic pain is one of the best known scientific articles in the history of pain research [1]. Their description is still extensively used in the teaching and writing about central pain.

Later milestones in the French literature on central pain are the works by Ajuraguerra [2], Garcin [3], and Mauguière and Desmeth [4].

Considering the impact on the opinions about CPS that Dejerine and Roussy's description of central pain has had, and still has, it is of interest to examine their thesis in the light of later research. They described six categories of symptoms and signs:
    1. Intractable pain. Central pain is truly intractable pain in almost all patients, and it is possible that thalamic lesions have a tendency to cause particularly severe pain [5].
    2. Light hemiparesis. Some patients do have light paresis, but about half of the patients with pain due to lesions that affect the thalamus have no paresis [5]. The paresis is explained by the fact that most cerebrovascular lesions (CVLs) that affect the thalamus extend laterally to include part of the posterior limb of the internal capsule. CVLs restricted to the thalamus do not result in paresis. In the three patients (out of the six described) in which Dejerine and Roussy did postmortem microscopy the lesions did extend laterally to the internal capsule.
    3. Hemihypesthesia including decreased deep sensibility. This is partly correct, partly incorrect, because all patients with central post-stroke pain caused by lesions in and around the thalamus have hemihypesthesia, with very few exceptions. However, it often

does not include deep sensibility loss, unless the ventroposterior thalamic region is involved.

4. Astereognosis. This does not appear to be a common finding in post-stroke central pain. It is probably dependent on a severe loss of tactile and proprioceptive sensibility.

5. Hemiataxia. Many patients do not have ataxia. In a mixed material with supratentorial lesions, ataxia was found in about 60% of the patients [5].

6. Choreoatetotic movements. In more recent materials this has rarely been observed, although it does occur in some patients.

It can be concluded that all symptoms and signs described by Dejerine and Roussy may be present in patients with true thalamic pain or, more generally, with central post-stroke pain, but all except the pain and the hypesthesia may be absent. Considering the lack of knowledge in the field at the time when they did their research, it is evident that Dejerine and Roussy´s description was a pioneering achievement. However, their description cannot be used today as criteria for the diagnosis of thalamic pain. Such criteria based on current knowledge have recently been worked out by the Special Interest Group on Central Pain of the IASP and published by Boivie [6].

Salient features of central pain

Dejerine and Roussy described patients with thalamic syndromes, including thalamic pain. The term thalamic pain was, up to recently, extensively used as a name for central pain in general. Current knowledge shows that this use of the term is incorrect, because it is now absolutely clear that most patients with central pain have lesions that do not involve the thalamus. Instead, it is recommended that the general term central pain is used. It has been defined by the International Assocation for the Study of Pain (IASP) as pain caused by a primary lesion or dysfunction in the central nervous system [7]. Thus, peripherally induced pain with central mechanisms is not central pain, even if the central mechanisms are prominent.

In the clinical research on central pain, six aspects are of particular interest: etiology, onset, spectrum of qualities, severity of the pain, coupling to sensory abnormalities and treatments.

The etiologies of CP are listed in Table I. The largest patient groups are those with CP caused by cerebrovascular lesions (central post-stroke pain = CPSP), multiple sclerosis (MS) and spinal cord injuries (SCI). The Table shows that many different kinds of lesions and disease processes can cause CP. It has been shown that CP can be caused by lesions at any level along the neuraxis, *i.e.* in the spinal dorsal horn, in the ascending sensory pathways, in the brainstem, in the thalamus, in the subcortical regions and in the cerebral cortex [6]. The disease processes that produce CP pain are both rapidly developing ones such as hemorrhages and cerebral infarcts, and slowly developing ones such as syringomyelia. It appears that the crucial feature of the lesions that cause CP is their location with regard to the sensory pathways and the projection zones of these (*see* below).

In recent years, it has become evident that many patients with Parkinson's disease experience pain and sensory symptoms [6]. Prevalence figures of around 45% have been given. The question has been raised if this is entirely secondary to the motor symptoms or if the pain to some extent might be a kind of central pain, *i.e.* pain directly caused by the neurodegenerative processes in the brain. If this would turn out to be the case, then this would represent entirely different mechanisms than those of the diseases listed in Table I. The major neurodegeneration in Parkinsons disease occurs in the basal ganglia, and it is known, from physiological experiments in the 1960-ies, that some of the somatosensory projection nuclei in the thalamus interact with the caudate nucleus. Hypothetically it is therefore possible that a dysfunction in the basal ganglia might result in somatosensory symptoms such as pain or paresthesia.

Table I. Major causes of central pain

Vascular lesions in the brain and spinal cord
infarcts, hemorrhages, vascular malformations
Multiple sclerosis
Traumatic spinal cord injury
Syringomyelia and syringobulbia
Tumours

From central post-stroke pain and CP after spinal cord injuries, it is known that the onset of CP is often delayed. The delay may be from weeks up to several years, but in many patients the pain starts almost immediately [6]. The explanation for this is unknown.

Central pain may appear in many guises. There is a wide spectrum of pain qualities among patients with CP, even among patients with the same kind of lesion [6, 8]. There is thus no pathognomonic character of any CP, but some pain qualities are more frequent than others. Most patients with CP experience more than one pain quality, for instance burning, aching and pressing pain, in the same or different body regions. The most common qualities are burning, aching, pricking, pressing, lacerating and lancinating.

Central pain is in almost all cases severe pain. The pain intensity as evaluated for instance with a visual analogue scale (VAS) will, in some patients, show relatively moderate or low values, but it is clear from talking to these patients that they suffer greatly from the pain. This may be explained by the fact that CP is mostly constant and has very irritating qualities.

Central pain is a symptom caused by dysfunctions in the CNS. It is therefore natural to ask if CP occurs together with some other neurological symptoms and signs. This is important in the search for mechanisms and for criteria for the diagnosis of central pain syndromes. In the two major groups of CP patients in which this has been systematically studied, namely in post-stroke CP and in MS, it is clear that the only symptoms and signs that regularly accompany CP are sensory abnormalities [5, 9, 10; this chapter]. No more than about half, or less than half of the patients with CP have or have had paresis, 40-60% have ataxia. Other neurological symptoms are rare.

In both CPSP and CP in MS, the sensory abnormalities are dominated by abnormal sensibility to temperature and pain, which is an indication of abnormal function in the spino-thalamic pathways, including their cortical projection zones [10, 17]. This conclusion has formed the basis for the hypothesis that only patients with lesions affecting the spinothalamic pathways may develop CP ([6]; *see* below).

Central pain is among the most difficult pain conditions to treat. Almost all patients have made the experience that analgesics do not relieve CP. This has been confirmed in opioid test in which the patients have been given high doses of strong opioids intraveneously. Only a small proportion of patients have responded with pain reductions in such test, and at very high doses (*see* below). A few patients with preserved dorsal column function may benefit from transcutaneous electrical nerve stimulation [11].

Tricyclic antidepressant drugs are the most effective drugs. About 50-70% of patients with CPSP find that tricyclics give relief, which in some cases is complete, in others more moderate [12]. In this chapter we report results from MS that indicate an effect on CP by amitriptyline also in MS. A few patients get relief from carbamazepine.

Apart from many basic questions about the mechanims underlying CP, there are still many unanswered questions regarding the clinical features of central pain syndromes. These questions can only be answered by systematic clinical research on well-defined groups of patients with CP. We have done such a study on MS-patients with CP and will report some of the results here (A Österberg, J Boivie, I Johansson, S Kalman, J Sörensen, K-Å Thuomas, in preparation).

Central pain in patients with multiple sclerosis

Patients and methods

All 429 patients with a diagnosis of definite multiple sclerosis (MS) in the patient register at the department of neurology were sent a questionnaire asking if they had experienced pain or sensory symptoms currently or previously during the course of the disease. The patients were asked to indicate the location on a pain diagram and to describe the quality of the pain. All patients admitting of pain were interviewed by telephone or at the outpatient clinic, where all patients suspected of having neurogenic pain were examined.

The diagnosis of MS was done according to the internationally accepted criteria, and was based on history, neurological examination, assays of the cerebrospinal fluid and magnetic resonance imaging (MRI).

After reminders, responses were recieved from 371 patients, *i.e.* a yield of 86%, which is a high figure for this kind of studies.

The examination of the MS patients suspected of having neurogenic pain included the following:
- A detailed history and a thorough neurological examination with particular emphasis on the features of the pain and sensory disturbances. The clinical sensory examination included test of touch by strokes of cotton wool, cold by applying the round surface of a tuning fork at room temperature (area 3.9 cm^2), and pinprick using a pin.
- Quantitative sensory testing (QST). In the QST, the sensibility to vibration, touch, warmth, cold, cold pain, and heat pain were analyzed. Thresholds to vibration were measured with a Vibrameter® (Somedic AB, Sweden) [13]. The threshold amplitude in μm was measured, with a constant probe pressure at a vibration frequency of 100 Hz. The means of three consecutive readings on each side of the body were recorded as the thresholds.
- The thresholds to touch were measured by applying graded punctate stimuli to the skin using a set of nylon filaments of varying bending pressures (von Frey hairs). The series of filaments represented stimuli from 10 mg to 300 g. The weakest stimulus that the patient identified more than 50% of the time was recorded as the perception threshold.
- A Thermotest® apparatus was used to quantitatively assess sensibility for non-noxious and noxious (cold pain, heat pain) temperatures. With this technique, the stimuli are given *via* a 25 x 50-mm plate that is placed on the skin. The plate consists of 36 peltier elements that can be heated or cooled in a controlled manner. The difference limen was used as the threshold for innoxious temperature [14]. The sensory testing was done on the feet, hands and cheeks.

The diagnosis of central pain was based partly on exclusion, partly on specific criteria. The most important determinants of this diagnosis were the following:
a) Pain with a regional distribution compatible with a CNS lesion. Trigeminal neuralgia (TN) is believed to be caused by a demyelinating lesion along the course of the nerve fibers in their passage to the trigemnial nuclei inside the brainstem. It is therefore considered as central pain, but results considering TN will be given separately, unless stated otherwise.
Pain arising from muscle spasms or other forms of spasticity were included in central pain.
b) Negative outcome of a thorough examination of the painful regions to find signs of nociceptive pain. Normal blood and other laboratory tests to exclude general non-neurologicalal disease. Pure back pain was not considered to be central pain, even if the examination failed to demonstrate a cause in musculoskeletal structures.

c) Negative outcome of a thorough neurological examination to find possible signs of peripheral neuropathy or rhizopathy, indicating the possibility of peripheral neurogenic pain.

d) Normal neurography, or abnormal results from neurography, but the pain did not conform with known forms of peripheral neurogenic pain.

e) No signs of psychiatric disease.

f) Vascular and tension headaches were not included in central pain.

Results

Table II shows the results from the survey of pain in 371 patients with MS. A majority of the patients reported pain of some kind (58%), including headache.

Table II. Prevalences of pain in 371 patients with MS. CP = central pain. TN = trigeminal neuralgia. The figure for CP does not include patients with only CP (*see* text).

No pain	42%
All pain	58%
Nociceptive pain	21%
Neurogenic pain not CP	2%
Uncertain pain type	3%
Central pain	24%
Trigeminal neuralgia	5%
All central pain	27%

Central pain has been divided into trigeminal neuralgia (TN) and more traditional central pain. In the following the term central pain refers to the latter unless otherwise stated. Altogether 100 MS patients had central pain, trigeminal neuralgia included, *i.e.* 27%. Eighteen of these patients had trigeminal neuralgia (including four patients in the major group), *i.e.* 5% of the whole population.

We have arrived at these figures after a critical review of the features of the pain in each patient. The figures are probably somewhat conservative. In addition to the 101 patients whose pain has been classified as central pain, another 16 patients (= 4.% of the study population) had pain that possibly or probably, but not certainly, was central pain. They have therefore not been included in the figures for central pain in Table II. If they are included, the figure for central pain in MS increases to 31%.

Women dominated among the central pain patients (70%; Table III), as they do among MS patients in general. It is not clear if women with MS have a relatively higher risk of developing central pain than men.

CENTRAL PAIN SYNDROMES

Table III. MS-patients with definite central pain. Four of the patients with trigeminal neuralgia also had common CP. Pts = patients. Ages, and disease and pain durations in years.

All CP, TN incl	100 pts
All trigeminal neuralgia	18 pts
Women	72%
Men	28%
Age - mean (range)	54 (28-79)
Disease duration - mean (range)	30 (7-54)
Pain duration - mean (range)	9 (1-34)
CP excl TN	86 pts
Women	70%
Men	30%
Age - mean (range)	52 (25-79)
Disease duration - mean (range)	19 (2-43)
Pain duration - mean (range)	12 (1/2-40)
CP sole first symptom	2 pts
CP first symptom together with others	7 pts

At the time of the investigation, the CP patients had a mean age of 52 years and a mean disease duration of 19 years. Two percent of the patients had CP as the sole first symptom of their disease, and in another seven percent, CP was part of a complex of symptoms at the onset of the disease. Thus, nine percent had pain as an initial symptom.

Except for the trigeminal neuralgia, almost all CP was constant. About one third of the patients reported that physical activities increase the pain, but otherwise the pain was not much affected by physical or emotional stimuli.

About half of the patients experienced the pain as both superficial and deep and about one fourth as deep pain (Table IV). In a large majority of the patients pain was experienced in the lower extremities (90%). Many of these also had pain in the upper part of the body, where central pain in general was less frequent.

Table IV. Percentages of pain qualities in 86 MS-patients with central pain.

1 pain quality	17
2 pain qualities	44
3 pain qualities	22
> 3 pain qualities	17
Burning	40
Aching	38
Pricking	24
Cutting	15

The trigeminal neuralgia had a rather uniform character, that did not appear to differ from what one finds in "idiopathic" TN. In this respect, the TN was different from CP in general, because 83% of these patients experienced more than one pain quality. The most common pain qualities are listed in Table V. In patients with pain in more than one body region the qualities could differ between the regions.

Table V. Location of CP in 86 MS-patients.

Superficial	10%
Deep	28%
Deep and superf.	52%
Could not tell	10%
Lower extremities	90%
Trunk	22%
Upper extremities	36%

From a clinical point of view, and also concerning mechanisms, it is of interest to find out if there is any connection between CP and other neurological symptoms and signs. With regard to CP in MS, three kinds of symptoms are of particular interest, namely paresis, ataxia and sensory disturbances. Table VI lists the prevalences of these symptoms and signs. Slightly less than half of the patients did not have paresis. About one fourth had moderate to severe paresis with a few being totally paraplegic. Less than one third had ataxia.

Table VI. Neurological symptoms and signs in 86 MS-patients with central pain at the time of the examination. Percentages.

Paresis - none	45
Paresis - light	32
Paresis - moderate to severe	25
Ataxia	29
Sensory abnormalities	96

As in other groups of CP patients, almost all MS-patients had sensory disturbances (96%). The results from the clinical and quantitative sensory testing are shown in Table VII. From the QST, it is evident that the sensibility to vibration, temperatures and pain (noxious temperatures) were severly affected with 61% showing total or severe loss of sensibility, whereas tactile sensibility was least affected with only 20% total or severe loss. The clinical examination of the sensibility is a much cruder and less sensitive technique than the QST. Thus it was not surprising to find that the results of these methods showed a lesser degree of sensory loss, than the QST.

CENTRAL PAIN SYNDROMES

Table VII Results of clinical and quantiative sensory testing in 52 MS-patients with non-paroxysmal central pain. Percentages of patients with decreased sensibility.

	Clinical testing			
	Normal	Mild-mod	Total loss	Hyperesthesia
Touch	30	43	13	14
Cold	28	29	20	23
Pinprick	34	34	9	19
	Quantitative sensory testing (QST)			
	Normal	Mild-mod	Severe	Total loss
Vibration	18	21	33	28
Touch	28	52	15	5
Innoxious temp.	10	29	27	34
Noxious temp.	20	56	34	

Response of CP in MS to morphine

There is still much debate about whether neurogenic pains respond to analgesics. The response to morphine i.v. has been tested in 13 of the MS patients with central pain.

Results of thirteen opioid naive patients can be reported here. Their mean age was 52 years and the duration of their pain averaged 11 years. The study was done single blind at the postoperative ward. The i.v. infusions started with two saline infusions, followed by morphine which was infused at a rate of 1 mg/kg/min. The morphine infusions started 30 minutes after the start of the saline infusions. The morphine infusions were stopped if a pain reduction of at least 50% was obtained, or if the patients became heavily sedated, had severe nausea or significant reduction of the breath frequency. Thirty minutes after the end of the morphine infusion, naloxone 0.4 mg was injected i.v. twice. The pain intensity was assessed by VAS ratings every 10 minutes.

Five patients responded with at least 50% pain intensity reductions after a mean of 43 mg morphine. The other eigth patients did not respond in this way, although they received 40 - 50 mg morphine. Two of the patients reporting > 50% pain reduction cannot be considered to be responders, because one of them was a placebo responder and the other was heavily sedated and could not be reliably evaluated. The remaining three appeared to be true responders, because they experienced a clear pain increase after the naloxone injections. However, it should be noted that these responses were obtained in opioid naive patients after infusions of extremely high doses of morphine over a short time.

Statistical analyses have been done of the plasma concentrations of morphine, and of the morphine metabolites M-3-G and M-6-G. No differences were found between the responders and non-responders with regard to these values.

Amitriptyline and carbamazepine in the treatment of CP in MS-patients

Some preliminary data can be reported from a study of the effect of amitriptyline and carbamazepine in the treatment of CP in MS-patients. The study was done double blind, cross-over as a three-phase study with placebo given as control treatment during the third phase. A one week interval between the treatment phases served as a wash-out period. The order of treatments was randomized. Tablets were given daily for four weeks at 8 AM and 8 PM using a double dummy procedure. The final daily dose of amitriptyline was 50 - 75 mg, and of carbamazepine 600 - 800 mg. When necessary, dose reductions were done by two independent neurologists, who were otherwise not involved in the study. Blood samples were taken after 2 and 4 weeks treatment.

The treatment effects were evaluated through daily ratings of pain intensity in the mornings and evenings using a 10 step categorical verbal scale, and through global ratings of the effects after each treatment period. Before and after each treatment, the patients were also assessed with the Comprehensive Psychopathological Rating Scale (CPRS) to find out if the patients were depressed and if reduced depression could be a possible explanation if the results would show reduced pain during the treatment.

Twenty-one patients with steady, constant pain and with a mean age of 55 years completed the controlled study. They had a mean pain duration of 13 years.

Table VIII shows preliminary results from the global ratings of the treament effects for each of the three treatments. Neither the statistical analyses nor the results of the daily pain intensity ratings or the plasma concentration assays have been completed and can therefore not be reported here.

Table VIII. Results of the global ratings of the effects of 4 weeks treatment with amitriptyline, carbamazepine and placebo in 21 MS-patients with non-paroxysmal CP.

	Amitript	Carbam	Placebo
Worse	2	8	2
Unchanged	8	11	18
Better	7	2	1
Much better	3	0	0
Pain free	1	0	0

On the basis of the data from the global ratings, one is inclined to conclude that amitriptyline was superior to carbamazepine and placebo, whereas carbamazepine did not appear to be beneficial to the patients. Thus 11 of 21 patients reported less pain during the amitriptyline treatment, compared to two and one patient, respectively, during the treatments with carbamazepine and placebo. It was also clear from the recordings of the side effects that carbamazepine gave more adverse effects than amitriptyline.

CENTRAL PAIN SYNDROMES

Conclusions about central pain in MS

From the present results, some conclusions can be made regarding central pain in patients with multiple sclerosis.
1. Pain is a major problem for patients with MS.
2. Around 27% of all MS-patients have central pain, including 5% with trigeminal neuralgia.
3. The CP dominates in the lower extremities. This might indicate that the pain is mainly caused by lesions in the spinal cord. It is well known that myelopathy is common in MS, but it has not, so far, been possible to show which lesions cause the central pain.
4. Apart from the trigeminal neuralgia, most of the CP is constant, steady pain.
5. The pain has many different qualities, the most common being burning, aching and pricking.
6. Almost all patients have severe abnormalities in temperature and pain sensibility, indicating that the spinothalamic pathways are affected in these patients. Many patients also have reduced vibration sensibility, whereas few have severely affected tactile thresholds. The majority of MS-patients with central pain have no paresis or ataxia.
7. Morphine only rarely relieves CP in MS, and only at extremely high doses.
8. Amitriptyline appears to have a relieving effect in some patients, whereas carbamazepine is not effective in the treatment of steady CP in MS.

Clinical perspectives on the mechanisms of central pain

In the clinical studies of CP, the questions with regard to the mechanisms have focused on the location of the lesions and their relationships to the somatosensory pathways. In the search for the answers to these questions, namely radiological imaging techniques, psychophysical methods to analyze the sensory abnormalities, and evoked potential techniques, whereas almost no postmortem studies have been done.

The examinations with magnetic resonance imaging (MRI) and computarized tomography (CT) have demonstrated lesions causing CP at all levels of the brain including various levels of the brainstem, the thalamus, the subcortical regions around the internal capsule, and in the primary and secondary somatosensory cortical regions [6]. With these techniques it has not yet been possible to show details about the exact location and extent of the lesions in the spinal cord that cause CP.

Throughout the years after Dejerine and Roussy's description of the thalamic syndrome much interest has focused around the question about thalamic involvements by the lesions that cause CP, mainly regarding CP after cerebrovascular lesions. One complicating factor in these discussions is the fact that many of the lesions that involve the thalamus extend laterally to include also the posterior limb of the internal capsule in which the thalamocortical projections pass. That makes it difficult to know if the pain is caused by the thalamic portion of the lesion.

There is evidence showing that no more than at the most 50% of all patients with central post-stroke pain have thalamic involvement by the lesions, but only a small proportion of these lesions are restricted to the thalamus [5, 15]. The results of two studies indicate that, in the thalamus, it is the ventroposterior nuclear region that is crucial for the development of CP [5, 16]. In a material of 40 patients with infarcts restricted to the thalamus, all three who developed CP had infarcts in this region (of 18 patients), whereas none of the 22 patients with infarcts in other parts of the thalamus developed CP [16].

From a functional point of view two major hypotheses regarding the mechanisms of CP have been discussed in the clinical litterature. One states that the crucial lesion is one that affects the dorsal column-medial lemniscal pathways. This hypothesis was favoured for many years. It implies that CP occurs because a lesion removes an inhibitory input to the spinothalamic projection zones from the dosal column pathway, thereby releasing abnormal nerve cell activity in the brain that leads to the experience of pain. This mechanism would thus be one of disinhibition.

If this hypothesis were correct one should be able to show a decrease in proprioception, and touch and vibration sensibility. However, the results of studies done with quantitative psychophysical methods in recent years have shown that this is not the case ([9, 10, 17] and present results from MS-patients). Many patients with CP have normal thresholds for these three modalities. Instead, they have turned out to have severe abnormalities in the sensibility to temperature and pain. These results, supported by clinical observations, have led to a dominance for the second hypothesis in the recent literature [6, 8, 18, 19]. This hypothesis states that only patients who have lesions that affect the spinothalamic pathways (indicated by abnormal sensibility to temperature and pain), including their thalamocortical projections, run the risk of developing CP. Results from evoked potential examinations in patients with central post-stroke pain support the hypothesis [20]. Fortunately only some patients with such lesions develop CP. The explanation to this is unknown.

Acknowledgements

The studies from which unpublished results are presented have been supported by grants from the Swedish Medical Research Council (grant nr 9058), the Bank of Sweden Tercentenary Foundation, the Swedish Association of the Neurologicalally Disabled, and the County Council of Östergötland. The authors wish to express their thanks to Mrs Gunnel Rosen and Mrs Gunn Johansson for excellent assistance.

References

1. Dejerine J, Roussy G. Le syndrome thalamique. *Rev Neurol (Paris)* 1906 ; 14 : 521-32.
2. Ajuraguerra DJ. *La douleur dans les affections du système nerveux central.* Paris : Doin, 1937.
3. Garcin R. Thalamic syndrome and pain central origin. In : Soulairac A, Cahn J, Charpentier J, eds. *Pain.* London : Academic Press, 1968 : 521-41.
4. Mauguiere F, Desmedt JE. Thalamic pain syndrome of Dejerine-Roussy. Differentation of four subtypes assisted by somatosensory evoked potentials data. *Arch Neurol* 1988 ; 45 : 1312-20.
5. Leijon G, Boivie J, Johansson I. Central post-stroke pain. Neurological symptoms and pain characteristics. *Pain* 1989 ; 36 : 13-25.
6. Boivie J. Central pain. In : Wall PD, Melzack R, eds. *Textbook of pain.* New York : Churchill Livingstone, 1994 : 871-902.
7. Mersky H, Bogduk N. *Classification of chronic pain.* Second edition. Seattle : IASP press, 1994.
8. Tasker R. Pain resulting from central nervous system pathology (central pain). In : Bonica JJ, ed. *The management of pain.* Philadelphia : Lea and Febiger, 1990 : 264-80.
9. Österberg A, Boivie J, Holmgren H, Thuomas K-Å, Johansson I. The clinical characteristics and sensory abnormalities of patients with central pain caused by multiple sclerosis. In : Gebhart GF, Hammond DL, Jensen TS, eds. *Progress in pain research and management.* Seattle : IASP Press, 1994 : 789-96.
10. Vestergaard K, Nielsen J, Andersen G, Ingeman-Nielsen M, Arendt-Nielsen L, Jensen TS. Sensory abnormalities in consecutive, unselected patients with central post-stroke pain. *Pain* 1995 ; 61 : 177-86.
11. Leijon G, Boivie J. Central post-stroke pain. The effect of high and low frequency TENS. *Pain* 1989 ; 38 : 187-91.
12. Leijon G, Boivie J. Central post-stroke pain; a controlled trial of amitriptyline and carbamazepine. *Pain* 1989 ; 36 : 27-36.
13. Goldberg JM, Lindblom U. Standardized method of determining vibratory perception thresholds for diagnosis and screening in neurological investigation. *J Neurol Neurosurg Psychiatry* 1979 ; 42 : 793-803.
14. Fruhstorfer H, Lindblom U, Schmidt WG. Method for quantitative estimation of thermal thresholds in patients. *J Neurol Neurosurg Psychiatry* 1976 ; 39 : 1071-5.
15. Lewis-Jones H, Smith T, Bowsher D, Leijon G. Magnetic resonance imaging in 36 cases of central post-stroke pain (CPSP). *Pain* 1990 ; suppl 5 : 278.
16. Bogousslavsky J, Regli F, Uske A. Thalamic infarcts: clinical syndromes, ethiology, and prognosis. *Neurology* 1988 ; 38 : 837-48.
17. Boivie J, Leijon G, Johansson I. Central post-stroke pain; a study of the mechanisms trough analyses of the sensory abnormalities. *Pain* 1989 ; 37 : 173-85.
18. Bowsher D, Lahuerta J. Central pain in 22 patients: clinical features, somatosensory changes and CT scan findings. *J. Neurol* 1985 ; : 232-97.
19. Pagni CA. Central pain due to spinal cord and brainstem damage. In : Wall PD, Malzack R, eds. *Textbook of pain.* Edinburg : Churchill Livingstone, 1989 : 634-55.
20. Casey KL, Boivie J, Holmgren H, Leijon G, Morrow TJ, Sjölund B, Rosen I. Laser-evoked cerebral potentials and sensory function in patients with central pain. *Pain* 1995 (in press).

18

Are there still indications for destructive neurosurgery at supra-spinal levels for the relief of painful syndromes ?

J. GYBELS [1], B. NUTTIN [2]

1. *Laboratory of Experimental Neurosurgery and Neuroanatomy,*
2. *Department of Neurosurgery,*
K.U.L. University of Leuven, Leuven, Belgium.

The question whether there are still indications for destructive neurosurgery at supraspinal levels for the relief of pain is a pertinent and timely one, but to answer it is difficult. We will first examine the data which were available up till 1989. At that time an exhaustive study of this problem was made [1]. We will then look at the answers to a questionnaire which was sent to all members of the European Society for Stereotactic and Functional Neurosurgery in 1994. The questionnaire was designed to find out what the actual neurosurgical practice was in the treatment of pain in malignancy and in the treatment of neuropathic pain. More particularly, the last item of this questionnaire was formulated as follows: "Do you think there are still indications for destructive neurosurgery at supra-spinal levels for the relief of painful syndromes? If yes, for which painful syndromes?" In a third section, we will comment a case history which will be published in "Controversies in Neurosurgery" and which underlines that an answer to the above-formulated question has to be approached with subtlety. Finally, we will have a new look to some old destructive interventions in the thalamus for neurogenic pain.

Clinical data up till 1989

A major difficulty arises when reporting results of interventions, although in recent years a trend can be observed where results are reported making use of multiple outcome measures and disinterested third party assessment. We [1] reported the results of the world literature guided by the degree of critical assessment of the original authors, the number of their cases, the availability of thoughtful reviews, the reputation of the authors and our own experience. Because of space limitation we have to summarize these results and we will do this by quoting the conclusions we reached for each intervention. This of course has a subjective character but is the best we can do. For rationale and results of the different supra-spinal lesion procedures we refer to [1].

Lesions in the brain stem

Bulbar trigeminal tractotomy and nucleotomy

This intervention is based on the anatomy of the nociceptive system in the trigeminal nerve. Several modalities of the procedure have been proposed with the level of incision as major proper characteristic: tractotomy according to Sjoqvist [2], bulbar trigeminal nucleotomy [3] and multiple lesions of the descending cephalic pain tract and nucleus caudalis "DREZ" lesions [4]. Our conclusion was: *"Trigeminal nucleotomy either at one or many levels needs further critical evaluation before its place can be decided. Intractable facial post-herpetic neuralgia is one of the most promising disorders to explore."*

Bulbar and pontine spinothalamic tractotomy

In this intervention, the spinothalamic tract is sectioned in the medulla oblongata [5] or in the pons [6] for intractable pain so high in the shoulder and neck that it cannot be alleviated by spinal anterolateral cordotomy. Our conclusion was: *"Published experience with this procedure is limited, but it may offer deep sustained high-level analgesia at a lesser risk than many other procedures."*

Stereotactic mesencephalotomy

Most neurosurgeons performing stereotactic mesencephalotomy aim at either the spinothalamic and quintothalamic pathways or the spinoreticular pathways, or both, and try to avoid the medial lemniscus. Our conclusions were: *"Two recent long-term follow-ups from Tokyo and Duke University describe satisfactory relief of central neurogenic pain by mesencephalotomies in about two thirds of 55 patients. The most widespread use of the procedure is pain of malignancies involving the head and neck. It competes with brain stimulation and intraventricular morphine."*

Thalamotomy

Since the first stereotactic thalamotomy in 1947, a number of targets have been selected such as the ventrocaudal nuclei (VPL-VPM), the intralaminar nuclei, the pulvinar, the dorsomedian nucleus and nuclei of the anterior group. Our conclusion was: *"Tasker's [7] conclusion, reasonable in our view, was that the risks of failure and complications are significantly greater for these procedures than for more peripheral operations so that these should usually be reserved for patients with cancer in the head and neck and certain other selected cases."*

Hypothalamotomy

On the assumption that ascending pain pathways reach the thalamic intralaminar nuclei by way of the hypothalamus, Fairman [8] proposed hypothalamotomy. Our conclusion was: *"Such important functions are concentrated in the hypothalamus that this has little appeal to most neurosurgeons as a stereotactic target, despite the low complication rate described today."*

Frontal lobe lesions

Interventions in the frontal lobe for persistent pain have been cingulotomy, inferior fronto-medial leukotomy and subcaudate tractotomy and they have demonstrated that some cerebral component of the limbic system is an appropriate target for this problem. Our conclusions were: *"Earlier conclusions were that the patients leukotomized for pain seem to suffer much more deficit than those leukotomized for psychosis [9]. This turns out to be wrong for appropriately placed and circumscribed lesions, which may be gratifyingly beneficial."*

Pre- and postcentral gyrectomy

Conclusions here were: *"Three cases of pre-and postcentral gyrectomy for pain relief are encouraging but too few on which to base a recommendation, especially when the successful surgeons have themselves described no more."*

Data from a 1994 poll

Two hundred fifteen questionnaires were sent to the members of the European Society of Stereotactic and Functional Neurosurgery in 1994. The number of completed questionnaires was 56. Five returned to sender without reaching the addressee and 5 members replied that interventions for pain were not performed in their unit. In the questionnaire it was asked whether a certain operation for pain in a given neurosurgical department was occasionally or often performed, and what the actual numbers were in 1993.

Table I gives the data for persistent pain in cancer, Table II for persistent neuropathic pain. In the third column there are indicated the total number of interventions performed in the 56 departments from which this information was obtained. This poll further revealed that for the 56 responders to the questionnaire the number of anterolateral cordotomies for cancer pain in 1993 was 86, for neuropathic pain 6, dorsal column stimulation for cancer pain 44 and for neuropathic pain 529, and intrathecal morphine administration in cancer pain 102, in neuropathic pain 69. It is probably fair to state that supraspinal destructive procedures for relief of painful syndromes are rarely performed.

When the question was asked: "Do you think that there are still indications for destructive neurosurgery at supra-spinal levels for the relief of painful syndromes?" 26 saw no indications for destructive neurosurgery at supra-spinal levels while 25 did. Of these 25, four indicated cranial nerve surgery in the posterior fossa which is not really the question we sought to answer. Therefore, the negative answers were the majority (26 no, 21 yes). The majority of the indications were pain in the face in cancer, rare indications were phantom pain, brachial plexus avulsion, and other "deafferentation" pains.

Table I. Results of a 1994 poll on the frequency of destructive neurosurgery at supra-spinal levels for relief of cancer pain.

Cancer pain	occasionally	often	number in 1993
Telencephalic operations			
Cingulotomy	5		
Others	1		
Hypothalamotomy	1		5
Thalamotomy			
Ventrocaudal thalamotomy (VPL-VPM)	3	1	15
Medial thalamotomy	3	2	10
Pulvinarotomy	3	1	8
Dorsomedian nucleus		1	8
Anterior thalamic nuclei		1	4
Operations in the brainstem			
Stereotactic bulb artrigeminal tractotomy and nucleotomy	2	1	3
Stereotactic bulbar and pontine spinothalamic tractotomy	4		2
Stereotactic mesencephalic tractotomy	8		7
Others			
Bulbar trigeminal tractotomy	1		
Not specified	1		1

Table II. Results of a 1994 poll on the frequency of destructive neurosurgery at supra-spinal levels for relief of neuropathic pain.

Neuropathic pain	occasionally	often	number in 1993
Telencephalic operations			
Cingulotomy	3		5
Postcentral gyrectomy			
Hypothalamotomy	1		4
Thalamotomy			
Ventrocaudal thalamotomy(VPL-VPM)	6	1	11
Medial thalamotomy	3	2	11
Pulvinarotomy	3		5
Dorsomedian nucleus	2		3
Anterior thalamic nuclei	2		3
Operations in the brainstem			
Stereotactic bulbar trigeminal tractotomy and nucleotomy	3		
Stereotactic bulbar and pontine spinothalamic tractotomy	2		
Stereotactic mesencephalic tractotomy	4	1	6
Open trigeminal tractotomy	1		3

A case history and two different views

The case: a 50 years old man underwent resection of a petroclival meningeoma. Three months after surgery, he began to have facial pain, which was persistent and increasing, associated with dysesthesia, and intractable to all forms of medical treatment. This pain deeply affected his life and performance.

Surgeon A: What should not be done in this case? No further peripheral denervation. My first choice of neurosurgical treatment would be radiofrequency lesions stereotactically placed in the nucleus caudalis of the Trigeminal system. I have performed over 200 nucleotomies. In a consecutive series of 141 patients with deafferentation pain, with follow-up from 1 to 16 years, abolition of the allodynia and a significant reduction, or less frequently, a complete abolition of the deep background pain was obtained in 72,6% of the cases without lasting side effects.

Surgeon B: It is very unlikely that this pain will respond to further peripheral denervation. Overall, the chance of a tractotomy or caudalis nucleotomy producing satisfactory relief is about 75%. Almost 100% of the patients will experience an undesired deficit of some sort, with debilitating limb ataxia in 10% and disabling contralateral limb sensory loss in 15% of the patients. One of the guiding principles for the management of difficult pain problems has to do with the Hippocratic oath "Primum non nocere". For all these reasons, this man should have a trial of Deep Brain Stimulation, prior to consideration of an ablative operation. The probability that Deep Brain Stimulation will help his pain is 50% and the risk to him is about 15%.

A new look at an old destructive supra-spinal procedure for the relief of persistent pain

As early as 1949 Hécaen et al. [10] suggested for the treatment of pain a lesion which interrupts, in addition to the ventrobasal complex, part of the diffuse thalamic projection system. Medial thalamotomy (essentially a lesion in the intralaminar nuclei) can bring pain relief without provoking a sensory deficit. The absence of severe complications made laminotomy at one time a popular intervention, but due to all too frequent recurrences of the original pain and the appearance of other treatment modalities such as neurostimulation and the intrathecal administration of drugs, the procedure was abandoned. The procedure has been taken up again by Jeanmonod and his colleagues [11]. These authors placed a lesion in the n. centralis lateralis (CL) in 45 patients with neurogenic pain. They report that, after a medial thalamotomy, 67% of the patients reached a 50% to 100% pain relief, without somatosensory deficits. Follow-up was short, ranging from 2 weeks to 38 months with a mean of 14 months. Pain was assessed pre-and postoperatively using:
 - 3 to 7 visual analogue determinations of pain intensity,
 - the patient's estimation in percent of the global postoperative improvement,
 - activities of daily living,
 - pain drug intake.

However, the data given in the publications of these authors do not allow the reader to assess for himself the amount of pain relief. Interestingly, microelectrode recordings of a total of 318 units in CL showed that half of the units exhibited lowthreshold calcium spike bursts. From their results, the authors propose a theory which states that neurogenic pain is due to an imbalance between central and ventroposterior nuclei, resulting in an overinhibition of both these nuclei by the thalamic reticular nucleus.

A cautious answer to a provocative question

With the data at our disposal — and needless to sa, these data are far from allowing to make a scientifically founded statement — we are of the opinion that for the time being, there are only very few indications for destructive neurosurgery at supra-spinal levels for the relief of pain. However, in neurological disease, nature demonstrates that long-standing "thalamic pain" caused by a stroke can subsequently and permanently be abolished by a new stroke (for description of a well documented case, see [12]). We agree therefore, for instance, with a respondent to the above-mentioned questionnaire when he replied to the question whether there were still indications for destructive supraspinal procedures: "Yes, median thalamotomy, if the work by Jeanmonod and colleagues in Zurich is confirmed".

Acknowledgements

The authors thank Dr Ron Kupers for valuable suggestions on the manuscript.

References

1. Gybels J, Sweet W. *Neurosurgical treatment of persistent pain*. Basel : Karger, 1989.
2. Sjoqvist O. Studies on pain conduction in the trigeminal nerve. *Acta Psychiat Neurol* 1938 ; 17 : 1-139.
3. Hitchcock E, Schvarcz J. Stereotaxic trigeminal tractotomy for post-herpetic facial pain. *J Neurosurg* 1972 ; 37 : 320-9.
4. Bernard E, Nashold B, Caputi F, Moossy J. Nucleus caudalis DREZ lesions for facial pain. *Br J Neurosurg* 1987 ; 1 : 81-92.
5. Schwartz H, O'Leary J. Section of the spinothalamic tract in the medulla with observations on the pathway for pain. *Surgery* 1941 ; 9 : 183- 93.
6. Hitchcock E. Stereotaxic pontine spinothalamic tractotomy. *J Neurosurg* 1973 ; 39 : 746-52.
7. Tasker R. Thalamic stereotaxic procedures. In : Schaltenbrand G, Walker A, eds. *Stereotaxy of the human brain*. Stuttgart : Thieme-Straton, 1982 : 484-97.
8. Fairman D. Neurophysiological basis for the hypothalamic lesion and stimulation by chronic implanted electrodes for the relief of intractable pain in cancer. *Adv Pain Res Ther* 1976 ; 1 : 843-7.
9. White J, Sweet W. *Pain and the neurosurgeon. A forty-year experience*. Springfield : Thomas, 1969.
10. Hécaen H, Talairach T, David M, Dell M. Mémoires originaux. Coagulations limitées du thalamus dans les algies du syndrome thalamique. *Rev Neurol* 1949 ; 81 : 917-31.
11. Jeanmonod D, Magnin M, Morel A. Thalamus and neurogenic pain: physiological, anatomical and clinical data. *Neuro Report* 1993 ; 4 : 475-8.
12. Soria E, Fine E. Disappearance of thalamic pain after parietal subcortical stroke. *Pain* 1991 ; 44 : 285-8.

19

Motor cortex stimulation for deafferentation pain relief in various clinical syndromes and its possible mechanism

T. TSUBOKAWA

University Research Center, Department of Neurological Surgery, Nihon University School of Medicine, Tokyo, Japan.

The term "deafferentation pain" has been used to refer to pain in which the flow of afferent nervous impulses has been partially or completely interrupted [1]. As such a definition implies, patients with deafferentation pain usually display sensory loss at the painful area. The symptom common to all patients is disturbance of the temperature and pain sensibilities, whereas the vibration and touch sensibilities are not always disturbed. It has been suggested that the causative neuronal damage in the patients is located in the neo-spinothalamic tract or the thalamocortical pathways [2-4], and that no lesion in the dorsal column medial lemniscal system is necessary for the manifestation of deafferentation pain, except deafferentation pain like a stump pain or phantom pain which can be classified as peripheral deafferentation pain [5].

Clinical observations of deafferentation pain have indicated that:
- deafferentation pain only occurs in 10-75% of cases who have interruption at the pain afferent pathways displaying the same magnitude and the same pathological findings [1],
- deafferentation pain occurs at several months after the onset of causative lesions at the pain afferent pathways [5, 6],
- deafferentation pain is located at the area of disturbance of pain sensation [1, 5, 6],

- deafferentation pain cannot be suppressed by the administration of morphine, but is inhibited by administration of barbiturate, ketamine or anticonvulsant [7],
- deafferentation pain can be temporarily alleviated by surgical thalamotomy [8] or ablation of the sensory cortex [9],
- any form of therapy including chronic thalamic stimulation, provides satisfactory pain control only in some limited cases [10],
- the pain-inducing mechanism of deafferentation is still incompletely understood [1, 5].

Recently, hyperactivity of neurons in the pain afferent pathways above the level of the interruptive lesions has been consistently observed in deafferented animals and patients suffering from deafferentation pain [11-14]. It is believed that such hyperactivities recorded at the sensory cortex and sensory thalamic nucleus could be one of the main factors leading to deafferentation pain, since destructive surgery of the area displaying remarkable hyperactivities is able to provide temporary relief of deafferentation pain [8, 9]. Further, it is possible for such hyperactivities at the sensory cortex and thalamus to be inhibited by motor cortex stimulation, in effective cases stopping deafferentation pain [15, 16].

Chronic motor cortex stimulation to relieve deafferentation pain in various clinical syndromes has been applied since 1989, based on the finding that hyperactivities at the sensory thalamus and sensory cortex after deafferentation could be inhibited by motor cortex stimulation in animal experiments [16, 17]. In this paper, the clinical effect of chronic motor cortex stimulation on deafferentation pain, and its possible underlying mechanism, will be discussed.

Experimental studies

Methods

Cats and rats were anaesthetized with metofane (rats) or ketamine (cats) and underwent right-side anterolateral spinal cord tractotomy (STT-tractotomy (cats)) or induction of a lesion at the right-side posterior ventrobasal thalamus (VB-lesion (rats)). At one to ten weeks after lesioning, the animals were anaesthetized with 1% halothane in a 67% N_2O - 33% O_2 gas mixture to carry out tracheotomy, arterial and venous cannulation and a small craniectomy. Following preparation for microrecording, artificial respiration without anaesthetic gas was instituted. As stimulating electrodes, a silver ball bipolar electrode was placed at the pre-central gyrus, and a silver wire electrode was applied to the left-side tibial nerve.

For the recording of single unit firing from the sensory cortex and thalamus, a glass micropipette filled with 3 M sodium chloride and pontamine sky blue was inserted into the target area through the small craniectomized hole. When single neuron activity was encountered, the receptive field was determined by application of non-noxious or noxious stimuli. The evoked firing and spontaneous firing rates were evaluated from the spike density curve and interspike interval histograms. In this experiment, the neurons were analyzed only when responding to left hind paw stimulation. Pre-central gyrus stimulation was applied to check on the changes in spontaneous and evoked firing patterns.

When a typical hyperactive neuron was recorded, the effect of administration of MK801, an N-methyl-D-aspartate (NMDA) receptor-coupled channel antagonist (0.5 - 1.0 mg/iv in rats, 4 - 16 mg/iv in cats), was observed.

After each experiment, both the recording site for single neuron activity and degenerative changes including the initial lesion were verified by histological methods.

Results

Hyperactive thalamic neurons following STT transection

In the posterior ventrobasal thalamic nucleus (VB) of 25 adult cats, 64 neurons responding to innocuous stimuli at the contralateral hind paw were recorded at 4-10 weeks after STT transection. Among them, 41 units were located within the core of the nucleus an 23 units were located at the shell area arbitrarily defined as the zone less than 500 mm distant from the margin of the nucleus (Figure 1). Only 5 of the 23 units recorded at the shell area still responded to peripheral noxious stimuli, even after STT transection. No such neuron was observed among the core-area neurons. The responses to noxious stimuli after STT transection may be mediated by a pathway other than these to the STT, since degeneration of the STT was confirmed.

All recorded neurons exhibited significant hyperactivity of both spontaneous firing rate and evoked firing at 3-4 weeks after STT transection (Figure 2). Significant increases in spontaneous firing rate and magnitude of the evoked firing were thus observed in both core and shell area neurons of the VB, respectively.

Motor cortex stimulation (10-100 Hz train stimulation) inhibited both spontaneous and evoked firings in all recorded hyperactive neurons during stimulation with a long-period (10 - 60 sec) after effect. However, there was no such inhibitory effect following post-central gyrus stimulation.

The effect of MK-801 on the hyperactive neurons after STT transection was examined in 5 neurons recorded in the shell area and 5 neurons recorded in the core area. MK801 significantly attenuated the spontaneous as well as evoked hyperactivity. A dose-dependent inhibition of the percent firing as compared to that before administration was observed (Figure 3). In contrast, no significant effects of MK-801 (8 mg/kg) were demonstrated on either the spontaneous or evoked firing recorded in sham-operated animals. Consistent with earlier studies [17], the present data indicated

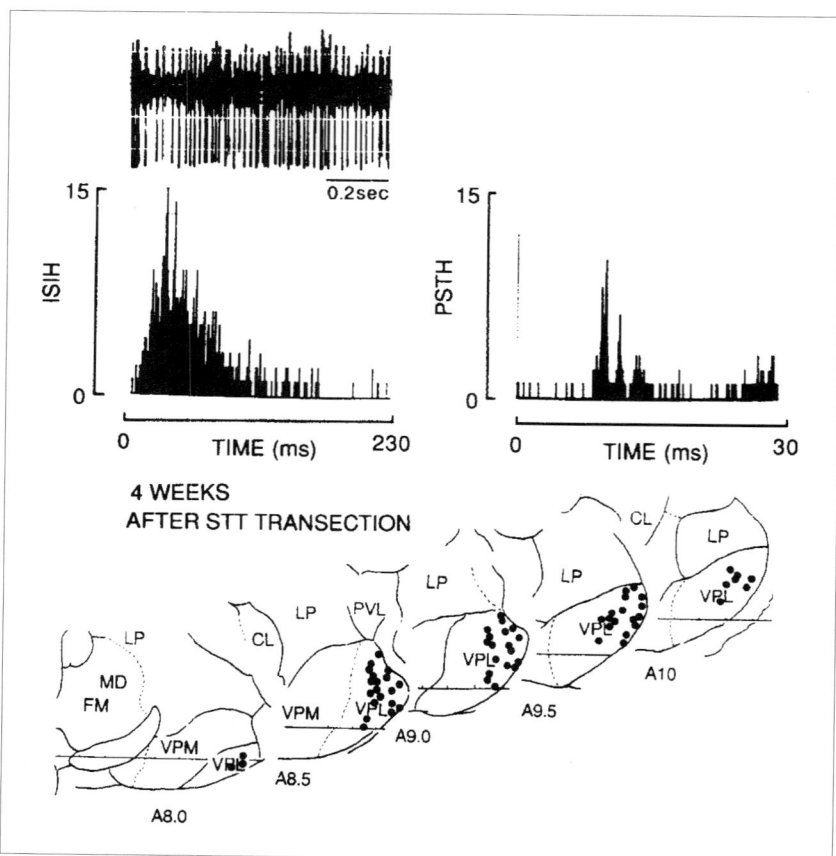

Figure 1. Example of a unit recorded 4 weeks after STT transection. Spontaneous firings show hyperactivity (upper) and both spontaneous firing rate and magnitude of the evoked firing are increased (middle). Location of recording site of 64 units are shown (lower).

that NMDA receptors are normally not responsible for either spontaneous or evoked firing of neurons within the somatosensory pathways in response to innocuous stimuli. It is possible that there was a group of neurons which had originally been silent and was activated at several weeks after deafferentation, or increased NMDA receptor, at regenerative neurons following lesion induction at the pain afferent pathway.

At the time of the regeneration period of deafferented neurons, activation of NMDA receptor at the regeneration site could be a critical component of the reorganized neural circuits responsible for the hyperactivities.

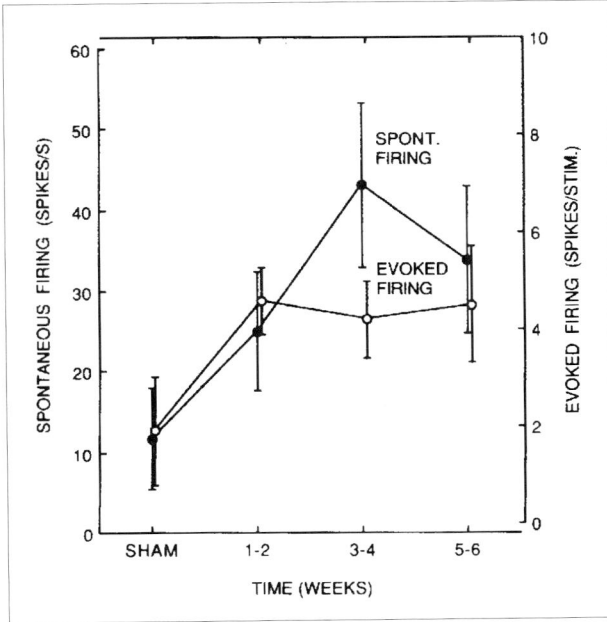

Figure 2. Time curse of neuronal activity after STT transection. Spontaneous and evoked firing show hyperactivity at 1-2 weeks after STT transection. The spontaneous firings progressively become maximum hyperactive 3-4 weeks.

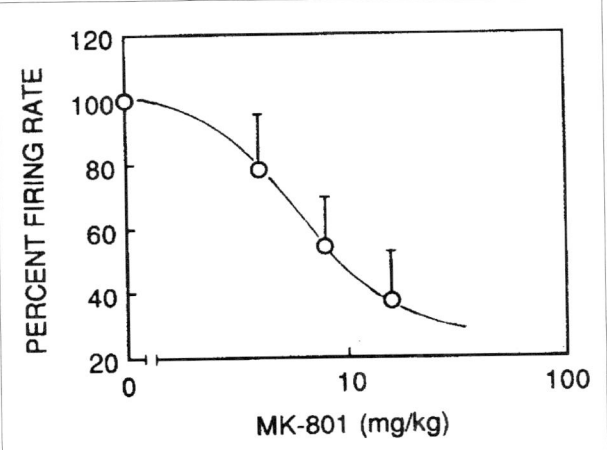

Figure 3. The spontaneous firings after STT transection are significantly attenuated by intravenous administration of MK-801.

Hyperactive neurons in the sensory cortex following lesioning at the thalamic posterior ventrobasal complex (VB)

At various periods ranging from one to 10 weeks after the induction of VB lesions, 72 neurons were recorded from the ipsilateral somatosensory cortex. Naturally, none of them responded to peripheral cutaneous stimuli, while 32 (44%) demonstrated non-bursting activity and 40 (56%) demonstrated bursting activity. In both groups of VB lesioned animals and sham control animals, neurons exhibiting spontaneous firing were encountered in layers II through VI (Figure 4).

The spontaneous firing rate of these neurons did, however, display a progressive increase as time elapsed following VB lesioning. As compared to the spontaneous firing rate of neurons in the sham-operated animals, the spontaneous spike density at 10 weeks after induction of the VB lesion reached a level which was significantly higher, and this tendency was widely evident among both bursting and non-bursting neurons in layers II through VI (Figure 4). Thus, neurons of the somatosensory cortex appeared to become hyperactive following thalamocortical deafferentation regardless of their gross spontaneous firing pattern and localization. In contrast to sham-operated animals, a significant decrease in spontaneous firing rate was noted following administration of MK801 in a dose-dependent manner at 4-10 weeks after VB lesioning. Train pulse stimulation at the pre-central gyrus could also inhibit the firing rate of these hyperactive neurons recorded at the post-central gyrus with a long poststimulation after-effect.

Clinical application of motor cortex stimulation and its outcome

Patient population

Thirty-eight patients with deafferentation pain evoked by various causative lesions have been selected as candidates for treatment by chronic motor cortex stimulation since 1989. Among the 38 patients, 32 had a causative lesion in the central nervous system and could be classified as central deafferentation pain: 14 patients had a thalamic lesion, 7 had a putaminal-internal capsule lesion, 6 had a brainstem lesion, caused by stroke, 3 had post-spinal cord injury, and 2 had postsurgical pain following medullary junction tumor. The other 6 cases suffered from peripheral deafferentation pain after amputation of the arm or leg or herpetic pain (Table I).

The interval between the onset of the original disease and the occurrence of pain ranged from 6 months to 1 year. The patients were treated by the administration of various kinds of medications, thalamotomy or spinal cord dorsal column stimulation. However, they continued to complain of severe spontaneous burning, tearing or deep boring pain at the area displaying hyposensibility by the pinprick test, and they maintained the painful area quiet and covered by using socks, gloves or a towel.

Their deafferentation pain did not respond to the morphine test but did effectively respond to the barbiturate or ketamine test [7].

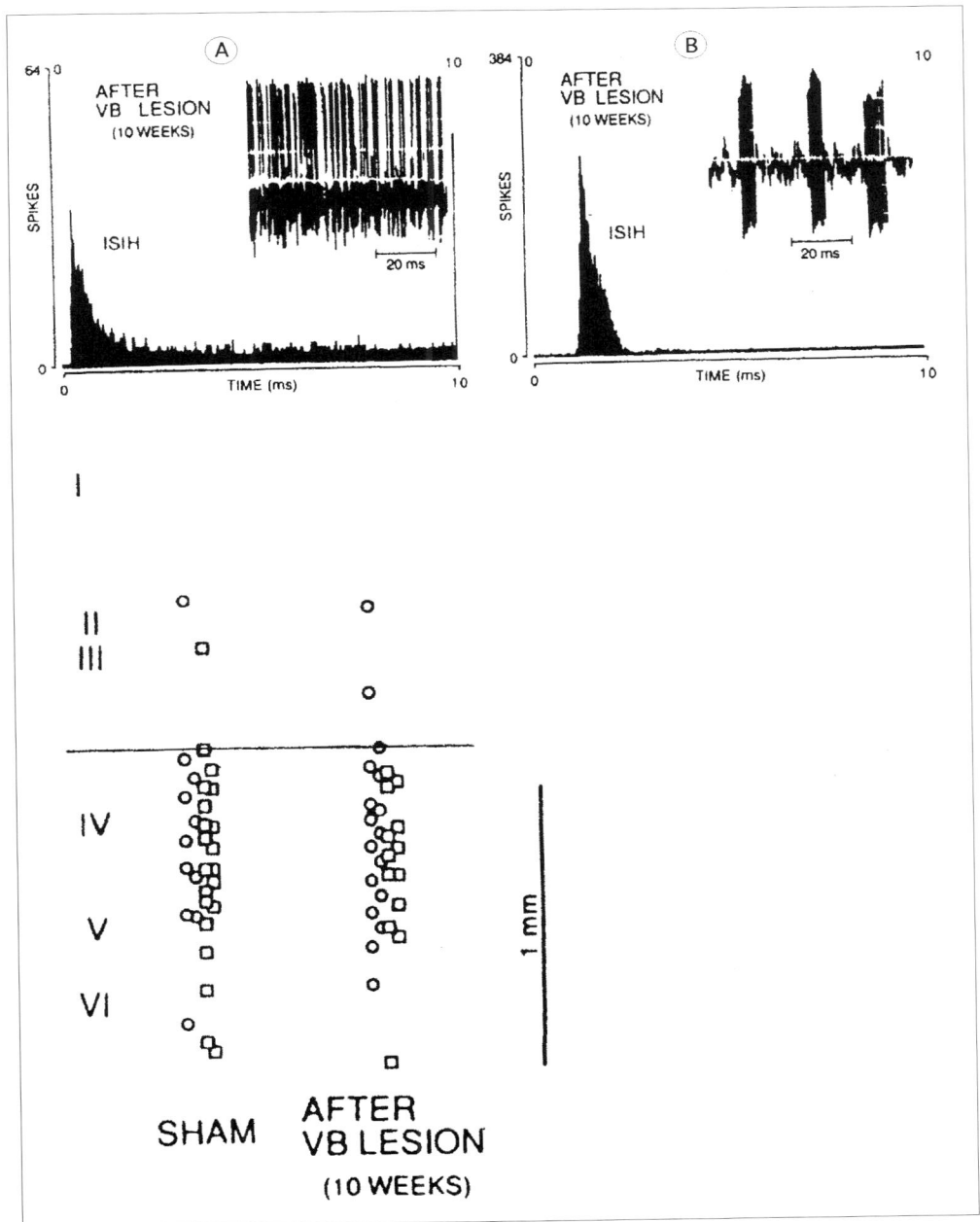

Figure 4. Example of interspike interval histogram obtained from non-bursting units (A) and bursting unit (B) recorded from cortex 10 weeks after BV lesion. C stocks laminar distribution of recording site (▫: Non bursting neuron, O: Bursting neuron)

Table I. Two years follow up results of motor cortex stimulation.

Pain	Causative lesion site	Number of treated cases	Effective cases (excellent-good)	Chronic implantation
Central deafferentation pain	putamen	7	5 (71%)	6 (1 fair)
	thalamus	14	10 (71%)	11 (1 fair)
	brainstem	6	5 (83%)	5
	medullo-spinal junction	2	2 (100%)	2
	spinal cord	3	1 (33%)	22 / 29 (76%) 1
Total		32 (2 → spinal stim.)	23 (72%)	25 (78%)
Peripheral deafferentation pain	stump pain	3	1 (33%)	1
	herpetic pain	2	1 (50%)	1
	peripheral nerve injury	1	0 (0%)	0
Total		6 (4 → thalamic stim.)	2 (33%)	2 (33%)

Surgical procedures

The location of the pre-central gyrus was estimated from bony landmarks employing the conventional method. Under local anaesthesia, a skin incision was made over the central sulcus and 1 to 4 cm lateral to the midline, depending on the location of the painful area. A small craniotomy, 3 to 4 cm in diameter, was carried out at the estimated area of the motor cortex. An electrode array (Model 3587, Medtronic Co.) with 4 plate electrodes of 0.5 cm in diameter, each separated by 10 mm, was inserted into the epidural space (Figure 5), usually placing the electrode array parallel to the mediolateral orientation of the pre-central gyrus. If the patients complaints involved both lower and upper extremities, two electrode arrays were used (Figure 6).

The location of the motor cortex was confirmed from phase reversal of the N20 wave of the somatosensory evoked potential recorded from the electrode, whenever the inserted electrode was moved from the post-central to pre-central gyrus. Various changes in N20 were observed in the present series of patients. The location of the motor cortex was also confirmed from muscle contraction in response to stimulation with the electrode, or the pyramidal evoked potential must be recorded [18].

Bipolar stimulation employing two appropriate electrodes was performed. It is most important to determine the best electrode-position based on motor responses at the painful area by using a stronger stimulation.

The electrode array was tightly sutured on the surface of the dura and this surface was carefully coagulated so as to prevent any clot formation and future growth of connective tissue. The stimulation system was internalized after a period of several days

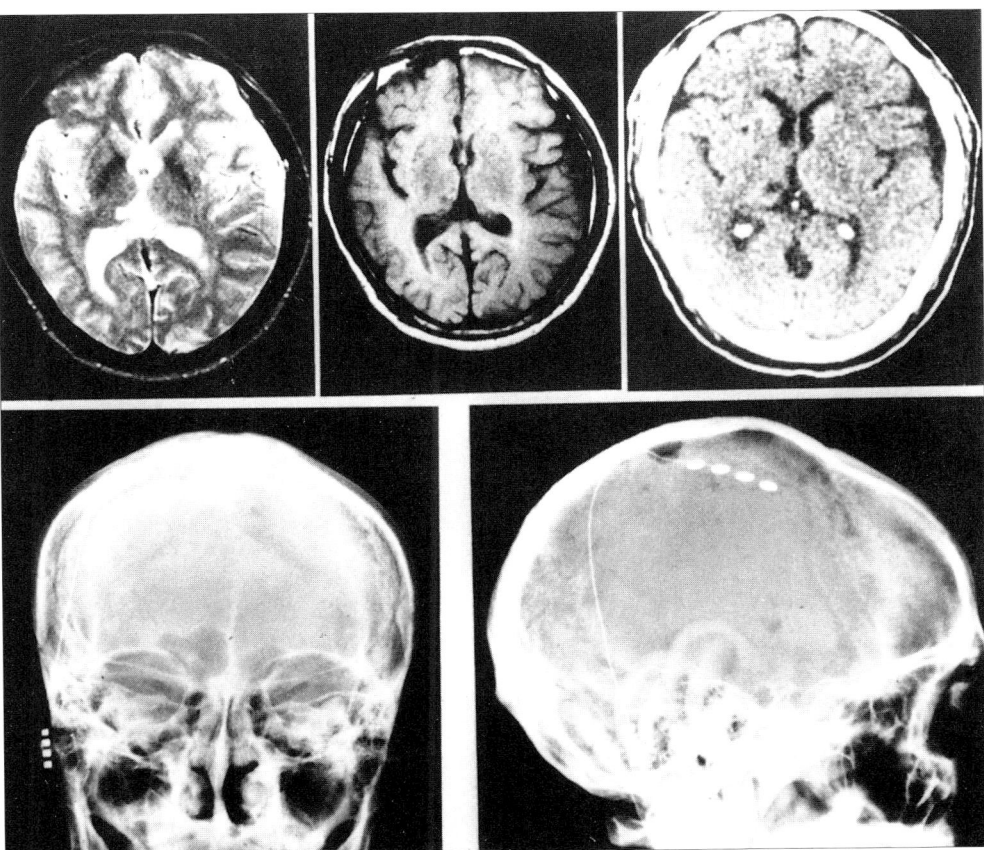

Figure 5. The patient with thalamic pain (as indicated by the causative lesion on CT and MRI) treated by motor cortex stimulation.

for test stimulation. During the period of test stimulation, a pair of electrodes providing the best pain inhibition is selected, and the effects of stimulation with various parameters and polarities are examined. Most of the patients usually select stimulation with an interpolar distance of 30 mm in order to cover a relatively broad motor area and 0.2 msec duration square pulse with a frequency of 25-50 Hz, and the stimulation strength is almost at the threshold to induce some sensation at the painful area.

Electroencephalographic recordings were repeatedly made, and diphenyl-hydantoin administrations were carried out in all treated cases.

Chronic stimulation procedure

Chronic stimulation was performed after internalization of the electrode using a wireless stimulation system (Model 3425, Medtronic Co.). Stimuli were delivered as

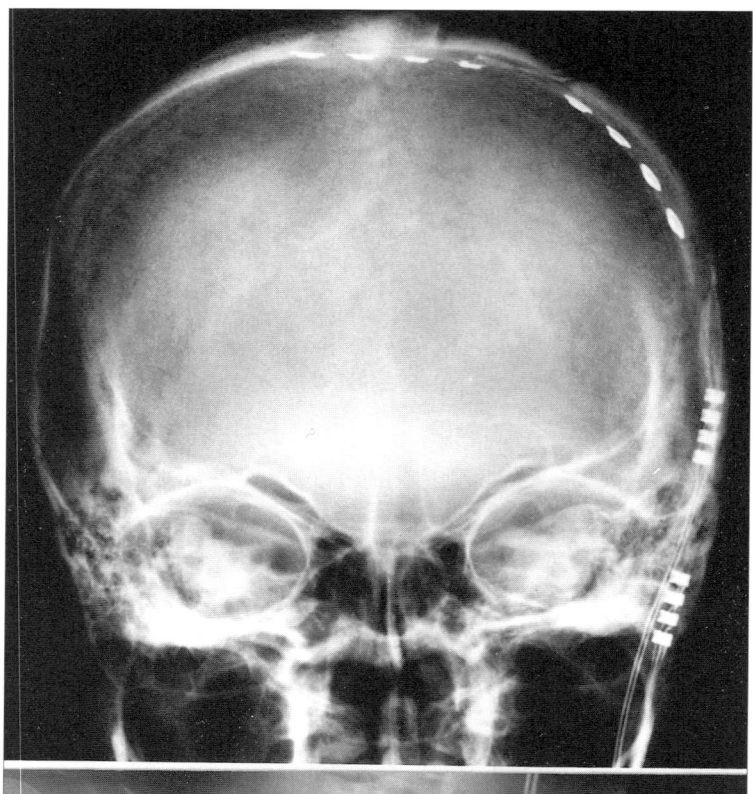
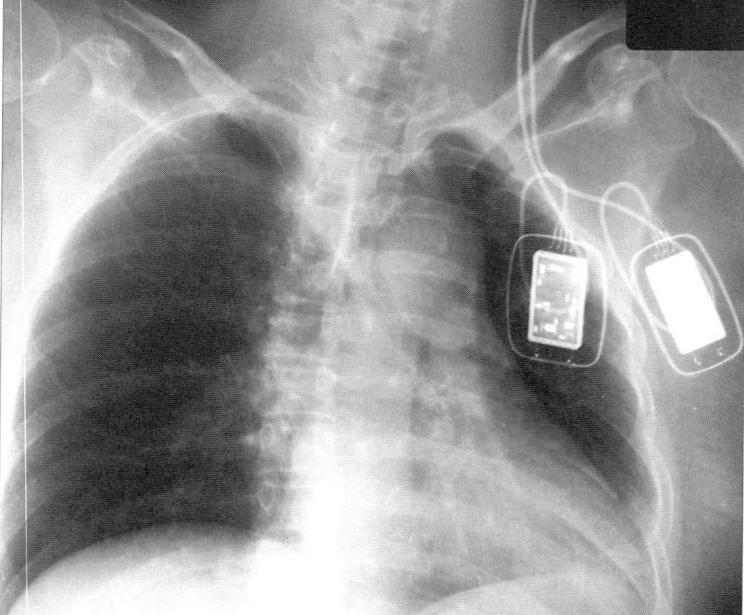

Figure 6. The patient with right side of the body deafferentation pain caused by thalamic bleeding treated by 2 sets of electrode which covered the leg, arm and face.

monophasic square pulses (duration, 0.1-0.5 msec). Stimulation was usually applied continuously for 5 to 10 minutes on each occasion, and no stimulation was given at night. The parameters for chronic stimulation were chosen so that the best pain relief was achieved, as estimated during the test stimulation. However, the frequency and intensity were restricted to a level slightly lower than the threshold for muscle contraction.

Results

The changes in pain severity of each patient were evaluated by a physician at a pain clinic independent of the neurosurgical service. Each patient was asked to describe the pain levels according to a visual analog scale. The effects of stimulation were classified into four categories: excellent (pain reduction by 80-100%), good (pain reduction by 60-79%), fair (pain reduction by 40-59%) and poor (pain reduction by less than 40%). In the patients evaluated as excellent or good, no use was made of any other supportive treatments.

In central deafferentation pain, 23 (72%) of the 32 cases were able to obtain satisfactory pain relief (excellent or good) following chronic motor cortex stimulation. The remaining 9 cases reported no effect or a less than 40% reduction in their pain (Table I).

The patients with causative lesions at the suprathalamic level to the brainstem with stroke, injury or post-surgical pain demonstrated remarkable improvement: 22 of the 29 patients (76%) were able to achieve satisfactory pain relief. However, among the patients with severe pain caused by spinal cord injury, only 33% (one of 3) showed satisfactory pain relief: in 2 cases, the stimulating electrode system had to be removed and spinal cord stimulation was performed.

In peripheral deafferentation pain, 3 cases had stump pain, 2 had post-herpetic pain, and one case had peripheral nerve injury pain. Chronic motor cortex stimulation was able to provide pain relief in only 2 cases (one excellent and one good case). In the other 4 cases, the stimulating system was removed and thalamic sensory relay nucleus stimulation was applied. For the relief of peripheral deafferentation pain, chronic thalamic sensory relay nucleus stimulation achieved excellent to good pain relief in 75% of the treated cases (Table II).

Thus in total, 32 cases were treated by chronic motor cortex stimulation (Table I) and they were followed up for more than 2 years.

The pain typically subsided within 5 minutes after the onset of motor cortex stimulation, and had completely faded away within approximately 10 minutes. This effect continued for one to 6 hours following termination of 10 minutes of stimulation. The pain inhibition usually occurred at intensities below the threshold for the production of muscle contraction. Whenever satisfactory pain relief was achieved, the

Table II. Two years follow up results of thalamic sensory relay nucleus stimulation.

Pain	Causative lesion site	Number of treated cases	Effective cases (excellent-good)	Chronic implantation
Central deafferentation pain		21	8 (38%)	8
Peripheral deafferentation pain	stump pain	7	6 (86%)	6
	herpetic pain	4	2 (40%)	2
	peripheral nerve injury	6	5 (83%)	5
	others	3	2 (67%)	2
Total		20	15 (75%)	15 (75%)

patients reported a sensation of light tingling or mild vibration projecting from the same area of distribution as their pain. Although the patients selected varying stimulation frequencies (5 to 120 Hz), they tended to apply a relatively lower frequency with a longer pulse duration.

During the follow-up period of 2 years, the patients maintained satisfactory pain relief by chronic motor cortex stimulation except in 3 cases, where a decrease in the effectiveness of pain relief was noticed and revision of the electrodes was required. Either growth of connective tissue above the dura or electrode dislocation was the reason for the decrease in effectiveness. However, following electrode revision, they again enjoyed the same pain relief as previously.

Interestingly, in most cases treated by chronic motor cortex stimulation, the total stimulation period *per* day to relieve the pain gradually decreased, and 2 cases among them were able to apply the stimulation just once in the morning without complaints of spontaneous deafferentation pain. Also, subjective improvement of motor deficits and abolished tremors were reported in the cases with thalamic and suprathalamic lesions as the causative lesion, but this improvement was not evidently objective. On the other hand, Woolsey *et al.* [19] found that, in severe Parkinson's disease, marked inhibition of tremor and rigidity was induced by pre-central stimulation but rarely by post-central stimulation.

There were no serious complications. None of our patients subjected to the above therapy developed either observable or electroencephalographic seizure activity. Thus, although possible development of seizure activity with intermittent chronic stimulation of the motor cortex had been the problem of greatest concern to us, no such complications actually resulted. Meyerson *et al.* [20] mentioned that most patients had one or two short-lasting generalized seizures during the test stimulation period; however, they encountered no patients who developed seizures during chronic motor cortex stimulation after internalization.

Discussion

Chronic motor cortex stimulation is an effective and safe treatment for the relief of central deafferentation pain. However, it is difficult to obtain suitable evidence to explain its underlying mechanism, although several animal experiments have been performed as described in this paper.

As a first possible mechanism, motor cortex stimulation could inhibit the hyperactivity of deafferented nociceptive neurons, and this inhibition might induce relief of pain, since, in patients with deafferentation pain, hyperactive neurons are situated at the cerebral synapses of the causative nociceptive neurons [21, 22], as observed in the above animal experiments, and removal of the hyperactive area can temporarily abolish the pain [9, 23-25]. These findings are consistent with the hypothesis that hyperactivity of deafferented nociceptive neurons gives rise to deafferentation pain. According to the experimental results, the hyperactivity occurred at the sensory cortex, and recording of the sensory relay thalamic nucleus is possible at 4-8 weeks after inducing lesions at the noxious afferent pathway. The hyperactivity is inhibited by motor cortex stimulation and also by administration of NMDA antagonist. Since NMDA receptor is not activated by nociceptive stimuli in normal animals [17], the hyperactivity is apparently caused by activated NMDA receptors which may be activated following deafferentation, or there may be an increase in density and a decrease in threshold of the receptors in the regenerative area following brain damage by the causative lesion. This interpretation is supported by the fact that:
- deafferentation pain occurs only in some limited cases even if the lesion itself has the same location and pathogenesis,
- the onset of deafferentation pain has a delay of several months after the onset of the causative lesion,
- chronic brain stimulation can induce an increase in nerve growth factor and glial cells within the regenerated area associated with the causative lesion in animal experiments [26].

It can be said therefore that motor cortex stimulation may not only inhibit the NMDA receptor activity induced by mal-adaptive regeneration, but also induce reorganization of the mal-adaptive regeneration. However, difficulties in explaining the effective mechanism of motor cortex stimulation by the above hypothesis still remain, because motor cortex stimulation cannot stop the central deafferentation pain of all treated patients and similar hyperactivity is also recorded at the medial and intralaminar thalamic neurons in patients with deafferentation pain [27].

As another possible mechanism, unusual new or damaged fiber connections between the noxious afferent system and non-noxious sensory system in the mal-adaptive regeneration area associated with the causative lesion could be related to the induction of deafferentation pain. Motor cortex stimulation may influence the pain inhibitory function of the system mediating activation of the non-noxious somatosensory neurons, as recognized in the gate control theory [28]. If the above hypothesis is true, motor cortex stimulation might activate unusual connections of non-noxious receptive neurons at the sensory cortex or the somatosensory thalamic nucleus, and this could inhibit the hyperactivity of noxious neurons which induce mal-adaptive regeneration associated with the causative lesion.

As a further possible mechanism, activation of the corticospinal tract might lead to pain inhibition, since good pain relief is achieved only when cortical stimulation is applied to the same area from which muscle contractions are induced by stronger stimulation [20, 29]. However, it seems unlikely that activation of corticospinal tract neurons is crucial for accomplishing pain inhibition, because pain inhibition by motor cortex stimulation is produced at an intensity below the threshold for muscle contraction. It could be hypothesized therefore that motor cortex stimulation selectively activates aberrant or unusual connections with the non-nociceptive neurons, and inhibits nociceptive neurons at various levels of the pain afferent system.

The mechanism of deafferentation pain control provided by motor cortex stimulation requires further studies involving both animal experiments and clinical observations of chronic motor cortex stimulation therapy.

Conclusion

Chronic motor cortex stimulation demonstrated central deafferentation pain control in almost 75% of treated patients without any serious complications. It represents the first choice of treatment, at least, for thalamic pain, suprathalamic pain and mesencephalobulbar pain caused by stroke or post-surgical lesions.

Based on the results of animal experiments and clinical observations, the underlying mechanism could be that motor cortex stimulation activates unusual regenerated connections with non nociceptive neurons to inhibit the nociceptive afferent neurons, and inhibits pathologically activated NMDA receptors of the damaged nociceptive neurons which are induced by mal-adaptive regeneration associated with causative lesions at the pain afferent system in the brain.

References

1. Tasker RR. Deafferentaion. In : Wall PD, Melzack R, eds. *Textbook of pain.* Edinburgh : Churchill Livingstone, 1984 : 119-32.
2. Dejerine J, Roussy G. Le syndrome thalamique. *Rev Neurol (Paris)* 1906 ; 14 : 521-32.
3. Leijon G, Boivie J, Johansson I. Central post-stroke pain: neurological symptoms and pain characteristics. *Pain* 1989 ; 36 : 13-25.
4. Holmgren H, Leijon G, Boivie J *et al.* Central post-stroke pain: somatosensory evoked potentials in relation to location of the lesion and sensory signs. *Pain* 1990 ; 40 : 43-52.
5. Pangi CA. Central pain and painful anaesthesia. *Prog Neurol Surg* 1906; 8 : 132-57.

6. Holmgren H, Leijon G, Boivie J, Johansson I, Ilievska L. Central post-stroke pain: somatosensory evoked potentials in relation to location of the lesion and sensory signs. *Pain* 1990 ; 40 : 43-52.
7. Yamamoto T, Katayama Y, Tsubokawa T, Koyama Y, Maejima S, Hirayama T. Usefulness of the morphine/thiamylal test for the treatment of deafferentation pain. *Pain Res* 1991 ; 6 : 143-6.
8. Tsubokawa T, Moriyasu N. Follow up results of centre median thalamotomy for relief of intractable pain. *Conf Neurol* 1975 ; 37 : 280-4.
9. Erickson TC, Bleckwenn WJ, Woolsey CN. Observations on the post-central gyrus in relation to pain. *Trans Am Neurol Assoc* 1952 ; 77 : 57-9.
10. Adams JE, Hosobuchi Y, Fields HL. Stimulation of internal capsule for relief of chronic pain. *J Neurosurg* 1974 ; 41 : 740-4.
11. Levitt M, Levitt J. Sensory hind-limb representation in the sensory cortex of the cat after spinal tractotomies. *Exp Neurol* 1968 ; 22 : 276-302.
12. Kjerulf TD, Loeser JD. Neuronal hyperactivity following deafferentation of the lateral cuneate nucleus. *Exp Neurol* 1973 ; 39 : 86-102.
13. Lenz FA, Kwan HC, Dostrovsky J, Tasker RR. Characteristics of the bursting pattern of action potentials that occurs in the thalamus of patients with central pain. *Brain Res* 1989 ; 496 : 357-69.
14. Tsubokawa T, Katayama Y, Hirayama T. Effects of thalamic sensory relay nucleus stimulation on trigeminal subnucleus caudalis neurons in the cat: inhibition of abnormal bursting hyperactivity after trigeminal rhizotomy. *Neurol Medicochir* 1987 ; 27 : 601-6.
15. Hirayama T, Tsubokawa T, Katayama Y, Yamamoto Y, Koyama S. Chronic changes in activity of thalamic relay neurons following spinothalamic tractotomy in cat: effects of motor cortex stimulation. *Pain* 1990 ; suppl 5 : 273.
16. Tsubokawa T, Katayama Y, Yamamoto T, Hirayama T, Koyama S. Chronic motor cortex stimulation for the treatment of central pain. *Acta Neurochir* 1991 ; suppl 52 : 137-9.
17. Tsubokawa T, Katayama Y, Yamamoto T, Hirayama T, Koyama S. Chronic motor cortex stimulation in patients with thalamic pain. *J Neurosurg* 1993 ; 78 : 393-401.
18. Katayama Y, Tsubokawa T, Maejima S, et al. Corticospinal direct responses in humans: identification of the motor cortex during intracranial surgery under general anesthesia. *J Neurol Neurosurg Psychiat* 1988 ; 51 : 50-9.
19. Woolsey CN, Erickson T, Gilson WE. Localization in somatic sensory and motor areas of human cerebral cortex as determined by direct recording of evoked potentials and electrical stimulation. *J Neurosurg* 1979 ; 51 : 476-506.
20. Meyerson BA, Lindblom U, Linderoth B, Lind D, Herregodts P. Motor cortex stimulation as treatment of trigeminal neuropathic pain. *Acta Neurochir* 1993 ; suppl 58 : 150-3.
21. Loeser JD, Ward AA Jr, White LE Jr. Chronic deafferentation of human spinal cord neurons. *J Neurosurg* 1968 ; 29 : 48-50.
22. Nashold BS Jr. Central pain: its origins and treatment. *Clin Neurosurg* 1974 ; 21 : 31 -22.
23. Horrax G. Experiences with cortical excisions for the relief of intractable pain. *Surgery* 1946 ; 20 : 593-602.
24. Lewin W, Phillips CG. Observation on partial removal of the post-central gyrus for pain. *J Neurol Neurosurg Psychiatry* 1952 ; 15 : 143-7.
25. White JC, Sweet WH. *Pain and neurosurgeon: a forty-year experience*. Springfield : Charles C Thomas, III, 1969.
26. Maejima S, Koshinaga M, Katayama Y, et al. Thalamic stimulation facilitates microglial and astroglial reactions in the cortex following spinal cord injury. *Adv Neurotrauma Res* 1993 ; 5 : 144-6.

27. Rinaldi PC, Young RF, Albe-Fessard D, *et al.* Spontaneous neuronal hyperactivity in the medial and intralaminar thalamic nuclei of patients with deafferentation pain. *J Neurosurg* 1991 ; 74 : 415-21.
28. Wall PD, Sweet WH. Temporary abolition of pain in man. *Science* 1967 ; 155 : 108-9.

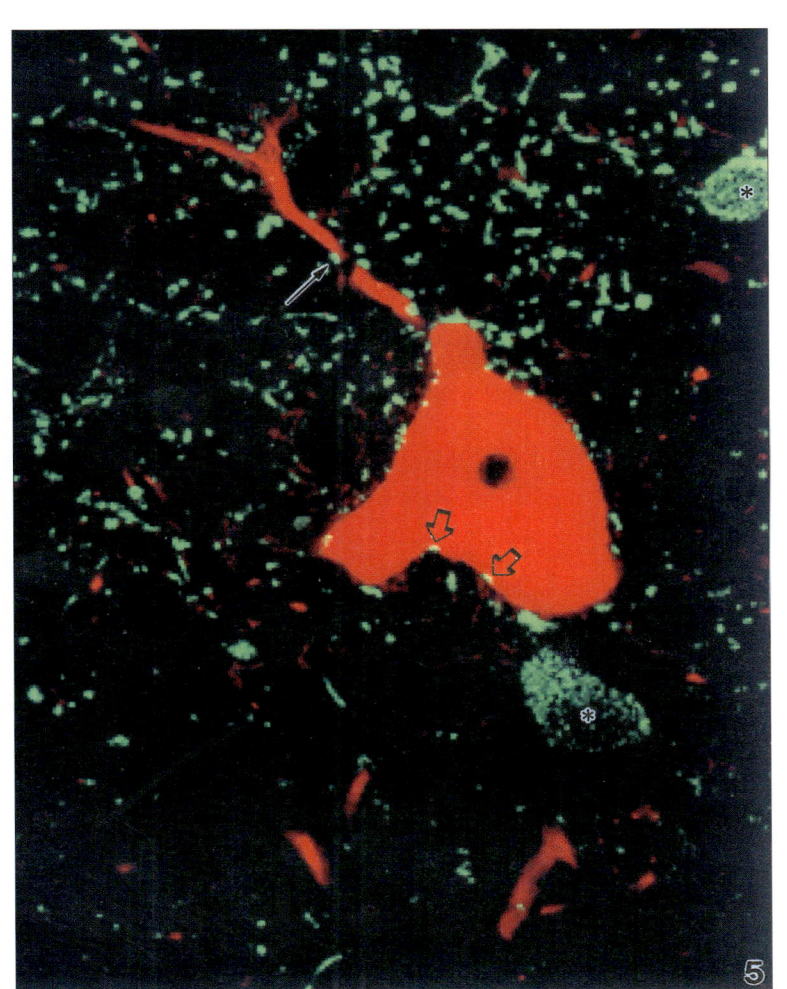

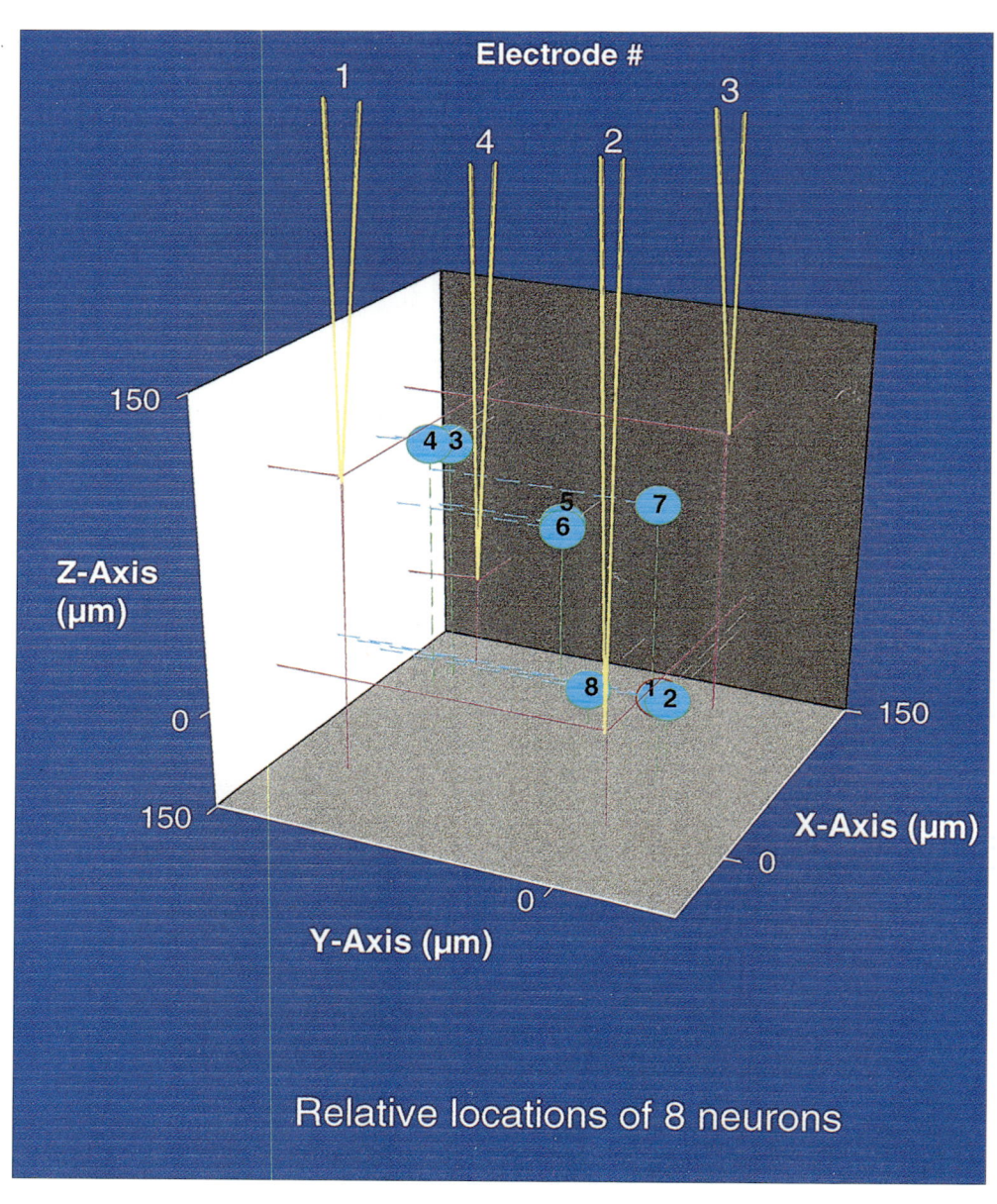

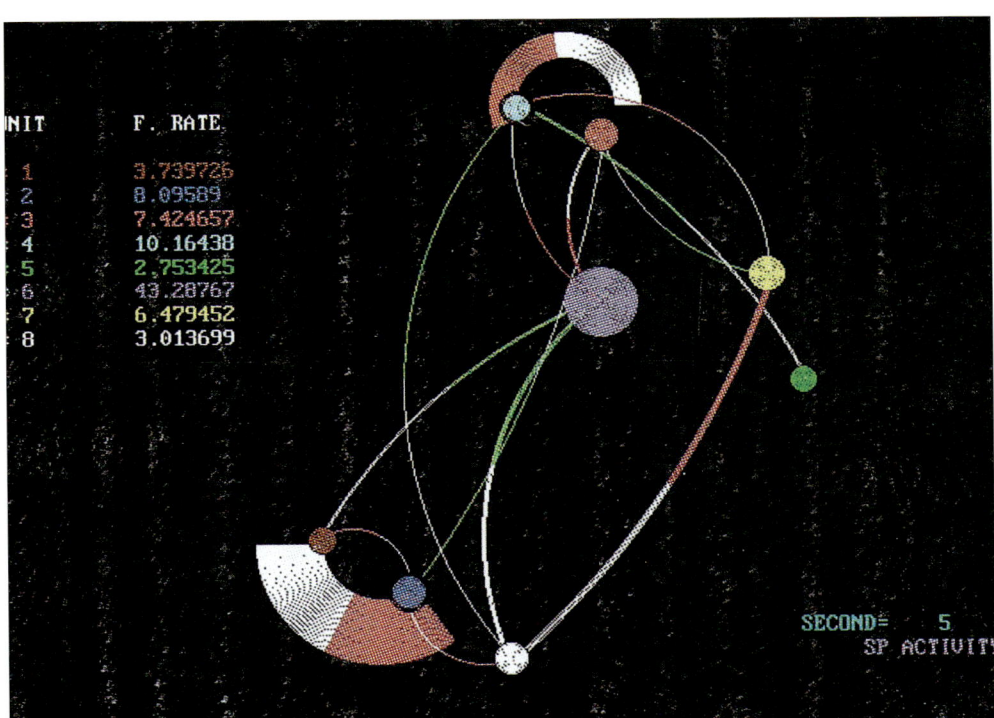

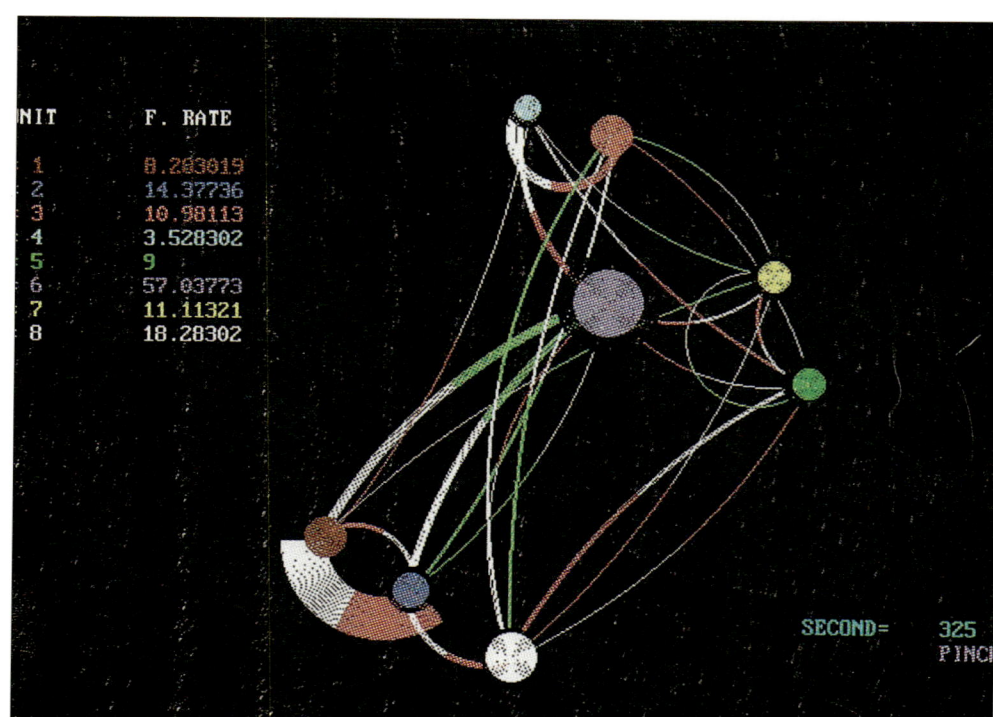

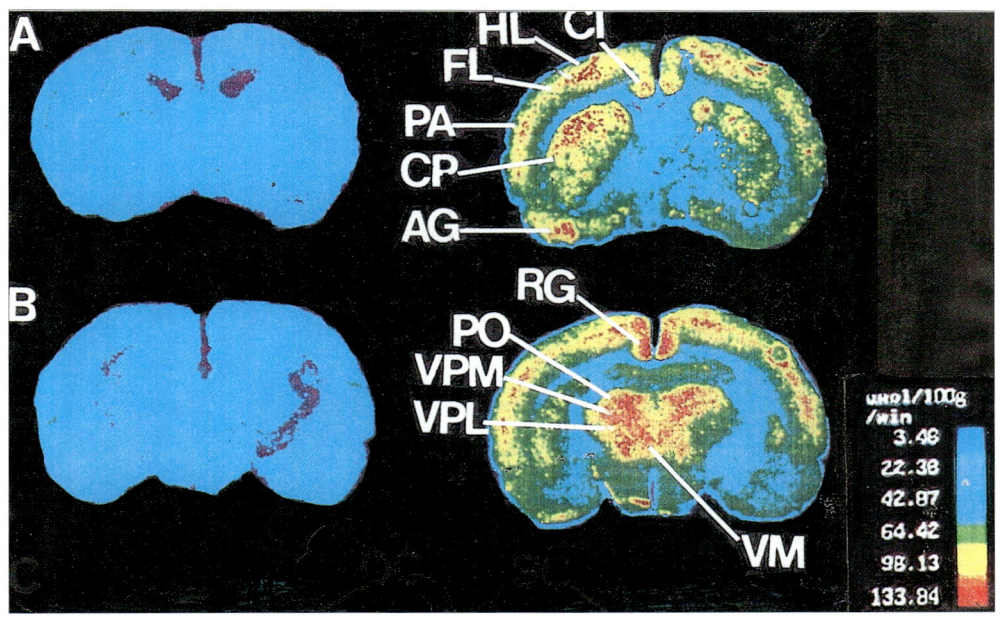

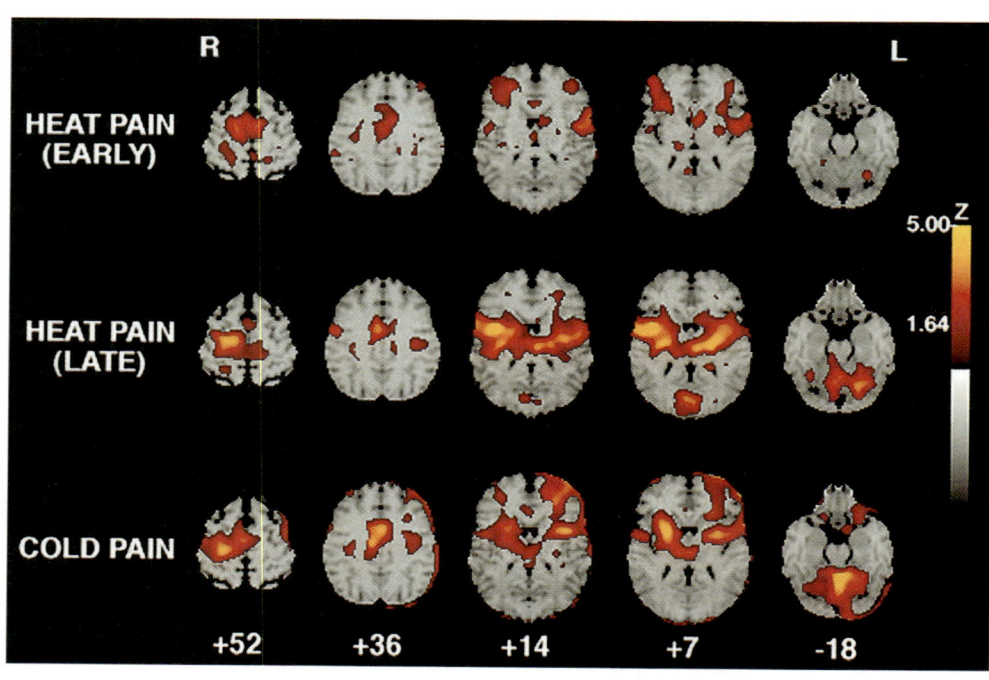

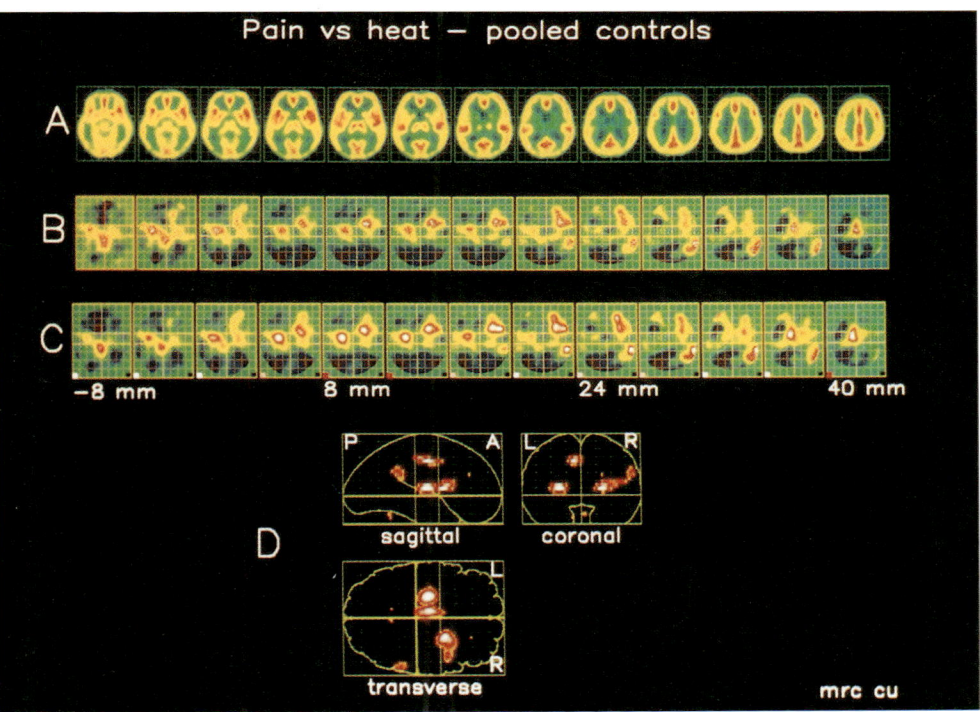

Imprimé par JOUVE, 18 rue Saint-Denis, 75001 PARIS
N° 232168 W- Dépôt légal : Décembre 1995